SPIRITUALITY
and the
THERAPEUTIC PROCESS

SPIRITUALITY
and the
THERAPEUTIC
PROCESS

A Comprehensive Resource From Intake to Termination

Edited by JAMIE D. ATEN *and* MARK M. LEACH

American Psychological Association ✦ Washington DC

Published by
American Psychological Association
750 First Street, NE
Washington, DC 20002
www.apa.org

To order
APA Order Department
P.O. Box 92984
Washington, DC 20090-2984
Tel: (800) 374-2721; Direct: (202) 336-5510
Fax: (202) 336-5502; TDD/TTY: (202) 336-6123
Online: www.apa.org/books/
E-mail: order@apa.org

In the U.K., Europe, Africa, and the Middle East, copies may be ordered from
American Psychological Association
3 Henrietta Street
Covent Garden, London
WC2E 8LU England

Typeset in Goudy by Circle Graphics, Inc., Columbia, MD

Printer: Book-mart Press, North Bergen, NJ
Cover Designer: Mercury, Rockville, MD
Technical/Production Editor: Tiffany L. Klaff

The opinions and statements published are the responsibility of the authors, and such opinions and statements do not necessarily represent the policies of the American Psychological Association.

Library of Congress Cataloging-in-Publication Data

Spirituality and the therapeutic process : a comprehensive resource from intake to termination / edited by Jamie D. Aten and Mark M. Leach. — 1st ed.
    p. ; cm.
  Includes bibliographical references and index.
  ISBN-13: 978-1-4338-0373-4
  ISBN-10: 1-4338-0373-9
  1. Psychotherapy—Religious aspects. 2. Psychotherapy patients—Religious life.
3. Psychotherapist and patient. 4. Spirituality. I. Aten, Jamie D. II. Leach, Mark M.
  [DNLM: 1. Psychotherapy—methods. 2. Professional-Patient Relations. 3. Spirituality.
WM 420 S7596 2009]

  RC489.S676S65 2009
  616.89'14—dc22

                                    2008016942

British Library Cataloguing-in-Publication Data

A CIP record is available from the British Library.

Printed in the United States of America
First Edition

CONTENTS

CONTRIBUTORS

Jamie D. Aten, PhD, Assistant Professor, Department of Psychology; Assistant Director of Health and Mental Health Research, Katrina Research Center, The University of Southern Mississippi, Hattiesburg

John J. Barrett, PhD, Associate Professor, Department of Psychology, Xavier University, Cincinnati, OH

Clark Campbell, PhD, Director of Training and Professor of Psychology, Graduate Department of Clinical Psychology, George Fox University, Newberg, OR

Barbara Couden Hernandez, PhD, Director, Loma Linda University Marriage and Family Therapy Clinic; Director of Clinical Education, Counseling and Family Sciences, Loma Linda University, Loma Linda, CA

Don E. Davis, doctoral student in counseling psychology, Department of Psychology, Virginia Commonwealth University, Richmond

Sondra Dowdle, doctoral student, Department of Counseling, Educational Psychology, and Special Education, Mississippi State University, Starkville

Lucy Flowers, master's student, Department of Counseling, Educational Psychology, and Special Education, Mississippi State University, Starkville

Randall Halberda, PsyD, Staff Psychologist, Battle Creek Veterans Affairs Medical Center, Battle Creek, MI

M. Elizabeth Lewis Hall, PhD, Associate Professor of Psychology, Rosemead School of Psychology, Biola University, La Mirada, CA

Todd W. Hall, PhD, Associate Professor of Psychology, Rosemead School of Psychology, Biola University, La Mirada, CA

William L. Hathaway, PhD, Director, Doctoral Program in Clinical Psychology; Professor of Psychology, School of Psychology and Counseling, Regent University, Virginia Beach, VA

Joshua N. Hook, doctoral student, Department of Psychology, Virginia Commonwealth University, Richmond

Ahmed Nezar Kobeisy, PhD, Chaplain, Syracuse University, Syracuse, NY

Elizabeth J. Krumrei, doctoral student, Department of Psychology, Bowling Green State University, Bowling Green, OH

Mark M. Leach, PhD, Professor, Department of Psychology, The University of Southern Mississippi, Hattiesburg

Michael W. Mangis, PhD, Associate Professor, Department of Psychology, Wheaton College, Wheaton, IL; Executive Director, Center for Rural Psychology, Elburn, IL

Andrea J. Miller, doctoral student, Department of Psychology, Virginia Commonwealth University, Richmond

Kari A. O'Grady, doctoral candidate, Department of Counseling Psychology and Special Education, Brigham Young University, Provo, UT

Kenneth I. Pargament, PhD, Professor, Department of Psychology, Bowling Green State University, Bowling Green, OH

Crystal L. Park, PhD, Associate Professor, Department of Psychology, University of Connecticut, Storrs

P. Scott Richards, PhD, Professor, Department of Counseling Psychology and Special Education, Brigham Young University, Provo, UT

Jennifer S. Ripley, PhD, Associate Professor of Psychology, School of Psychology and Counseling, Regent University, Virginia Beach, VA

David A. Safran, PhD, Licensed Clinical Psychologist, private practice, Staten Island, NY

Steven J. Sandage, PhD, Associate Professor of Marriage and Family Studies, Bethel University, St. Paul, MN

Lewis Z. Schlosser, PhD, Assistant Professor, Department of Professional Psychology and Family Therapy, Seton Hall University, South Orange, NJ

Jeanne M. Slattery, PhD, Professor, Department of Psychology, Clarion University of Pennsylvania, Clarion

Brent T. Tucker, PhD, Assistant Professor of Counseling and Psychology, Director of Community Counseling Program, College of Education, Troy University, Dothan, AL

Nathaniel G. Wade, PhD, Assistant Professor of Psychology, Department of Psychology, Iowa State University, Ames

Marsha I. Wiggins, PhD, Professor, Counseling Psychology and Counselor Education, University of Colorado at Denver and Health Sciences Center, Denver

Everett L. Worthington Jr., PhD, Professor, Department of Psychology, Virginia Commonwealth University, Richmond

J. Scott Young, PhD, Associate Professor, Department of Counseling, Educational Psychology, and Special Education, Mississippi State University, Starkville

Brian J. Zinnbauer, PhD, Staff Psychologist, Cincinnati Veterans Affairs Medical Center, private psychotherapy practice, Cincinnati, OH

SPIRITUALITY
and the
THERAPEUTIC PROCESS

INTRODUCTION

JAMIE D. ATEN AND MARK M. LEACH

Spirituality is a powerful dimension of human experience, with growing
importance and diversity in today's changing world.
—Froma Walsh

In our clinical work, supervision, teaching, and discussions with other
mental health providers, we have seen and heard of the profound impact spirituality can have on clients. Several years ago I (Jamie D. Aten) worked with
a client who engaged in frequent self-injurious behaviors. At the time of our
termination, it had been nearly 6 months since he had engaged in self-
inflicted injury. When asked which aspect of therapy had been most helpful,
he replied, "Your encouragement to reconnect with my spirituality and a
spiritual community of believers. I found healing in my spirituality." More
recently I supervised a beginning therapist whose client reported seeking
counseling because of her fear of damnation. As therapy progressed, the
client brought in a journal that she wanted to share with my supervisee. In
the journal was a detailed daily record of what she believed to be sinful behaviors and thoughts. This journal turned out to be one of many such journals
she had maintained for over 18 years. Any exploration or discussion of the
client's spirituality only led to more ruminations and deeper feelings of guilt
and fear. The client ended up terminating prematurely from therapy.
Although representing two polar experiences, these two case examples speak
to the influence and power of spirituality. They also highlight how important
it is for therapists to have an awareness of spiritual matters and the knowledge

and skill set that will enable them to address these concerns in counseling and psychotherapy.

As a means of filling this need, we have brought together a diverse group of therapists and researchers from various mental health fields (counseling and clinical psychology, counselor education, and marriage and family therapy) to create this book. The authors represent numerous spiritual backgrounds and worldviews (e.g., Christian, Jewish, Islamic, agnostic) and have expertise in integrating spirituality into their clinical work and teaching. They have all come together around one goal: to provide readers with a "start-to-finish" approach to integrating spirituality across the various stages of the therapeutic process in counseling and psychotherapy. In this book, the chapter authors provide practical strategies, techniques, and examples of how to implement spirituality at each stage of treatment, from before the clinical intake (starting with an understanding of ethical practice guidelines and therapist self-awareness) through termination. Personal self-reflection questions, diverse spiritual case examples, and a multiple-session case study chapter are provided to further enhance readers' understanding and ability to incorporate spirituality into counseling and psychotherapy.

CHAPTER-BY-CHAPTER OVERVIEW

In chapter 1, we offer readers a contextual introduction to spirituality and mental health. Specifically, we highlight (a) diverse definitions of spirituality, (b) research on positive and negative effects of spirituality on mental and physical health, (c) historical issues surrounding psychology and spirituality, (d) cultural findings pertaining to spirituality, (e) clinical issues related to spirituality, and (f) training on spirituality.

In chapter 2, Hathaway and Ripley discuss the growing literature on ethical, legal, and effective therapeutic practices when assessing and treating clients with spiritual concerns. Beginning with an overview of applied ethics and their relationship to representative ethical codes, the authors introduce the reader to professional and practice guidelines and legal precedents. They present preliminary practice guidelines for working with spiritual clients that grew from an ad hoc committee of the American Psychological Association and their relationship to evidence-based practices. They end with a series of well-conceived vignettes highlighting some of the dilemmas and challenges encountered in treatment, including ethical and legal commentary.

In chapter 3, Wiggins provides a number of unique strategies for helping therapists gain self-awareness and insight into how their experiences with spirituality may affect therapy with spiritual clients and issues. More specifically, readers learn how to construct a spiritual genogram and a spiritual autobiography, do guided journaling, and practice mindfulness. Common impediments to working with clients' spiritual issues that are interrelated to therapist self-awareness are also addressed. The diverse case studies in this chapter represent therapists from a wide range of spiritual traditions. Questions are also posed throughout the chapter to help readers gain a deeper level of self-understanding and ultimately apply the material presented. Recommendations for overcoming potentially negative experiences with spirituality and biases toward spirituality are offered.

In chapter 4, Leach, Aten, Wade, and Hernandez discuss how therapists can integrate spirituality into the clinical intake process by facilitating spiritual acceptance early in treatment. How agency climate and referral sources can influence clients' responsiveness and understanding of the role of spirituality in therapy are noted. Recommendations are also made for creating intake forms that allow clients to make informed decisions about their treatment and that can help set the stage for discussing the spiritual. Sample excerpts from an agency informed consent that addresses spirituality, an informed consent for spiritually oriented interventions, and a professional self-disclosure form on spirituality are provided. Implicit and explicit methods for inquiring about spirituality during the clinical interview are also outlined. A detailed case study pulls together the various components of this chapter.

In chapter 5, Pargament and Krumrei outline a three-stage approach to assessing spirituality in clinical practice, including an initial spiritual assessment, extensive spiritual assessment, and implicit spiritual assessment. Suggestions for how therapists can create an atmosphere conducive to spiritual assessment are also addressed. The authors provide strategies for exploring how spirituality can influence the lives of clients, from being a source of strength to confounding problems. Likewise, the authors propose a model that can help therapists understand how clients search for the sacred, and they discuss the implications of such an endeavor during the assessment phase. Helpful probing questions and assessment instruments are highlighted in a practical approach that is further enhanced through case vignettes, tables, and figures.

In chapter 6, Park and Slattery propose a meaning systems approach to conceptualizing spirituality in counseling and psychotherapy. The authors help readers see how clients utilize spirituality to make meaning of their experiences. Moreover, therapists are shown how to create conceptualizations that incorporate clients' worldviews. The role of spirituality in case conceptualizations, as well as how this approach can be used to inform other theoretical orientations, is presented. Common spiritual stressors, strengths, and barriers that warrant consideration in the case conceptualization process are discussed. Tables, exhibits, figures, case material, and a detailed meaning-based case conceptualization and analysis walk readers through this important stage of the therapeutic process.

In chapter 7, Zinnbauer and Barrett highlight how spirituality can be incorporated into treatment planning. Overall, the authors encourage therapists to take a multiculturally sensitive approach to working with clients' spirituality. They also provide a novel seven-component model for accomplishing this task, which includes (a) identifying presenting complaints, (b) using the ADDRESSING model to incorporate cultural assessment, (c) developing a problem list and strengths list, (d) identifying the desired final outcome, (e) setting goals and resolving measurement issues, (f) selecting and implementing interventions, and (g) incorporating periodic review of progress. Several sample treatment plans that address various encounters with clients' spirituality are presented. How to and how not to incorporate spirituality into the treatment planning phase are also highlighted.

In chapter 8, Young, Dowdle, and Flowers provide six principles to guide therapists in their attempt to establishing strong therapeutic alliances with clients presenting with spiritual issues and spiritually oriented clients: (a) build a strong therapeutic alliance, (b) trust clients' view of the therapeutic alliance, (c) utilize relational experiences of the spiritual perspective, (d) respect clients' spiritual ideals, (e) use a less judgmental approach, and (f) explore client resistance. The chapter also highlights a number of insights based on the current psychotherapy literature into how therapists may approach spirituality when building a relationship with clients. Case examples, along with a detailed case study that systematically highlights each of outlined therapeutic alliance building principles, further help make the material applicable to clinical practice. The authors also provided a novel contribution by asking a diverse group of therapists to reflect on and share their experiences and thoughts on each of the guiding principles noted.

In chapter 9, Schlosser and Safran provide recommendations for integrating spirituality into the treatment implementation phase of the therapeutic process. They discuss the commonalities between mental health practices and the sacred, bringing attention to areas of intersection. Treatment implementation considerations, such as client issues, therapist issues, and contextual factors, are noted. The authors use in-depth case examples that demonstrate how spirituality can be integrated into common theoretical approaches, such as cognitive–behavioral, interpersonal, psychodynamic, and humanistic therapies. Readers are introduced to spiritually accommodative and spiritually oriented approaches to therapy. Considerations and suggestions for using spiritual interventions, along with helpful tables for implementing spiritual interventions, are also given.

In chapter 10, Aten et al. give insight into how spirituality may surface and can be utilized during psychotherapy termination. The authors help prepare readers for common spiritual issues that frequently arise in termination, even if spirituality had not been a focus in previous sessions. Strategies for addressing spirituality in this underexamined phase of treatment are also outlined, ranging from exploring clients' existential questions to referring to spiritual leaders. Means for therapists to resolve potential spiritual differences that can present during termination are also discussed. An in-depth case study is provided that ties together the various strategies and topics presented in the chapter.

In chapter 11, O'Grady and Richards present a multiple-session case study that covers the breadth of the therapeutic process and bridges the aforementioned chapters. The authors describe and highlight how to integrate spirituality throughout the course of the therapeutic process. For example, they discuss how they typically approach spiritual issues while also reflecting on suggestions provided throughout the text, describe how the therapist in the case study worked with the client at each stage of treatment, and follow with author commentary. The authors also provide a brief introduction to their primary theoretical orientation for working with the spiritual: theistic–integrative psychotherapy. Overall, this chapter combines the ideas and material presented in the other chapters while also adding to the diversity of ideas and thoughts presented earlier. This chapter will help readers, regardless of their own spiritual traditions or theoretical orientations, to apply the material presented across the therapeutic process.

In chapter 12, Worthington et al. present one of the most comprehensive models to date for incorporating spirituality into clinical training. The authors argue that changes need to be made in the way most training programs currently address spirituality and train therapists in this area. They offer a number of unique training strategies that range from advising and mentoring activities to postdegree strategies that, if implemented, will facilitate a more comprehensive training experience for therapists-in-training and professional therapists. Steps are also provided to help training programs identify how they currently approach spirituality in training; this is followed by programmatic recommendations for enhancing spirituality training. An initial research agenda for studying effective strategies for integrating spirituality into clinical training is also posed.

CONCLUSION

On the basis of their clinical work, research, and personal experiences, the chapter authors summarize how spirituality can be integrated into the therapeutic process, offering a review of proven strategies outlined in the literature as well as offering new and innovative perspectives and approaches. Our interest in spirituality and mental health has always been driven by curiosity. In fact, that is how this book first began, with a question, "What would a step-by-step approach to integrating spirituality into counseling and psychotherapy look like?" I (Jamie D. Aten) can remember first pondering this question in graduate school seated in a night class on theories of counseling as we discussed and scrutinized the therapeutic process. This one question soon started multiplying. "How can I be more self-aware about spiritual issues?" "How can I integrate spirituality in the clinical intake?" "How can I integrate spirituality in assessment?" And so on. Later I would find out that my coeditor (Mark M. Leach) had been asking many of these same questions, which led to this collaboration. In many ways, this book is a direct response to the questions we have been asking, that our colleagues have been asking, that our students have been asking, that countless other mental health professionals have been asking and grappling with for years. We feel fortunate to have had the opportunity to pose these questions to the wonderful collection of authors who have made contributions to this book.

1

A PRIMER ON SPIRITUALITY
AND MENTAL HEALTH

JAMIE D. ATEN AND MARK M. LEACH

Clearly there is a connection between spiritual beliefs and healing in the traditional cultures of the world, and it is currently emerging within Western psychology.

—Mary Fukuyama and Todd Sevig

It is our belief that theory, research, and practice should be interconnected, especially when working with spiritual issues in therapy. In this chapter, we provide an overview of spirituality and mental health definitions, trends, and research to orient readers to the evolving body of professional psychology literature on spirituality. Although by no means exhaustive, this primer was written to lay a foundation for interpreting and applying the theoretical propositions and clinical practice strategies offered in the following chapters.

SPIRITUAL CONTEXT

The meaning of the word *spirituality* has been the source of great debate among mental health professionals, as numerous definitions have been proposed, compared, and critiqued (Zinnbauer, Pargament, & Scott, 1999). Zinnbauer and Pargament (2005) proposed that "spirituality is defined as a personal or group search for the sacred. Religiousness is defined as a personal or group search for the sacred that unfolds within a traditional sacred context" (p. 35). Spirituality is regarded as a broader construct than religion, although both are multidimensional and have common characteristics. Reflected in these definitions is a sense of interconnectedness or similarity between the constructs of spirituality and religion, which mental health professionals have traditionally embraced while using the terms interchangeably (Spilka, Ladd, & McIntosh, 1996). Psychology of religion researchers have also explored how participants define spirituality and religion and have found that a majority of those sampled either embrace similar or overlapping definitions of spirituality and religion or consider themselves to be both spiritual and religious (e.g., Corrigan, McCorkle, & Schell, 2003). Despite advances to differentiate between spirituality and religion (e.g., Zinnbauer et al., 1999), the differences in language and measures researchers have used to operationalize and study spirituality and religion have largely been superficial (e.g., Hill et al., 2000).

In fact, it has only been in the last few decades that a distinction between spirituality and religion has begun to gain momentum (Hill et al., 2000). It has been suggested that cultural values, such as the value placed on individualism (Spilka, Hood, & Hunsberger, 2003) and the self (Sperry & Shafranske, 2005) in the United States, have prompted greater interest in spirituality because of the emphasis on individual experience versus the communal experience frequently associated with organized religion. For instance, in a 2003 Gallup (2002) poll, researchers found that participants viewed spirituality as "personal and individual" rather than "organized religion and church doctrine." Similar views have also been expressed in the mental health literature that suggest that although spirituality and religion may be interconnected in the lives of individuals, it is possible to embrace spirituality and religion separate from one another. For example, Richards and Bergin (1997) noted, "It is possible to be religious without being spiritual and spiritual without being religious" (p. 13). They added,

> We view religious as a subset of the spiritual. Religious has to do with theistic beliefs, practices, and feelings that are often, but not always, expressed institutionally and denominationally as well as personally. . . . Spiritual experiences tend to be universal, ecumenical, internal, affective, spontaneous, and private. (p. 13)

For instance, a colleague of ours recently shared that, as a lesbian, she found religion to be oppressive and even harmful at times, but she has been able to find renewed purpose and meaning in spirituality. This example is not used to say that religion is harmful or that spirituality is "better" than religion but rather is used as an illustrative point to highlight that spirituality and religion can represent dichotomous expressions of the sacred.

Although we believe that it is helpful to recognize the nuances between spirituality and religion as noted earlier, we would disagree with those who have equated spirituality only with positive connotations (e.g., transcendence) while equating religion with more negative connotations (e.g., dogmatic). Zinnbauer and Pargament (2005) also cautioned against further polarizing the definitions and meanings associated with spirituality and religion, noting that "narrow definitions of the terms or polarizations of the two [spirituality and religion] as incompatible opposites are likely to hinder inquiry within the psychology of religion" (p. 27). We would also suggest that such categorical characterizations will likely hinder therapists' therapeutic effectiveness with the spiritual and religious in counseling and psychotherapy. To adopt the stance that all things religious are negative could place us at risk for repeating history by revisiting our field's early stigmatization of religion and religious clients; we argue for a more balanced approach to defining spirituality and religion.

Thus, for the purposes of this book, when referring to spirituality or the spiritual we have chosen to use the definition offered by Frame (2003), which we believe offers a balanced conceptualization of the many components of spirituality: "*Spirituality* includes one's values, beliefs, mission, awareness, subjectivity, experience, sense of purpose and direction, and a kind of striving toward something greater than oneself. It may or may not include a deity" (p. 3). As noted at the beginning of this chapter, there are many ways of viewing spirituality; this is only one of many perspectives. Yet, we have chosen this definition because we think that it highlights the similarities between spirituality and religion while also addressing the unique characteristics of spirituality for mental health professionals.

RESEARCH CONTEXT

Researchers and theorists have identified various ways of being spiritual or religious, with intrinsic, extrinsic, and quest orientations being the three most commonly cited ways of expressing or living out one's faith (e.g., Salsman & Carlson, 2005). Those for whom spirituality is an internal, guiding, and significant influence on everyday living may be conceptualized as exhibiting an intrinsic orientation. Extrinsic spirituality plays a more peripheral role to how people live, whereby spirituality and spiritual involvement are often guided by more external influences or needs (e.g., the need for community; Allport & Ross, 1967). Seeking individuals who are struggling with the complexities, tensions, and paradoxes of spirituality can be categorized as operating from a quest orientation (e.g., Baston, 1976). A number of different models have also been presented to help explain how spirituality develops (e.g., Fowler, 1991). Although each model posits a unique perspective on spiritual development, the models appear to share several common underpinnings. Most of the models propose that individuals in the early stages of spiritual development often adopt a more literal, exclusive, and static belief system (e.g., Genia, 1995). Individuals at the early stages of spiritual development are also more likely to adopt beliefs similar to familiar attachment figures (e.g., parents) and frequently internalize images of a spiritual being or make attributions to a spiritual being that reflect these attachments. Yet, as individuals progress, a more universal perspective marked by openness may emerge (e.g., Oser, 1991). This does not mean that core spiritual beliefs are abandoned but rather that similarities and differences between spiritual traditions are appreciated (e.g., Washburn, 1988).

Studies have also shown that spirituality can have a profound positive impact on client functioning (e.g., Miller & Thoresen, 2003). A number of reviews have brought attention to the positive impact spirituality can have on health, from lower blood pressure rates to enhanced physical functioning (e.g., Koenig & Cohen, 2002). Spiritual rituals and practices (e.g., prayer and meditation) have also been shown to improve both mental and physical health in outcome studies (e.g., Argyle, 2002). Clients report feeling as though spiritual rituals and practices help to strengthen and maintain their relationship with the sacred. Tedeschi and Calhoun (1996) noted that survivors of natural disasters frequently report positive gains related to spirituality despite the insurmountable circumstances they encounter. That is, spiritual beliefs can directly influence the way people interpret their experiences and make meaning that can facilitate positive mental health outcomes (Park, 2005). For example, researchers (e.g., Pargament, Desai, & McConnell, 2006) have found that spiritual beliefs can facilitate healthy coping by individuals who face hardships such as a personal illness or loss. Overall, Koenig (2004) established that more than 500 studies in the 20-year span from 1980 to 2000 found positive relationships between spirituality and general mental health, well-being, and a reduction in substance abuse.

Involvement in a spiritual community can also have a positive impact on clients by leading to the reestablishment of social norms that can facilitate acceptance, nurturing, and approval from others (e.g., Koeing & Cohen, 2002; Morgan, Marsden, & Lacey, 2000). Similarly, getting connected with a spiritual community can be pivotal in providing a social support system for clients who feel powerless or marginalized (Watlington & Murphy, 2006). Researchers have also documented higher levels of self-satisfaction and well-being among clients who maintain a belief in a spiritual being or power (e.g., Hart, 1999). Clients frequently enter therapy feeling demoralized, as if they have no control over what is happening to them or their life. A relationship with the Divine can offer a sense of control to spiritually committed clients. The relationship with a transcendent spiritual being or power may also give clients a sense of wonder and of the supernatural, leading to an improved sense of well-being (e.g., Siegel & Schrimshaw, 2002; VandeCreek, Janus, & Pennebaker, 2002).

There is a growing body of literature that highlights the positive effects of spirituality and religion on mental and physical functioning. Still, therapists need to be aware that spirituality and religion are not always sources of growth for clients and, for some, may actually be a source of strain or exacerbate preexisting symptomatology. As Exline and Rose (2005) noted, "Casual consumers of this research might embrace a simplistic view of religion and spirituality as a panacea for life's troubles. But although people typically report more comfort than strain in their religious lives, strain is common" (p. 316).

Researchers have made great strides over the last 2 decades in this area of study, which have led to a more sophisticated understanding of the potential negative effects related to spirituality and religion. For example, negative spiritual and religious coping strategies, such as blaming God, have been correlated with negative mental health outcomes (e.g., Pargament, Koenig, & Perez, 2000). Likewise, researchers have found that religious strain (e.g., having anger toward God) was related to higher levels of depression in participants (e.g., Exline, Yali, & Lobel, 1999; Exline, Yali, & Sanderson, 2000). Substance abuse problems have also been linked in some instances with spirituality and religion that facilitates guilt or suppressive behaviors (e.g., Zuckerman, Austin, Fair, & Branchey, 1987). Likewise, those who use spirituality and religion for self-gain or purely extrinsically motivating reasons are more at risk for a wide range of psychological problems (e.g., Koenig, 1998). Researchers have also shown that scrupulosity or religious obsessive–compulsive symptoms (e.g., fixating on perceived sinful behavior) are common in samples of individuals with obsessive–compulsive disorder (Ciarrocchi, 1995; Nelson, Abramowitz, & Whiteside, 2006). Conversely, Hathaway (1999) added another interesting conceptual layer, suggesting that individuals' mental disorders can affect their religious and spiritual functioning, resulting in "a reduced ability to perform religious/spiritual activities, achieve religious/spiritual goals, or experience religious/spiritual states because of a psychological disorder" (Hathaway, Scott, & Garver, 2004, p. 97).

The aforementioned studies are important because they help provide therapists and researchers with a broader and more balanced perspective for understanding how people use spirituality and religion. The studies have also led to new conceptualizations of spirituality and religion in the mental health fields. It would seem that in most cases it is not the spirituality and religion that are necessarily healthy or unhealthy; rather, mental and physical health outcomes are correlated with how people internalize, interpret, make meaning, and use their spirituality and religion (e.g., Koenig, 1998; Koenig, McCullough, & Larson, 2001).

HISTORICAL CONTEXT

Before the rise of psychology, spiritual and religious leaders were responsible for their community's spiritual and mental health (Sevensky, 1984).

It would not be outrageous to suggest that the extraordinary preoccupation with psychology in America . . . owes something to the heritage of experiential piety; that America became a nation of psychologists in part because it had once been a land of Pietists. (Holifield, 1983, p. 65)

Yet, from a historical perspective, the relationship between leaders in spiritual and mental health communities has been one of mistrust, misunderstanding, and missed opportunities, leading to a schism between these two groups. In fact, some of these disputes have been played out in highly public arenas, with representatives from both sides making egregious claims about the other (Richards & Bergin, 2000). One of the first major conflicts to arise between spiritual and mental health leaders in North America occurred over the Emmanuel movement (Caplan, 1998).

In 1906, Harvard Medical School professor Dr. James Jackson Putnam and Episcopalian minister Dr. Elwood Worcester brought together Boston physicians and Episcopalian ministers to care for the impoverished. What started as a public health experiment in Boston quickly grew into a national movement known as the Emmanuel movement. Those involved with the Emmanuel movement provided health and religious education, medical examinations, and minister-employed psychotherapy. Caplan (1998) stated, "more than any other single factor, the Emmanuel movement not only raised the American public's awareness of psychotherapy but also compelled the American medical profession to enter a field that it had long neglected" (p. 118).

Although the Emmanuel movement brought positive attention to the general public about the benefits of psychotherapy, the movement had come under scrutiny and was being publicly criticized by the American medical profession. Leaders in the field of medicine stated that clergy were not properly trained or equipped to provide psychotherapy and that the scope of such practices should be limited to medical providers. A year later, Freud delivered a series of lectures at Clark University bringing psychoanalysis to the United States. Already under pressure by the American medical profession, the Emmanuel movement ended with the rise of psychoanalysis. As psychoanalysis flourished in the United States, so did Freud's beliefs and teachings on the harmful effects of religion and spirituality. Freud's colleagues and successors continued to promote spirituality and religion as a universal neurosis, undeniably affecting the way mental health providers perceived religious and spiritual clients (Blazer, 1998; Caplan, 1998; Webster, 1995).

With time, psychoanalysis would no longer be the only "force" in psychology. Clinical modalities such as behaviorism, cognitive therapy, and humanism grew in popularity among academic and applied circles; mental health professionals were beginning to expand their view of the human condition. However, many of the leading voices from these theoretical camps, such as B. F. Skinner and Albert Ellis (it should be noted that Ellis later modified his position), also shared Freud's disdain for religion and spirituality

(Brown & Srebalus, 1996). Overall, numerous influential historical figures in the field of psychology thought that spirituality and religion contributed to, if not caused, psychopathology. Another common view held by many early mental health professionals was that spirituality and religion were little more than defense mechanisms that people used to manage anxiety, avoid facing existential questions, justify personal behavior, or control the behavior of others (Blazer, 1998). Combined with the fact that science distanced itself from spirituality and religion, spiritual and religious clients were still largely seen in a negative fashion, despite the efforts of researchers and theorists such as James (1902/1961), Jung (1938), May (1953), Allport (1950, 1955), and Frankl (1962), all of whom wrote extensively on the positive nature of spirituality and religion (Plante, 1999). Eventually, mental health professionals began to conceptualize religion and spirituality in a more positive light, and by the mid-1980s to early 1990s a renewed interest in this area was evident.

This positive upsurge in mental health professionals' view of religion and spirituality has continued through the 1990s to the present (Worthington, Kurusu, McCullough, & Sandage, 1996). The advancement of diverse psychological and counseling theories, an upsurge in multicultural sensitivity and awareness, research demonstrating the positive effects of religion and spirituality on mental health (e.g., Bergin & Jensen, 1990), and contributing societal trends (e.g., America's "spiritual awakening") represent several factors that accounted for this shift in perspective (Plante, 1999). Mental health professionals have become increasingly aware of the need for multicultural sensitivity when working with clients from a wide variety of cultural backgrounds, including spiritual backgrounds (Watts, 2001). Some researchers believe that mental health professionals have also become more open to considering the role of spiritual beliefs in clients' mental health (e.g., Miller, 1999; Zinnbauer & Pargament, 2005).

The many studies that document the positive effects and therapeutic benefits of spirituality exemplify this renewed interest and acceptance (e.g., Koenig, Larson, & Matthews, 1996). Books on spirituality and mental health have also increased in number (e.g., Walker, Gorsuch, & Tan, 2004). Peer-reviewed psychological journals dedicated to spiritual topics have similarly flourished, including *Counseling and Values; International Journal for the Psychology of Religion; Journal of Psychology and Christianity; Journal of Psychology and Theology; Journal of the Scientific Study of Religion; Mental Health, Religion, and Culture;* and *Research in the Social Scientific Study of Religion.* Methods and strategies for improving relationships or collaboration between spiritual leaders and mental health professionals have also been investigated (e.g., Aten, 2004; McMinn, Aikins, & Lish, 2003). Studies have also shown a noticeable increase in the percentage of mental health professionals who hold spiritual beliefs (e.g., Miller, 1999; Shafranske & Malony, 1990) and who think that spiritual competencies are important to clinical practice (Young, Frame,

Cashwell, & Belaire, 2002). Mental health professionals' participation in professional activities and groups that interface spirituality with psychology (e.g., Division 36—Psychology of Religion of the American Psychological Association and Association of Spiritual, Ethical, Religion, and Values division of the American Counseling Association) has risen. The "Ethical Principles of Psychologists and Code of Conduct" of the American Psychological Association (2002) included new language that addresses spirituality and religion and encourages psychologists to attend to these topics with cultural sensitivity. The American Counseling Association's (2005) code of ethics now also embraces spirituality as a component of diversity (see this volume, chap. 2). The addition of spiritual problems to the fourth edition of the *Diagnostic and Statistical Manual of Mental Disorders* (American Psychiatric Association, 1994) as a V-code further reflects mental health professionals' new appreciation and efforts to understand and work with client spirituality as well. For a more detailed account on the history and relationship between mental health professionals and spirituality, see Delaney and DiClemente (2005) and Kemp (1996).

CULTURAL CONTEXT

Melton (2002) identified more than 2,300 different religious and spiritual groups in the United States consisting of the following (from largest to smallest): Christian groups; Eastern groups; spiritualist, psychic, and New Age groups; Ancient Wisdom groups; Magick groups; Middle Eastern groups; and unclassified spiritual groups, the last of which continue to grow. On the basis of Gallup (1997) poll findings, 95% of Americans believe in a Higher Power, 87% state that God answers prayers, 84% try to live according to their spiritual beliefs, and 93% identify with a specific spiritual group. Keller (2000) wrote, "among clients [who present] for therapy, those in the United States are likely to be directly active in a religious organization" (p. 29). According to Eck (2002), these statistics indicate that the majority of clients seeking therapy "have a spiritual or religious orientation that is important to them" (p. 268). It has been estimated that between 50% and 90% of clients in therapy are spiritually committed (Eck, 2002).

In a national study of spiritual transformation, Smith (2006) reported that half of all Americans have had at least one, if not multiple, spiritual change experiences. Furthermore, several studies have brought attention to the powerful role spirituality can play among various cultural groups. For instance, personal spirituality and affiliation with a spiritual community are recognized as being very important to many African Americans, who have historically viewed spirituality as a source of inspiration, encouragement, and hope (Leong, Wagner, & Tata, 1995). Ethnic identity among American

Indians also appears to be influenced by spirituality, with spirituality playing a prominent role in everyday life, rituals, and ceremonies (Choney, Berryhill-Paapke, & Robins, 1995). Williams and Lawler (2000) found that interfaith couples can also benefit from sharing their spirituality with one another, leading to larger social circles, increased intimacy, and greater respect for diversity.

CLINICAL CONTEXT

Researchers who examined the perceptions and practices of spiritual and religious clients have reported that large numbers of clients seek help from clergy before they seek treatment from mental health providers. Fifty-three percent of clients report that they would seek help from a pastoral care center if one were available (Worthington et al., 1996). Spiritually committed clients' distrust of mental health professionals may be one plausible explanation for why these clients tend to underuse mental health services (e.g., Richards & Bergin, 1997). Despite the notion that many spiritually committed clients view psychotherapy as a secular process with philosophical underpinnings that may vary from their own spiritual beliefs, it would appear that many are open to therapy that is sensitive to their belief systems (Jones, 1994; Rose, Westefeld, & Ansley, 2001). Similarly, clients report that they prefer therapy that includes their spiritual belief system, with 78% stating that spiritual values should be addressed in therapy. There is also evidence that spiritually committed clients prefer entering into a therapeutic relationship with a mental health professional who shares their spiritual tradition (e.g., Ripley, Worthington, & Berry, 2001). Spiritually committed clients seem to prefer therapists who use prayer, scripture, and explicit spiritual themes in therapy (e.g., McCullough, 1999; Wade, Worthington, & Vogel, 2007), and these clients view mental health professionals who integrate spiritual interventions (e.g., quote a sacred text) into therapy more optimistically and as more competent (Erickson, Hecker, & Kirkpatrick, 2002).

However, as noted earlier, historically mental health professionals have held a less positive view of spirituality and religion, underscoring the importance and potential value of attending to the spiritual needs and issues of their clients. This perspective often resulted in a skewed and narrow case conceptualization of the presenting problem and may have led to inadequate treatment planning, as powerful sources of gain were largely overlooked (e.g., Gerson, Rhianon, Gold, & Kose, 2000). Although more mental health professionals are becoming more accepting of spirituality, there are those who still think that spirituality should not be addressed in psychotherapy. Examples of documented reasons for opposition include (a) fear of imposing personal values; (b) bias or negative attitudes toward religion; (c) lack of theoretical model and training; (d) trained to minimize or disregard the importance of spirituality in the lives of their clients; and (e) view of the spiritual as outside of their scope of practice, reserving such dialogue for clergy (e.g., Miller & Thoresen, 2003). Studies have also shown that mental health professionals tend to view spiritual clients more pessimistically than nonspiritual clients, such as over-pathologizing spiritual clients or feeling less equipped to work with spiritual clients (e.g., Gerson et al., 2000; Tucker et al., 2002). Notwithstanding these findings, a great deal of progress has been made, as there has been an increased interest and acceptance of spirituality by a substantial number of mental health professionals over the last 25 years (Benes, Walsh, McMinn, Domingues, & Aikins, 2000).

TRAINING CONTEXT

Although mental health professionals are becoming more aware of the potential benefits of attending to the spiritual and religious beliefs and needs of their clients, few have received the proper training to work with these issues (e.g., Schulte, Skinner, & Claiborn, 2002). According to Pate and High (1995), spirituality topics "are addressed when they arise in practicum and internship seminars, but typically they are not formally introduced" (p. 2). Kelly (1994) reported that less than 25% of counselor education programs covered spirituality as a course component in their curriculum. This percentage dropped significantly when religious programs were excluded from consideration. In their study of the Council for Accreditation of Counseling and Related Educational Programs (CACREP), Young et al. (2002) found that "only 28% of respondents viewed their colleagues as similarly capable of addressing [spiritual] issues as a component of counselor preparation" (p. 22). Likewise, the majority of participants reported that more intentional and specific training was needed in counselor education on spirituality. It has also been estimated that 5% of clinical psychologists receive training on spiritual matters (Shafranske & Malony, 1990). Another study indicated that approximately 13% of clinical psychology programs offer a course that focuses on spirituality (Brawer, Handal, & Fabricatore, 2002). Brawer et al. (2002) pointed out that the specifics, variability, and frequency of how often these courses are offered seemed unclear. Eighty-two percent of counseling psychology training directors reported that their programs do not offer a course specifically designed to address spirituality. Likewise, few counseling psychologists are engaged in spirituality research in their training programs (Schulte et al., 2002). A survey study by Russell and Yarhouse (2006) also found a lack of spirituality training opportunities for predoctoral interns in clinical and counseling psychology.

SUMMARY

This chapter highlighted spirituality in the contexts of research, history, culture, clinical practice, and training. Therapists are encouraged to take the ideas and findings covered in this chapter into consideration when working with spiritual issues and clients. Although many questions remain that warrant additional attention and study in the professional psychology literature, there are numerous insights to be gained from the current body of knowledge for effectively integrating spirituality into the therapeutic process.

REFERENCES

Allport, G. W. (1950). *The individual and his religion*. New York: Macmillan.

Allport, G. W. (1955). *Becoming: Basic considerations for a psychology of personality*. New Haven, CT: Yale University Press.

Allport, G. W., & Ross, J. (1967). Personal religious orientation and prejudice. *Journal of Personality and Social Psychology, 5*, 432–443.

American Counseling Association. (2005). *Code of ethics and standards of practice*. Alexandria, VA: Author.

American Psychiatric Association. (1994). *Diagnostic and statistical manual of mental disorders* (4th ed.). Washington, DC: Author.

American Psychological Association. (2002). Ethical principles of psychologists and code of conduct. *American Psychologist, 57*, 1060–1073.

Argyle, M. (2002). State of the art: Religion. *Psychologist, 1*, 22–26.

Aten, J. D. (2004). Improving understanding and collaboration between campus ministers and college counseling center personnel. *Journal of College Counseling, 7*, 90–96.

Baston, C. D. (1976). Religion as prosocial: Agent or double agent? *Journal for the Scientific Study of Religion, 15*, 29–45.

Benes, K. M., Walsh, J. M., McMinn, M. R., Domingues, A. W., & Aikins, D. C. (2000). Psychology and the church: An exemplar of psychologist–clergy collaboration. *Professional Psychology: Research and Practice, 31*, 515–520.

Bergin, A. E., & Jensen, J. P. (1990). Religiosity of psychotherapists: A national survey. *Psychotherapy, 27*, 3–7.

Blazer, D. (1998). *Freud vs. God: How psychiatry lost its soul and Christianity lost its mind*. Downer Grove, IL: InterVarsity Press.

Brawer, P. A., Handal, P. J., & Fabricatore, A. N. (2002). Training and education in religion/spirituality within APA-accredited clinical psychology programs. *Professional Psychology: Research and Practice, 33*, 203–206.

Brown, D., & Srebalus, D. (1996). *Introduction to the counseling profession*. Needham Heights, MA: Allyn & Bacon.

Caplan, E. (1998). *Mind games: American culture and the birth of psychotherapy*. Los Angeles: University of California Press.

Choney, S. K., Berryhill-Paapke, E., & Robbins, R. R. (1995). The acculturation of American Indians: Developing frameworks for research and practice. In J. G. Ponterotto, J. M. Casas, L. A. Suzuki, & C. M. Alexander (Eds.), *Handbook of multicultural counseling* (pp. 73–92). Thousand Oaks, CA: Sage.

Ciarrocchi, J. W. (1995). *The doubting disease: Help for scrupulosity and religious compulsions*. Mahwah, NJ: Paulist Press.

Corrigan, P., McCorkle, B., & Schell, B. (2003). Religion and spirituality in the lives of people with serious mental illness. *Community Mental Health Journal, 39*, 487–499.

Delaney, H. D., & DiClemente, C. C. (2005). Psychology's roots: A brief history of the influence of Judeo-Christian perspectives. In W. R. Miller & H. D. Delaney (Eds.), *Judeo-Christian perspectives on psychology: Human nature, motivation, and change* (pp. 31–56). Washington, DC: American Psychological Association.

Eck, B. E. (2002). An exploration of the therapeutic use of spiritual disciplines in clinical practice. *Journal of Psychology and Christianity, 21*, 266–280.

Erickson, M. J., Hecker, L., & Kirkpatrick, D. (2002). Clients' perceptions of marriage and family therapists addressing the religious and spiritual aspects of clients' lives: A pilot study. *Journal of Family Psychotherapy, 13*, 109–125.

Exline, J. J., & Rose, E. (2005). Religious and spiritual struggles. In R. F. Paloutzian & C. L. Park (Eds.), *Handbook of the psychology of religion and spirituality* (pp. 315–330). New York: Guilford Press.

Exline, J. J., Yali, A. M., & Lobel, M. (1999). When God disappoints: Difficulty forgiving God and its role in negative emotion. *Journal of Health Psychology, 4*, 365–379.

Exline, J. J., Yali, A. M., & Sanderson, W. C. (2000). Guilt, discord, and alienation: The role of religious strain in depression and suicidality. *Journal of Clinical Psychology, 56*, 1481–1496.

Fowler, J. W. (1991). Stages in faith consciousness. *New Directions for Child Development, 52*, 27–45.

Frame, M. W. (2003). *Integrating religion and spirituality into counseling: A comprehensive approach*. Pacific Grove, CA: Brooks/Cole.

Frankl, V. (1962). *Man's search for meaning*. New York: Simon & Schuster.

Gallup, G. H., Jr. (1997). *The Gallup poll: Public opinion 1997*. Wilmington, DE: Scholarly Resources.

Gallup, G. H., Jr. (2002). *The Gallup poll: Public opinion 2001*. Wilmington, DE: Scholarly Resources.

Genia, V. (1995). *Counseling and psychotherapy of religious clients: A developmental approach*. Westport, CT: Praeger.

Gerson, J., Rhianon, A., Gold, J., & Kose, G. (2000). Multiple belief systems in psychotherapy: The effects of religion and professional beliefs on clinical judgment. *Journal of Contemporary Psychotherapy, 30*, 27–33.

Hart, K. E. (1999). A spiritual interpretation of the 12-steps of Alcoholics Anonymous: From resentment to forgiveness to love. *Journal of Ministry in Addiction and Recovery, 6,* 25–39.

Hathaway, W. L. (1999, August). Impairment in religious functioning as a clinically significant issue for diagnosis. In W. L. Hathaway (Chair), *Clinically significant religious impairment: Diagnostic and practice issues*. Symposium conducted at the 107th Annual Convention of the American Psychological Association, Boston, MA.

Hathaway, W. L., Scott, S. Y., & Garver, S. A. (2004). Assessing religious/spiritual functioning: A neglected domain in clinical practice? *Professional Psychology: Research and Practice, 35,* 97–104.

Hill, P. C., Pargament, K. I., Hood, R. W., McCullough, M. E., Swyers, J. P., Larson, D. B., & Zinnbauer, B. J. (2000). Conceptualizing religion and spirituality: Points of commonality, points of departure. *Journal for the Theory of Social Behavior, 30,* 51–77.

Holifield, E. B. (1983). *A history of pastoral care in America: From salvation to self-realization*. Nashville, TN: Abingdon Press.

James, W. (1961). *The varieties of religious experience*. New York: Collier Books. (Original work published 1902)

Jones, S. L. (1994). A constructive relationship for religion with the science and profession of psychology: Perhaps the boldest model yet. *American Psychologist, 49,* 184–199.

Jung, C. G. (1938). *Psychology and religion*. New Haven, CT: Yale University Press.

Keller, R. R. (2000). Religious diversity in North America. In P. S. Richards & A. E. Bergin (Eds.), *Handbook of psychotherapy and religious diversity* (pp. 27–55). Washington, DC: American Psychological Association.

Kelly, E. W. (1994). The role of religion and spirituality in counselor education: A national survey. *Counselor Education and Supervision, 33,* 227–237.

Kemp, H. V. (1996). Historical perspective: Religion and clinical psychology in America. In E. P. Shafranske (Ed.), *Religion and the clinical practice of psychology* (pp. 71–112). Washington, DC: American Psychological Association.

Koenig, H. G. (1998). *Handbook of religion and mental health*. San Diego, CA: Academic Press.

Koenig, H. G. (2004). Religion, spirituality and medicine: Research findings and implications for clinical practice. *Southern Medical Journal, 97,* 1194–1200.

Koenig, H. G., & Cohen, H. J. (Eds.). (2002). *The link between religion and health: Psychoneuroimmunology and the faith factor*. Oxford, England: Oxford University Press.

Koenig, H. G., Larson, D. B., & Matthews, D. A. (1996). Religion and psychotherapy with older adults. *Journal of Psychology and Theology, 24,* 155–185.

Koenig, H. G., McCullough, M. E., & Larson, D. B. (2001). *Handbook of religion and health*. Oxford, England: Oxford University Press.

Leong, F. T. L., Wagner, N. S., & Tata, S. P. (1995). Racial and ethnic variations in help-seeking attitudes. In J. G. Ponterotto, J. M. Casa, L. A. Suzuki, & C. M.

Alexander (Eds.), *Handbook of multicultural counseling* (pp. 415–438). Thousand Oaks, CA: Sage.

May, R. (1953). *Man's search for himself*. New York: Norton.

McCullough, M. E. (1999). Research on religion-accommodative counseling: Review and meta-analysis. *Journal of Counseling Psychology, 46,* 92–98.

McMinn, M. R., Aikins, D. C., & Lish, R. A. (2003). Basic and advanced competence in collaborating with clergy. *Professional Psychology: Research and Practice, 34,* 197–202.

Melton, J. G. (2002). *Encyclopedia of American religions* (7th ed.). Detroit, MI: Gale Research.

Miller, W. R. (Ed.). (1999). *Integrating spirituality into treatment: Resources for practitioners.* Washington, DC: American Psychological Association.

Miller, W. R., & Thoresen, C. E. (2003). Spirituality, religion, and health: An emerging research field. *American Psychologist, 58,* 24–35.

Morgan, J. F., Marsden, P., & Lacey, J. H. (2000). "Spiritual starvation?": A case series concerning Christianity and eating disorders. *International Journal of Eating Disorders, 28,* 476–480.

Nelson, E. A., Abramowitz, J. S., & Whiteside, S. P. (2006). Scrupulosity in patients with obsessive–compulsive disorder: Relationship to clinical and cognitive phenomena. *Journal of Anxiety Disorders, 20,* 1071–1086.

Oser, F. K. (1991). The development of religious judgment. In F. K. Oser & W. G. Scarlett (Eds.), *Religious development in childhood and adolescence* (pp. 5–25). San Francisco: Jossey-Bass.

Pargament, K. I., Desai, K. M., & McConnell, K. M. (2006). Spirituality: A pathway to posttraumatic growth or decline? In L. G. Calhoun & R. G. Tedeschi (Eds.), *Handbook of posttraumatic growth: Research and practice* (pp. 121–137). Mahwah, NJ: Erlbaum.

Pargament, K. I., Koenig, H. G., & Perez, L. M. (2000). A comprehensive measure of religious coping: Development and initial validation of the RCOPE. *Journal of Clinical Psychology, 56,* 519–543.

Park, C. L. (2005). Religion and meaning. In R. F. Paloutzian & C. L. Park (Eds.), *Handbook of the psychology of religion and spirituality* (pp. 295–314). New York: Guilford Press.

Pate, R. H., & High, H. J. (1995). The importance of client religious beliefs and practices in the education of counselors in CACREP-accredited programs. *Counseling and Values, 40,* 2–5.

Plante, T. G. (1999). A collaborative relationship between professional psychology and the Roman Catholic church: A case example and suggested principles for success. *Professional Psychology: Research and Practice, 30,* 541–546.

Richards, P. S., & Bergin, A. E. (1997). *A spiritual strategy for counseling and psychotherapy.* Washington, DC: American Psychological Association.

Richards, P. S., & Bergin, A. E. (2000). Toward religious and spiritual competency for mental health professionals. In P. S. Richards & A. E. Bergin (Eds.), *Hand-*

book of psychotherapy and religious diversity (pp. 3–26). Washington, DC: American Psychological Association.

Ripley, J. S., Worthington, E. L., & Berry, J. W. (2001). The effects of religiosity on preferences and expectations for marital therapy among married Christians. American Journal of Family Therapy, 29, 39–58.

Rose, E. M., Westefeld, J. S., & Ansley, T. N. (2001). Spiritual issues in counseling: Clients' beliefs and preferences. Journal of Counseling Psychology, 48, 61–71.

Russell, S. R., & Yarhouse, M. A. (2006). Training in religion/spirituality within APA-accredited psychology predoctoral internships. Professional Psychology: Research and Practice, 37, 430–436.

Salsman, J. M., & Carlson, C. R. (2005). Religious orientation, mature faith, and psychological distress: Elements of positive and negative associations. Journal for the Scientific Study of Religion, 44, 201–209.

Schulte, D. L., Skinner, T. A., & Claiborn, C. D. (2002). Religious and spiritual issues in counseling psychology training. The Counseling Psychologist, 30, 118–134.

Sevensky, R. L. (1984). Religion, psychology, and mental health. American Journal of Psychotherapy, 38, 73–86.

Shafranske, E. P., & Malony, H. N. (1990). Clinical psychologists' religious and spiritual orientations and their practice of psychotherapy. Psychotherapy, 27, 72–78.

Siegel, K., & Schrimshaw, E. (2002). The perceived benefits of religious and spiritual coping among older adults living with HIV/AIDS. Journal for the Scientific Study of Religion, 41, 91–102.

Smith, T. W. (2006). The National Spiritual Transformation Study. Journal for the Scientific Study of Religion, 45, 283–296.

Sperry, L., & Shafranske, E. P. (2005). Spiritually oriented psychotherapy. Washington, DC: American Psychological Association.

Spilka, B., Hood, R. W., & Hunsberger, B. (2003). The psychology of religion: An empirical approach. New York: Guilford Press.

Spilka, B., Ladd, K. L., & McIntosh, D. N. (1996). The content of religious experience: The roles of expectancy and desirability. International Journal for the Psychology of Religion, 6, 95–105.

Tedeschi, R. G., & Calhoun, L. G. (1996). The Posttraumatic Growth Inventory: Measuring the positive legacy of trauma. Journal of Traumatic Stress, 9, 455–471.

Tucker, B., Boyer, M., Aten, J., Jones, S., Price, A., & Johnson, T. (2002, June). Therapists' diagnostic impressions of religious clients. Poster presented at the Association for Women in Psychology Conference, Vancouver, British Columbia, Canada.

VandeCreek, L., Janus, M., & Pennebaker, J. (2002). Praying about difficult experiences as self-disclosure to God. International Journal for the Psychology of Religion, 12, 29–39.

Wade, N. G., Worthington, E. L., Jr., & Vogel, D. L. (2007). Effectiveness of religiously tailored interventions in Christian therapy. Psychotherapy Research, 17, 91–105.

Walker, D. F., Gorsuch, R. L., & Tan, S. Y. (2004). Therapists' integration of religion and spirituality in counseling: A meta-analysis. Counseling and Values, 49, 69–80.

Watlington, C. G., & Murphy, C. M. (2006). The roles of religion and spirituality among African American survivors of domestic violence. *Journal of Clinical Psychology, 62,* 837–857.

Washburn, M. (1988). *The ego and the dynamic ground.* Albany: State University of New York Press.

Watts, R. E. (2001). Addressing issues in secular counseling and psychotherapy: Response to Helminiad's (2001) views. *Counseling and Values, 45,* 207–217.

Webster, R. (1995). *Why Freud was wrong: Sin, science, and psychoanalysis.* New York: Basic Books.

Williams, W. P., & Lawler, M. G. (2000). The challenges and rewards of interchurch marriages: A qualitative study. *Journal of Psychology and Christianity, 19,* 205–218.

Worthington, E. L., Jr., Kurusu, T. A., McCullough, M. E., & Sandage, S. J. (1996). Empirical research on religion and psychotherapeutic processes and outcomes: A 10-year review and research prospectus. *Psychological Bulletin, 119,* 448–487.

Young, J. S., Frame, M. W., Cashwell, C. S., & Belaire, C. (2002). Spiritual and religious competencies: A national survey of CACREP-accredited programs. *Counseling and Values, 47,* 22–33.

Zinnbauer, B. J., & Pargament, K. I. (2005). Religiousness and spirituality. In R. F. Paloutzian & C. L. Park (Eds.), *Handbook of the psychology of religion and spirituality* (pp. 21–42). New York: Guilford Press.

Zinnbauer, B. J., Pargament, K. I., & Scott, A. B. (1999). The emerging meanings of religiousness and spirituality: Problems and prospects. *Journal of Personality, 67,* 889–919.

Zuckerman, D. M., Austin, F., Fair, A., & Branchey, L. (1987). Associations between patient religiosity and alcohol attitudes and knowledge in an alcohol treatment program. *International Journal of Addictions, 22,* 47–53.

2

ETHICAL CONCERNS AROUND SPIRITUALITY AND RELIGION IN CLINICAL PRACTICE

WILLIAM L. HATHAWAY AND JENNIFER S. RIPLEY

The ethical instinct, although not the most prominent, is the most constant and persistent factor in the religious life.

—E. D. Starbuck

This chapter examines common ethical concerns arising from clinical practice with religious and spiritual issues. Fortunately, a professional encountering such issues has a growing body of professional guidance from which to draw in determining an ethical response (Johnson, 2001; Johnson, Ridley, & Nielsen, 2000; Josephson & Peteet, 2004; Miller, 2003; West, 2000; Yarhouse & VanOrman, 1999). Before we enumerate and explore the different types of ethical concerns, consider issues raised by the following case.[1]

Ankita is a 35-year-old Hindu woman who grew up in India. She was married to an older man when she was 15 through an arranged marriage. She explained that the marriage was not consummated until she was 18 and lasted only a few years after that time. She later got a divorce, much to the disapproval of her family, and moved to Europe. She met and married an Australian businessman who was several years older than her and moved into an apartment he provided for her in

---

[1]For the cases presented in this chapter, pseudonyms and sometimes composite cases are used, and identifying details have been altered for confidentiality.

a large western U.S. city. Ankita eventually decided to end the relationship although she still described it as "friendly" during the initial interview.

Ankita entered counseling at a Christian practice because she wanted to talk through a number of issues with someone who might understand "spiritual concerns." She stated that in India her family members would often talk to each other to get help with their problems. She did know a few other Hindus residing in her current community but stated that she had trouble relating to them because they were in conventional Hindu marriages. When the therapist asked Ankita to describe what she meant by a therapist who understood spiritual concerns, she paused for a minute and then replied, "I guess by that I mean someone who believes there is a spiritual side to life, a way we should live and path we should walk. I mean . . . well, I think we should try to be successful in life . . . to try to become the persons we should be, and that is why I have made some choices that have been against the wishes of my family. But I don't feel this was completely right either . . . I thought you might understand that as a religious therapist."

Ankita's case represents the complex considerations that often arise when spirituality presents as an issue in therapy. Spirituality was important for Ankita and led her to choose a therapy context that was explicitly identified with a religious tradition. Ankita referenced "spirituality" almost as an aside, without spontaneous elaboration. When clients raise issues of spirituality in therapy, it is not unusual for them to feel that their words have a clear meaning to the therapist, yet this is often not the case. There are many potential meanings for terms such as *spirituality*, *religion*, *faith*, or *belief* (Zinnbauer, Pargament, & Scott, 1999).

The therapist wondered about Ankita's choice of a Christian counselor. It is a characteristic feature of Hinduism to be open to expressions of spirituality from other faiths (Huyler, 1999). Yet, Ankita's personal life choices had also put her at odds with her family of origin and other communal obligations she felt from her Hindu faith. Later sessions would reveal that part of the reason Ankita sought out the Christian therapist was to avoid the rejection that she feared from other Hindu women who had pursued a more conventional relational path.

Ankita's presentation of "spiritual concerns" raises numerous ethical issues that should be attended to by therapists. These include practicing in a manner that is respectful of religious and spiritual diversity, avoiding bias, doing good, doing no harm, not imposing therapist values on the client, respecting client autonomy, practicing in a competent manner, being mindful of role-related obligations that arise from professional identity, and seeking consultation as needed to help realize these ideals. We now turn to a more detailed discussion of these ethical issues and how they are woven into the context of contemporary mental health professions.

PROFESSIONAL ETHICS AND PROFESSIONAL PRACTICE

The promulgation of ethics codes has become a hallmark characteristic of contemporary professions (Baker, 1999; Hathaway, 2006). There are several distinctive features associated with such contemporary codes. Rather than being merely honorific professions, as in the Hippocratic Oath, these codes now reflect corporate commitments to exemplify specific ethical principles in concrete aspects of practice. Although this development represents a convergence of several important strands of applied ethics, three are particularly relevant to our discussion: principlism, specification, and casuistry.

Principlism is the general term for any approach to ethics that is guided by explicit and preselected ethical principles. During the last few decades, many health care-related professions have become increasingly influenced by a particular model of principlism advocated by the biomedical ethics gurus Beauchamp and Childress (1979, 2001). They have championed the "Georgetown mantra," arguing that professional ethics should be guided by an attempt to exemplify the principles of nonmaleficence, autonomy, benevolence, and justice. Professionals familiar with the American Psychological Association's "Ethical Principles of Psychologists and Code of Conduct" (hereafter referred to as the Ethics Code; APA, 2002; see also http://www.apa.org/ethics/code2002.pdf) will recognize the similarity between the Georgetown mantra and three of the five principles from the current Ethics Code: beneficence and nonmaleficence (Ethical Principle A), justice (Ethical Principle D), and respect for people's rights and dignity (Ethical Principle E).

Whereas principlism is a common feature of more recent approaches to biomedical ethics, perhaps the most distinctive aspect of contemporary professional ethics has been its penchant for specification of behavioral duties. The phrases *professional ethics* and *medical ethics* first appeared in Thomas Percival's (1803) groundbreaking text that became the model for subsequent professional codes. A key departure of Percival's approach to medical ethics from the earlier brief, honorific oaths in medicine was the detailed and highly specific delineation of specific behavioral expectations for health care (Baker, 1999). In contrast to the predominantly generic duties reflected in the Hippocratic Oath, Percival's text went into great detail about concrete aspects of practice, such as the need for physicians do their rounds early and often to maximize the effectiveness of the health care system or the need of an aging physician to be open to peer feedback and consultation to ensure that patient care is not compromised. The specified duties in such a code of conduct are often presented or discussed within professions as applications of the profession's ethical principles. The APA Ethics Code (2002) reflects this Percivalian motif.

If this were the whole story of contemporary professional ethics, then we would be following a highly regimented approach to ethical decision making similar to the following:

1. A profession commits itself to a set of principles.
2. The profession then reflects on the specific implications of those principles for how its professionals should conduct themselves in concrete situations that characterize its professional practice.
3. These implications are spelled out in a code of conduct.
4. When the set of principles adopted by a profession seem to pull a professional in competing directions, either some rule is created that clarifies the considerations that should take precedence or a strategy tells how to make proper compromises between the principles.

If only ethical paths were so easily navigated! A growing group of critics in bioethics have dissented from this principlism model of ethical decision making. For instance, Jonsen and Toulmin (1990) argued that principlism does not do justice to the historical role of clinical judgment in response to the idiosyncratic complexities of concrete cases. In contrast to a model that emphasizes the top-down application of universal principles, they argued for one that is more attuned to subtle but idiosyncratic features of the ethical dilemmas that often present themselves with specific cases. They also argued for a greater appreciation of the classical approach to professional jurisprudence and ethics known as casuistry. Casuistry tries to mine the wisdom of case examples by reflecting on how exemplars wisely handled analogous situations.

It is beyond the scope of this chapter to arbitrate these divides between principlism and its antiprinciplist critics. What we will do is alternate between a principle-focused and case-generated discussion of how therapists should handle the spiritual and religious issues they encounter in practice.

Professional guidance on clinical practice with spiritual and religious issues has been burgeoning in recent years. Most of this guidance has been derived from ethical and theoretical considerations (Cashwell & Young, 2005; Griffith & Young, 2004; Hawkins & Bullock, 1995; Richards & Bergin, 2005). It has occasionally been the focus of mainstream psychology journals but more often has appeared in niche publications primarily purveyed by practitioners with special interests in spirituality (Johnson et al., 2000; Lomax, Karff, & McKenny, 2002; McClemore & Court, 1977; Tan, 1994). An empirical clinical psychology of religion is just beginning to emerge, but numerous commentators have found substantive implications from professional codes for this practice domain (Tan & Johnson, 2005; Worthington & Sandage, 2001, 2002).

SOURCES OF ETHICAL GUIDANCE
FOR SPIRITUALITY IN PRACTICE

Therapists have a variety of sources of ethical guidance when they encounter issues of spirituality and religion in practice. In addition to relevant principles and standards from professional ethics codes or jurisprudence, there are also relevant practice guidelines and policy statements promulgated by professional bodies, liability and risk management considerations, evidence-based practice findings, and the practice habits of clinical psychology of religion exemplars. Table 2.1 summarizes some authoritative sources of ethical guidance that explicitly address spiritual or religious issues for practice.

Practice Guidelines

A number of practice guidelines adopted as recommended "best practices" by different professional organizations explicitly address spiritual and religious considerations. Practice guidelines regarding child custody and child protection evaluations recommend particular attention to how religion may bias the outcome of such evaluations (APA, 1994; APA, Committee on Professional Practice and Standards, 1999). The American Psychiatric Association (1989) provided an early set of guidelines "enjoining respect for . . . patients beliefs" and disapproving of psychiatrists imposing their beliefs on clients or substituting religious practices or concepts for accepted therapeutic practices.

Legal Precedents

Another source of explicit guidance regarding clinical practice with spiritual and religious issues arises from court decisions. *Bruff v. North Mississippi Health Services, Inc.* (2001) provides a clear example of such a precedent. The plaintiff, Sandra Bruff, was a hospital counselor who was dismissed in 1996, a firing she claimed was a result of her religious objections to homosexuality. Hermann and Herlihy (2006) gave a helpful analysis of the legal and ethical implications of this case for therapists. They characterized the court's decisions as follows:

> In March 2001, the United States Court of Appeals for the Fifth Circuit held that an employer's statutory obligation to make reasonable accommodations for employees' religious beliefs does not include accommodating a counselor's request to be excused from counseling homosexual clients on relationship issues. . . . The counselor who filed the lawsuit claimed that her employer's failure to allow her to refrain from counseling clients on issues inconsistent with her religious beliefs violated federal law. The court disagreed and found that the counselor's allegations had no merits. (Hermann & Herlihy, 2006, p. 414)

TABLE 2.1
Examples of Sources of Explicit Ethical Guidance for Spiritual Issues in Practice

Source	Category	Example
APA (2002) "Ethical Principles of Psychology and Code of Conduct"	Professional code	Ethical Principle E. Respect for People's Rights and Dignity: "Psychologists are aware of and respect cultural, individual, and role differences, including those based on . . . religion. Psychologists try to eliminate the effect on their work of biases based on these factors, and they do not knowingly participate in or condone activities of others based upon such prejudices" (p. 4). Standard 3.01. "In their work-related activities, psychologists do not engage in unfair discrimination based on . . . religion" (p. 5).
American Counseling Association (2005) Ethics Code	Professional code	C.5. Nondiscrimination: "Counselors do not condone or engage in discrimination based on . . . religion/spirituality" (p. 10). E.8. Multicultural Issues/Diversity in Assessment: "Counselors recognize the effects of . . . religion, spirituality . . . on test administration and interpretation, and place test results in proper perspective with other relevant factors" (p. 13).
APA (1994) "Guidelines for Child Custody Evaluations in Divorce Proceedings"	Practice guidelines	Guideline 6. "The psychologist engaging in child custody evaluations is aware of how biases regarding . . . religion . . . may interfere with an objective evaluation and recommendations. The psychologist recognizes and strives to overcome any such biases or withdraws from the evaluation" (p. 678).
APA (2000) "Guidelines for Psychotherapy With Lesbian, Gay, and Bisexual Clients"	Practice guidelines	"Key issues for practice include an understanding of . . . the "coming out" process and how variables such as . . . religion may influence this process . . . struggles with spirituality and religious group membership" (p. 1442).
American Psychiatric Association (1989) Guidelines Regarding Possible Conflict Between Psychiatrists' Religious Commitments and Psychiatric Practice	Practice guidelines	I. Psychiatrists should maintain respect for their patients' beliefs. A. It is useful for clinicians to obtain information on the religious or ideologic orientation and beliefs of their patients so that they may properly attend to them in the course of treatment. B. If an unexpected conflict arises in relation to such beliefs, it should be handled with a concern for the patient's vulnerability to the attitudes of the psychiatrist. Empathy for the patient's sensibilities and particular beliefs is essential.

(continues)

TABLE 2.1
Examples of Sources of Explicit Ethical Guidance for
Spiritual Issues in Practice   *(Continued)*

Source	Category	Example
		C. Interpretations that concern a patient's beliefs should be made in a context of empathic respect for their value and meaning to the patient. II. Psychiatrists should not impose their own religious, antireligious, or ideologic systems of beliefs on their patients, nor should they substitute such beliefs or ritual for accepted diagnostic concepts or therapeutic practice. A. No practitioner should force a specific religious, antireligious, or ideologic agenda on a patient or work to see that the patient adopts such an agenda. B. Religious concepts or ritual should not be offered as a substitute for accepted diagnostic concepts or therapeutic practice.
Bruff v. North Mississippi Health Services, Inc. (2001)	Legal precedent	"An employee has a duty to cooperate in achieving accommodation of his or her religious beliefs, and must be flexible in achieving that end" (p. 503).

Note. APA = American Psychological Association.

Although correct on the general facts, Herman and Herlihy may be mischaracterizing some subtle but important aspects of the decision. Recall that they characterized the appellate court's findings as giving no merit to Bruff's allegations. In fact, the court stated that "Bruff established her prima facie case of religious discrimination." The court then shifted the burden of proof to Bruff's employer to demonstrate why they did not accommodate her religious beliefs and preferences.

Bruff's employer noted that the relevant law requires such accommodation unless it creates more than a *de minimis* cost and thus creates an "undue hardship" for the employer. The court concluded that Bruff's employer had demonstrated that her requested accommodations would result in an undue hardship. The reader is referred to Foltin and Standish (2004) for a more thorough discussion of the use of the *de minimis* standard in considering when religious accommodations pose such undue employer hardships. It is not entirely clear that the court would have ruled in the same way if it had been possible to accommodate Bruff's requests without creating an undue hardship. The court did not challenge the initial burden of the employer to otherwise accommodate an employee's religion.

Hermann and Herlihy (2006) also explored the ethical issues raised by Bruff's refusal to provide relational counseling for her homosexual client. Bruff alleged that her desire to refer homosexual clients who desire relational counseling to other therapists was consistent with ethical standards that call for practice within one's domain of competence. In contrast, Hermann and Herlihy contended that this obligation must be balanced against every counselor's obligation to avoid discrimination, avoid value imposition, respect client autonomy, pursue fairness (justice), do good, and avoid harm. These tensions are particularly salient in this case because Bruff was one of only three counselors in a program that had to provide a general range of services to all eligible recipients. Herman and Herlihy's discussion illustrates the relevance of the professional codes and the complexities of managing the varieties of ethical considerations that arise from spiritual and religious considerations in the multifaceted and diverse context of practice.

Exemplar Guidance

As we noted earlier, there is now a growing body of literature generated by practitioners, researchers, and instructors who specialize in clinical work with spiritual and religious issues. Although there is no formally recognized specialty in this practice niche, several doctoral programs provide specially designed curriculum to cultivate skills in this area, continuing education workshops on working with spiritual and religious issues in practice have been successful parts of professional conferences for several years, and the training texts published by primary mental health associations have been well received (Cashwell & Young, 2005; Josephson & Peteet, 2004; Richards & Bergin, 2005; Shafranske, 1996).

APA Division 36 (Psychology of Religion) has been devoted to the psychology of religion for decades, and the American Counseling Association has its Association for Spiritual, Ethical, and Religious Values in Counseling (ASERVIC). Both of these professional bodies have been developing guidance for professional practice with spiritual and religious issues. Members of ASERVIC, for example, have published a list of spiritual competencies for counseling, including being sensitive to clients' expressed religious and spiritual preferences and being able to describe client religion and spiritually in light of its cultural context (Cashwell & Young, 2005).

An ad hoc committee of APA Division 36 formed in 2004 has been exploring the development of practice guidelines for clinical work with religious and spiritual issues. In 2005, the committee generated 26 preliminary practice guidelines for working with religious and spiritual issues (Hathaway, 2005). The guidelines were developed inductively by the committee after reflecting on convergent thematic suggestions from semistructured interviews with 25 nationally known experts in the practice area. The preliminary guidelines focus on assessment, therapy, and diversity considerations. They are presented in Appendix 2.1. It is important to note that the preliminary guidelines are just that—preliminary. They have not been formally adopted by APA Division 36 or any other authoritative body. They represent the sorts of common best practice recommendations from exemplar clinicians who specialize in addressing religious and spiritual issues in practice. They are also primarily derived from the application of standard ethical considerations to this practice domain.

Evidence-Based Practice

The last source of guidance for ethical professional practice comes from the evidence-based practice movement. In 2005, APA formally adopted a resolution that supports evidence-based practice in psychology. Evidence-based practice "is the integration of best research evidence with clinical expertise and patient values" (Institute of Medicine, 2001, p. 147). Note that this is a broader notion than empirically validated treatment. Evidenced-based practice also explicitly considers client values and clinical knowledge from practice.

Evidence-based practice considerations can provide important ethical guidance for clinical practice with religious and spiritual issues. APA Ethical Standard 2.01b, Boundaries of Competence, states the following:

> Where scientific or professional knowledge in the discipline of psychology establishes that an understanding of factors associated with . . . religion . . . is essential for effective implementation of their services . . . psychologists have or obtain the training, experience, consultation, or supervision necessary to ensure the competence of their services, or they make appropriate referrals. (APA, 2002, pp. 4–5)

Ensuring competent care in such cases is vital to prevent harm and to maximize treatment benefit.

Although this source of guidance holds promise for informing better practice with spiritual and religious issues in the future, at present most of the evidence provides only anecdotal or indirect guidance for clinical work with spiritual and religious issues. Some reviews of relevant research have generally found that spiritually or religiously congruent therapy practices were as effective as practices that excluded spiritual accommodations. The reviews did not find any robust evidence of an incremental treatment outcome benefit from inclusion of spiritual components (e.g., Tan & Johnson, 2005; Worthington & Sandage, 2002). Yet they did note that spiritually accommodative approaches appeared to be comparable in efficacy with secular approaches and may be conducive to other benefits. For instance, religiously committed clients may obtain higher levels of spiritual well-being from spiritually accommodative therapy

(Worthington & Sandage, 2001). These clients also tend to prefer such accommodations as a personal value, one of the dimensions that the APA (2005) evidence-based practice policy recommends clinicians consider. Much more empirical work needs to be done to explore the effectiveness of such spiritually focused and accommodative therapy. The current evidence suggests that spiritually accommodative practice does not reduce treatment benefit, may be more respectful of spiritually oriented client values, and may produce other sorts of benefits for such clients.

CASE REFLECTIONS

We now turn to a discussion of several vignettes that illustrate how wisdom from these varied sources might shed ethical light on some of the challenges that can often arise from working with spiritual and religious issues in practice. The vignettes are inspired by case situations encountered by us, our supervisees, or colleagues. However, the details of each vignette are drawn from an aggregate of multiple cases or otherwise altered to protect the identity and privacy of clients. The cases collectively indicate the sorts of ethical issues that routinely present in practice when addressing religious and spiritual concerns. Although not every issue is relevant to every case, issues of avoiding bias and value imposition, respecting client autonomy and self-determination, appreciating the role of multiple overlapping diversity factors, self-awareness, respecting confidentiality, practicing within one's domain of competence, seeking appropriate consultation, and informed consent resurface in a majority of the vignettes.

Vignette 1—The Gradys: Protecting Against Bias

The Gradys are a couple in their 40s, both in their second marriage. Diane enthusiastically converted to a conservative evangelical Christian religion 5 years ago. She is heavily involved in leading women's outreach groups at their local church. Quinton considers himself a Christian but is not highly committed, attending church about once a month. Diane's pastor recommended they see a therapist, who is known in the community as a Christian. Diane is highly concerned that her husband drinks alcohol, about two drinks a day. She considers this to be a sin. Diane entered therapy with the presenting problem of her husband's drinking.

Several factors make this case particularly prone to problematic triangulations in which the therapist may counterproductively align with one member of the dyad (Stratton & Smith, 2006). The couple has important differences in how they understand their own religious identities, despite their shared general affiliation as Christians. The Christian therapist was referred by the pastor of Diane's church. Consequently, it is possible that Quinton will enter therapy already suspecting that he is on the "other side" from the therapist, whom he will likely see as allied with his wife's religious outlook. A more troubling possibility is Quinton might be right! What if the therapist is biased against Quinton's religious outlook and shares Diane's attitude toward alcohol consumption based on religious convictions? Imagine further that the therapist proceeded with the counseling, concurring with Diane's goal of reducing Quinton's alcohol consumption without any other evidence of alcohol-related problems.

The therapist in this case would appear to be imposing his or her own religious biases on at least one of the individuals in the dyad, inconsistent with Principle E of the APA (2002) code calling for psychologists to "try to eliminate the effect on their work of biases based on . . . religion" (p. 4). Similar prohibitions are found in the American Counseling Association (2005) ethics code and the American Psychiatric Association (1989) guidelines. Furthermore, by participating in this problematic triangulation with Diane against Quinton, the therapist is likely reducing the chances of a positive outcome for the marital therapy and may be contributing to an adverse outcome. This could potentially lead to a violation of cardinal principles of "doing good" and "doing no harm" embodied in all relevant professional codes. It is important to note that although both Diane and Quinton self-identify as Christians, Christianity is a sociologically diverse faith tradition. The fact that the therapist and both members of the couple are Christian does not mean that they have congruence on all of the clinically relevant spiritual issues or values, including whether alcohol consumption is appropriate for a Christian.

If the therapist instead followed a practice pattern similar to the one recommended by APA's Division 36 preliminary practice guideline M-2 (see Appendix 2.1), a different state of affairs may have resulted:

> Psychologists strive to be self-aware of their own perspectives, attitudes, history, and self-understandings of religion and spirituality. Psychologists should be mindful of how their own background on religious/spiritual matters might bias their response and approach to clients of differing background.

The following alternative strategies would have been more congruent with this advice and less likely to lead to the ethical perils noted earlier: On finding out that the couple was referred by the pastor and that religious themes were a concern for Diane, the therapist could have done a more careful assessment of each person's individual spiritual and religious outlook. In most practice contexts, imposition of a religious or spiritual prohibition about non-pathological behaviors, such as Quinton's normal-range alcohol consumption, would be difficult to justify. A spiritually self-aware therapist would take steps to avoid imposing this religious outlook on Quinton. It may also be advisable to explore each client's fears or expectations regarding whether the therapist would take sides because of religious differences. This will require the therapist to have engaged in self-reflection regarding his or her own religious and spirituals beliefs, attitudes, and values (Hagedorn, 2005).

Vignette 2—Mary: A Case for Collaboration?

Mary is an African American married mother of four diagnosed with major depression. Through the influence of a sibling, she has begun to attend a small local church, which has been generally supportive and helpful to her. However, Mary complained that when she talked about her depression with her minister's wife, the minister's wife gossiped by telling several church members about her problems. Mary felt betrayed, and her depression worsened. She has displayed increased signs of suicidality. She requested that her therapist work with her minister but specifically forbade working with the minister's wife. It is unclear if the minister will respect Mary's confidentiality with regard to his wife. However, the minister could also be a significant support for Mary especially as hospitalization appears to be imminent.

Although clergy may have a moral obligation and popularly perceived role expectation to maintain confidentiality, there is a great deal of variability in whether such a duty is actually embraced in particular faith traditions. There is also no consistent nonecclesiastical regulatory authority that would provide oversight when alleged beaches of ministerial confidentiality have occurred despite suggestions that such a legal duty should be developed for clergy (Griffith & Young, 2004). Consequently, a therapist cannot count on confidentiality being protected or understood in the same way within a religious community that it might be among mental health professionals. Because of these sorts of uncertainties, therapists may often avoid collaborating with spiritual or religious professionals.

APA (2002) Ethical Standard 4.01 states that "psychologists . . . take reasonable precautions to protect confidential information" (p. 7). Assuming that the therapist obtained a release from Mary to discuss the information with the minister, the psychologist may be absolved of legal culpability for breaching confidentiality even if the minister subsequently discusses it with his wife. Yet even if the therapist was not technically guilty of this violation, the effect on therapy may be the same. Mary's trust in her therapist would likely erode and further exacerbate her troubling situation.

Still, as this vignette suggests, there is often much to be gained from effective collaboration with religious communities (see chap. 10, this volume). Mary found significant support from her religious community. There are helpful models of constructive collaboration between mental health professionals and members of the clergy (McMinn & Dominguez, 2005). In Mary's case, it would be important to have a careful and respectful discussion about what she may want to be shared with the minister, understanding that the therapist may not be able to guarantee the confidentiality of such information once it is disclosed. Once Mary understands the nature of the communication and collaboration with her minister that is being suggested by her therapist, it will be important to obtain permission from her for the agreed-on arrangement. As the holder of the privilege to the confidential information, Mary must formally release the therapist to engage in any disclosures with her minister (Sperry, 2007). Whereas formal release may occur through an explicit verbal acknowledgment, the more typical standard of practice is to have Mary sign an explicit, time-limited document that spells out the nature of the information that will be disclosed, its purposes, and other relevant details of the arrangement. Although not routinely part of such a release or authorization, it would be wise to include a clear statement acknowledging the degree to which the minister is or is not legally bound by the confidentiality parameters of the therapy.

Vignette 3—Nasser: Competence and Autonomy

> Nasser is a recent immigrant from the Philippines who is pursuing a college degree. He is also a Muslim who embraces many Westernized values and lifestyle patterns. One of Nasser's primary concerns is anxiety about his sexual activity, as he's struggling with having a sexual relationship with a European American girlfriend but feeling some guilt about it. He frames this as primarily a religious problem. Nasser's therapist grew up Catholic and has not had any scholarly training in Islamic religion. In their small college town, there are no known Muslim therapists for referral, and Nasser reports that he rarely attends the local mosque because it is very conservative.

Nasser's case reflects the challenges and opportunities religious pluralism presents for therapists. Most therapists will encounter a wide spectrum of spiritual and religious faith traditions in their client population. Often these will be quite different from the therapists' personal traditions. In addition to these between-groups differences, there is also considerable variation within each faith tradition. In Nasser's case, we have someone whose multicultural background creates added complexities: He is a Filipino immigrant who self-identifies as Muslim, yet he is also religiously divergent from other Muslims in his current community. In this case, there is a real possibility that the therapist will fail to appreciate clinically important nuances of the client's particular convergence of multiple diversity backgrounds.

When therapists have questionable competence for working with a client of a particular background, it is important that they take adequate steps to ensure that the client's clinical care is not compromised. This is an issue of practicing within one's range of competence. APA (2002) Ethical Standard 2.01c states that "psychologists planning to provide services . . . involving populations, areas, techniques . . . new to them undertake relevant education, training, supervised experience, consultation, or study" (p. 5). Nassar's therapist would likely need to obtain consultation from a therapist competent in working with Nassar's constellation of issues. If it becomes clear that consultation alone is insufficient for competent therapy, then referral may be indicated.

Vignette 4—Custody Evaluation: A Case of Religious Bias?

> Dr. Bob, a psychologist in a rural Midwest location, was asked to do a custody evaluation of Mr. Smith's 8-year-old daughter. Mr. Smith is an active member of a conservative Baptist church where his daughter has also been active in the youth group since they moved to the region 2 years ago. Mr. Smith and his wife are now going through a divorce, and both parents are contesting for custody. His daughter has visited her mother periodically since the separation. Mrs. Smith has relocated to the Northeast where she grew up before the couple met at a Midwestern college. In a report to the court, Dr. Bob indicated that although both parents appear to have certain strengths, it would be better for the daughter to be raised by her father. He reasoned this because the daughter expressed religious faith and the mother was an agnostic. He asserted that, all things being equal, it is better to have a child raised in a home that is faith congruent. Mrs. Smith felt that the court was being hostile toward her because of her agnosticism. Dr. Bob and the family court judge both attended a church in the same denomination as Mr. Smith.

The case of Dr. Bob again raises issues of bias and value imposition. However, it has the added complication of child welfare and legal issues. Because deeply held worldviews, values, spiritual outlooks, and other such characteristics often shape the way one perceives individuals, the child custody situation is particularly susceptible to the effect of religion or spiritual bias. When psychologists identify spiritually with one parent in a child custody dispute more than the other, they are at heightened risk for letting this bias their judgment. In Dr. Bob's case, there are little scientific data to support his judgment that the parent with a faith congruent to the child's would be the better custodian of the child. Consequently, it is much more likely that this judgment reflects a proreligious bias on the part of Dr. Bob that predisposed him against Mrs. Smith. Unfortunately, this scenario has played out before in child evaluation settings. That is why the APA (1994) guidelines on child custody evaluations specifically state that a "psychologist engaging in child custody evaluations is aware of how biases regarding . . . religion . . .

may interfere with an objective evaluation and recommendations. The psychologist recognizes and strives to overcome any such biases or withdraws from the evaluation" (p. 678).

As with our earlier case illustrating concerns about bias, the cultivation of self-awareness is an important first corrective step. Other strategies might include consulting with another professional proficient in child custody evaluations who has a divergent spiritual perspective from the therapist; participating in team evaluations with other professionals who represent a diverse set of personal backgrounds; checking out the research bases for one's biases (e.g., Are there any empirical data that parent–child faith congruence produces better child outcomes?); or, finally, resorting to the strategy recommended by the guidelines, simply withdrawing from such cases.

Vignette 5—Tim: Autonomy or Internalized Prejudice?

Tim is a 25-year-old man who has experienced same-sex attraction since early adolescence. However, he is also an adherent of a religious tradition that views homosexual behavior as immoral. He entered therapy to resolve the conflict he was experiencing between his same-sex attraction and his religious beliefs.

Similar to Nasser's case, often clients present not with just one defining dimension of diversity but with several. In some cases, the client may be conflicted over how and whether to integrate these multiple diversity dimensions. Haldeman (2004) eloquently outlined the conflict facing such clients:

The practical and ethical ramifications for the sexually/spiritually conflicted client are considerable. For example, if gay identity is expressed to the exclusion of a conservative religious background, the potential losses of family and community are not easily replaced, especially for the individual unfamiliar with the gay community. And these losses may pale in contrast with the profound existential loss of a religious institution whose doctrine provided meaning and comfort but whose doors are not open to noncelibate, same-sex-attracted individuals. Similarly difficult challenges face the individual who chooses religious expression instead of same-sex attraction. The repression of same-sex feelings for the individual seeking to live in a heterosexual or celibate manner can exact a great psychic toll. (p. 713)

Therapist diversity considerations further complicate the picture. Imagine that this client was being seen by a conventionally religious therapist whose religious tradition echoed the same beliefs as the client's about homosexuality. This therapist–client pattern would risk a premature foreclosure on their shared religious attitude toward homosexual behavior and may generate a suboptimal or even iatrogenic treatment plan to address this area of mutual concern. For example, the therapist may use pathological connotations to describe at least some aspects of homosexuality despite the fact that the major mental health organizations have taken stands incongruent with such views (APA, 2000; Haldeman, 2004). Alternatively, imagine a different therapist treating the client who holds consistently gay-affirming attitudes and beliefs. In this therapist–client match the risk is that the therapist may be inadequately respectful toward the client's religious values and beliefs. Such attitudes could range from undervaluing the salience of the religious perspective to the client to an outright hostile rejection of the client's religious beliefs and values.

Both Haldeman (2004) and Yarhouse (1998) provided extensive discussions of just these sorts of cases. Haldeman (2004) noted that the likely ethical challenges to arise in treating sexual minority clients "include informed consent about treatment, alternative treatments, disseminating accurate clinical and scientific information about sexual orientation, respect for individual autonomy, and protection from bias on the part of the practitioner" (p. 692). Tim's case vignette highlights the issue of client autonomy. This principle present in the professional codes for the mental health professions calls for respecting the dignity and worth of individuals, including their "right of self-determination" (APA, 2002, p. 4). Therapists do not have to personally embrace the choices made by the client, but they do have to acknowledge and support the client's right to make them. At the same time, the APA's (2000) Guidelines for Psychotherapy With Lesbian, Gay, and Bisexual Clients enjoins practitioners to be mindful of the sociocultural context in the client's self-understandings regarding his or her sexual identity development. The client might be operating under misinformation or interpersonal influences that interfere with his or her ability to engage in well-informed, autonomous decision making.

Vignette 6—Sondra: Therapist Disclosure of Spirituality

Sondra has always seen herself as a "just" and "typical" person throughout her life. She completed her educational goals at a local college without any fanfare and is a certified public accountant. She was raised in an "irreligious" family and describes herself as not religious or spiritual. Sondra made an appointment with a mental health professional after a brief but disconcerting experience on a recent hiking trip with her friend. While she was walking ahead by herself on a scenic section of a mountain trail, she had a sudden awareness of the "connectedness" of her life with everything around her. This event was unlike anything she had previously experienced, and she was not aware of anything that may have precipitated it. It seemed to pull her outside of her mundane life, but it also was quite disorienting, leading her to question how she was going about her life. She did not know how to make sense of the event or even whether to think of it as positive or negative. The psychologist determined that Sondra did not meet the criteria for a *DSM–IV–TR* (*Diagnostic and Statistical Manual of Mental Disorders*, 4th ed., text rev.) Axis I or II disorder but classified her with a "spiritual problem." Toward the end of the session, Sondra noticed that the psychologist had a statue of the Buddha on her desk and was curious about what this might signify, so she asked the psychologist to "tell me what this would mean to you in your spiritual path?"

Sondra's case fits the category of a "Religious or Spiritual Problem V-code" from the influential *DSM–IV–TR* of the American Psychiatric Association (2000) psychiatric classification system for mental disorders. This category describes religious or spiritual issues that warrant the focus of a clinical attention without indicating the presence of a disorder. Individuals conceptualizing Sondra's case from a transpersonal perspective may conclude that she is undergoing a "spiritual emergence." Lukoff (1998) explained that in emergence "there is a gradual unfoldment of spiritual potential with minimal disruption in psychological/social/occupational functioning, whereas in spiritual *emergency* there is significant abrupt disruption in psychological/social/ occupational functioning" (pp. 38–39).

Sondra's apparent freshly stimulated "spiritual interests" coupled with curiosity about the therapist's personal spirituality resulted in an inviting opportunity for therapist disclosure of spirituality. Indeed, having the statue of the Buddha, or any other religious artifact, will likely be seen as self-disclosure by clients regardless of therapist intent. The combination of a relatively low risk but potentially spiritually intriguing clinical presentation might tempt a therapist to lower his or her defenses and become more disclosing than the therapist might otherwise be. The session could turn into an encounter in which the therapist self-indulges his or her own spiritual interests by, for instance, relaying personal peak experiences or sharing a religious testimony for no deliberate clinical reason. As long as the client had unimpaired mental health, there would likely be little adverse consequence from such a therapist disclosure. Yet by its very nature such an encounter could be exploitive. The therapist would be functioning not for the client's benefit but for his or her own. The risks from such a therapist behavior would not be limited to improper therapist intent. It could pressure the client to present in certain ways that the client might not have otherwise presented as a result of a "halo effect" produced by the therapist spiritual disclosures.

The American Psychiatric Association's (1989) guidelines make it clear that any therapist spiritual self-disclosure that represents an imposition of the therapist's spirituality on the client is never appropriate. APA's Division 36 preliminary practice multicultural guideline M-4 (see Appendix 2.1) provides further direction on when such disclosures might be appropriate:

> Psychologists are mindful of factors that influence the appropriateness of their own religious/spiritual self-disclosure to a client. These include but are not limited to disclosures that are
> (a) congruent with the treatment orientation or approach used,
> (b) consistent with other general background self-disclosures offered to a client at the outset of treatment,
> (c) facilitative of the treatment, and
> (d) necessary to address a potential value conflict that might impede treatment.

Tjeltveit (1999) cautioned, however, that as therapists we can never remove our biases entirely. In light of this limitation, he recommended pursuing enhanced self-awareness, doing what we can to minimize value imposition, and using well-crafted therapist disclosures of religious or spiritual backgrounds when obtaining consent for treatment. Such disclosures should be sufficient to make the client aware of the worldview of the therapist that might guide the therapist's approach to practice or cardinal values without going beyond what is clinically relevant for the benefit of the client's informed choice. Miller (2003) provided examples of such advanced inform consents that address therapist spiritual or religious background, as well as the manner in which religious and spiritual issues or techniques might be brought into therapy.

Vignette 7—Mira: Spiritual Techniques or Pastoral Care?

> Mira is 23-year-old woman who is a regular participant in the Spanish worship team at her charismatic, nondenominational church. She is fluent in English. She has been struggling with widespread and free-floating worries about many different things since her teenage years. These worries seem to have intensified in the last few years although Mira could not describe any specific precipitant for this change. Mira does not believe that she should struggle with worry at this level because she should be able to just trust God to take care of things. She was referred to her psychologist because someone in her church thought he might be a Christian. When she arrived for the first session, she described her problems and then requested to only use "Bible counseling" and "prayer" to help her get over them. She also stated that she did not want to "use secular counseling" to get better.

Recall from our earlier discussion that the current evidence is that accommodating religious and spiritual interventions in clinical practice does not reduce the benefit of such treatment. Mira's case presents a more challenging scenario. She requested treatment using only spiritual or religious techniques. Although there is research related to the mental health correlates of facets of spirituality such as religious coping patterns (Pargament, 1997), prayer or meditation, or attendance at religious services (Hebert, Dang, & Schultz, 2007), there is no well-designed research on the exclusive use of such spiritual techniques to treat psychological dysfunction.

According to APA's Division 36 preliminary intervention guideline I-7 (see Appendix 2.1),

> When psychologists use religious/spiritual techniques in treatment, such as prayer or devotional meditation, they
> (a) clearly explain the proposed technique to the client and obtain informed consent,
> (b) do so in a competent manner that is respectful of the intended religious and spiritual function of the technique in the client's faith tradition, and
> (c) adopt such techniques only if they are believed to facilitate a treatment goal.

Although spiritual or religious techniques may have a beneficial effect on anxiety, there is a real risk that adoption of such "sacred disciplines" for clinical treatment will represent a co-option of their religious or spiritual purpose (Tan, 1994, 2003).

APA (2002) Ethical Standard 10.01(b) states that

> when obtaining informed consent for treatment for which generally recognized techniques and procedures have not been established, psychologists inform their clients/patients of the developing nature of the treatment, the potential risks involved, alternative treatments that may be available, and the voluntary nature of their participation. (p. 13)

Mira's request might be thought of as a request for an unproven treatment. If this is a correct characterization of her situation, then the expectations outlined in APA Ethical Standard 10.01(b) might be sufficient. Yet, using such exclusively spiritual approaches in the absence of standard treatments for generalized anxiety may risk harming the client or at least risk the loss of the potential benefit from well-supported treatments.

There are numerous case discussions in the literature of the use of religious and spiritual interventions as an appropriate adjunct to standard treatments (Richards & Bergin, 2005). A wise course of action in Mira's case may be to further discuss her anxiety issues and her concerns about "secular therapy" and describe for her what would be a spiritually accommodative course of treatment, augmenting standard treatments for generalized anxiety disorder. If she continues to insist on only a spiritual technique approach, it is likely a pastoral counselor may be a more appropriate and competent provider for this option and an appropriate referral could be made. If she agrees to an integrative approach that combines spiritual techniques with standard secular treatments, then the sorts of informed-consent issues discussed in Sondra's case should be used.

Vignette 8—Peter: Competent Spiritual Assessments?

> Peter is a nonreligious new therapist under supervision during his intern-ship year. Peter has an intake with a highly religious Jewish client. The client talks with pressured speech, considerable anxiety, and some illogical thought patterns. Peter believes the client may be in a manic phase of a bipolar disorder. The client uses religious language throughout his intake, discussing God speaking to him and how God has a special plan for his life. Peter believes the client may be hallucinating and is ready to diag-nose the client as bipolar with psychotic features.

We have given a number of examples of how spiritual or religious thera-pist biases may interfere with ethical clinical practice. It is also possible that biases from a secular or nonreligious outlook may have this same adverse out-come. In Peter's case, his nonreligious background may have left him without a frame of reference to evaluate whether religious and spiritual experiences or beliefs indicate a psychotic process or a normative feature of the client's faith group. The same principles and standards that call psychologists to avoid bias based on religion apply here. APA's Division 36 preliminary practice guideline A-5 (see Appendix 2.1) indicates that helpful spiritual assessment is aimed at "determining how normative the client's religious/spiritual life is for the client's religious reference group." If Peter lacks the necessary knowledge to accomplish this task, then it will be important for him to gain assistance through consulta-tion from suitably qualified professionals or key informants in the client's faith community.

CONCLUSION

The relative ubiquity of spiritual and religious issues in the human con-dition makes their clinical encounter inevitable. Because professional codes have been developed to provide guidance for the entire field of practice, they advance ethical principles and standards that have relevance for any clinician who desires to carve out a practice niche with religion and spirituality. There is a growing body of literature from existing niche practitioners, researchers, and clinical training faculty that provides more nuanced and useful specific guid-ance for this practice area. There is evidence that the mental health professions are warming up to a more routine and explicit focus on spiritual and religious issues in practice (Richards & Bergin, 2005; Sperry & Shafranske, 2005). If this warming trend continues, the streams of guidance will likely flow with greater speed, force, and in more direct courses.

Still, it is important to note that these changes in professional climate speak more to a perceptual neglect among professionals than any change in the prevalence of spiritual and religious issues in the lives of clients. Percival (1803) observed a similar myopia in the medical students of his own day. He was concerned that an increasing secularity and callusing of religious concern appeared to be an artifact of their modern medical training. Consequently, his pioneer code of conduct for medical ethics contained prescriptions to strengthen the spiritual life of the medical students. The various ethical principles, standards, and guidelines of the contemporary mental health professions do not prescribe personal spiritual development as either a professional duty or even an aspiration. However, if the predominant secular attitude of our training models leads us to a dim vision of spiritual and religious issues that are often of overriding concern to our clients, it may be time for us to take another page from Percival's book.

PRELIMINARY PRACTICE GUIDELINES FOR WORKING WITH RELIGIOUS AND SPIRITUAL ISSUES

RELIGIOUS/SPIRITUAL ASSESSMENT GUIDELINES

A-1. Psychologists are mindful that religion/spirituality is a vital and important aspect of many clients' lives.

A-2. Psychologists are attentive to indications that clients have religious/spiritual concerns and take steps to convey to the client that expressing such concerns is appropriate if present.

A-3. Psychologists are encouraged to routinely incorporate brief screening questions to assess for the presence of clinically salient religious/spiritual client concerns.

A-4. The need for more extensive spiritual assessments is suggested when clients indicate that religious/spiritual factors are personally and clinically salient to their presenting concern.

A-5. Spiritual assessment is most helpful when aimed at gaining an understanding of the clinically relevant dimensions of the client's religious/spiritual life. Such assessment should be directed toward the following goals:

    (a) determining how normative the client's religious/spiritual life is for the client's religious reference group,

    (b) exploring whether clinical problems are adversely impacting religious/spiritual functioning, and

    (c) evaluating how aspects of the client's religion/spirituality might constitute either constraints on treatment or productive resources for coping.

A-6. Psychologists are sensitive to biases that arise from religious/spiritual factors in the way in which clients complete psychological tests.

A-7. Psychologists are cautious to avoid interpreting client reports of attitudes or behaviors that are normative for a client's religious community as indicative of pathology.

A-8. Psychologists strive to be attentive to individual differences in religion/spirituality and avoid stereotypic inferences based the client's identification with a spiritual tradition.

RELIGIOUS/SPIRITUAL INTERVENTION GUIDELINES

I-1. Psychologists obtain appropriate informed consent from clients before incorporating religious/spiritual techniques and/or addressing religious/spiritual treatment goals in counseling.

I-2. Psychologists accurately represent to clients the nature, purposes, and known level of effectiveness for any religious/spiritual techniques or approaches they may propose using in treatment.

I-3. Psychologists do not use religious/spiritual treatment approaches/techniques of unknown effectiveness in lieu of other approaches/techniques with demonstrated effectiveness in treating specific disorders or clinical problems.

I-4. Psychologists attempt to accommodate a client's spiritual/religious tradition in congruent and helpful ways when working with clients for whom spirituality/religion is personally and clinically salient.

I-5. Religious/spiritual accommodations of standard treatment approaches/protocols are done in a manner that
   (a) does not compromise the effectiveness of the standard approach or produce iatrogenic effects,
   (b) is respectful of the client's religious/spiritual background,
   (c) proceeds only with the informed consent of the client, and
   (d) can be competently carried out by the therapist.

I-6. Psychologists are mindful of contraindications for the use of spiritually/religiously oriented treatment approaches.
   (a) Generally, psychologists are discouraged from using explicit religious/spiritual treatment approaches with clients presenting with psychotic disorders, substantial personality pathology, or bizarre and idiosyncratic expressions of religion/spirituality.
   (b) Psychologists should discontinue such approaches if iatrogenic effects become evident.

I-7. When psychologists use religious/spiritual techniques in treatment, such as prayer or devotional meditation, they
   (a) clearly explain the proposed technique to the client and obtain informed consent,
   (b) do so in a competent manner that is respectful of the intended religious/spiritual function of the technique in the client's faith tradition, and
   (c) adopt such techniques only if they are believed to facilitate a treatment goal.

I-8. Psychologists appreciate the substantial role faith communities may play in the lives of their clients and consider appropriate ways to harness the resources of these communities to improve clients' well-being.

I-9. Psychologists avoid conflictual dual relationships that might arise in religious/spiritually oriented treatment or in adjunctive collaborations with faith communities.

I-10. Psychologists set explicitly religious/spiritual treatment goals only if
   (a) they are functionally relevant to the clinical concern,
   (b) can be competently addressed within the treatment,
   (c) can be appropriately pursued within the particular context and setting in which treatment is occurring, and
   (d) are consented to by the client.

I-11. Psychologists commit to a collaborative and respectful demeanor when addressing client aspects of a client's religion/spirituality the psychologist deems maladaptive or unhealthy. The preferred clinical goal in such cases is to promote more adaptive forms of the client's own faith rather than to undermine that faith.

RELIGIOUS/SPIRITUAL MULTICULTURAL PRACTICE AND DIVERSITY GUIDELINES

M-1. Psychologists make reasonable efforts to become familiar with the varieties of spirituality and religion present in their client population.

M-2. Psychologists strive to be self-aware of their own perspectives, attitudes, history, and self-understandings of religion and spirituality. Psychologists should be mindful of how their own background on religious/spiritual matters might bias their response and approach to clients of differing background.

M-3. Psychologists do not seek to proselytize or otherwise impose their worldview on the client.

M-4. Psychologists are mindful of factors that influence the appropriateness of their own religious/spiritual self-disclosure to a client. These include but are not limited to disclosures that are
   (a) congruent with the treatment orientation or approach used,
   (b) consistent with other general background self-disclosures offered to a client at the outset of treatment,
   (c) facilitative of the treatment, and
   (d) necessary to address a potential value conflict that might impede treatment.

M-5. Psychologists are encouraged to gain competence in working with clients of diverse religious/spiritual backgrounds through continuing education, consultation, and supervision.

M-6. The need for clinical referral based on religious/spiritual factors is suggested when

(a) the client expresses a strong preference for a therapist with a different religious/spiritual background and this preference persists after reasonable attempts are made to establish rapport with the client,

(b) the presenting problem requires an understanding of the client's religious/spiritual background that exceeds the psychologist's competence regardless of relevant consultation or supervision, and

(c) a religious/spiritual difference between the client and the psychologist impedes treatment.

M-7. Psychologists respect religion/spirituality as an important diversity domain and are mindful of the complex ways this domain relates to other areas of diversity such as ethnicity, race, age, gender, or sexual orientation.

REFERENCES

American Counseling Association. (2005). *Code of ethics and standards of practice*. Alexandria, VA: Author.

American Psychological Association. (1994). Guidelines for child custody evaluations in divorce proceedings. *American Psychologist, 49*, 677–680.

American Psychological Association. (2002). Ethical principles of psychologists and code of conduct. *American Psychologist, 57*, 1060–1073.

American Psychological Association. (2005). *Policy statement on evidence-based practice in psychology*. Retrieved from http://www.apa.org/practice/ebpstatement.pdf

American Psychological Association, Committee on Professional Practice and Standards, Board of Professional Affairs. (1999). Guidelines for psychological evaluations in child protection matters. *American Psychologist, 54*, 586–593.

American Psychological Association, Division 44/Committee on Lesbian, Gay and Bisexual Concerns Joint Task Force on Guidelines for Psychotherapy with Lesbian, Gay and Bisexual Clients. (2000). Guidelines for psychotherapy with lesbian, gay, and bisexual clients. *American Psychologist, 55*, 1440–1451.

American Psychiatric Association. (1989). *Guidelines regarding possible conflict between psychiatrists' religious commitments and psychiatric practice*. Washington, DC: Author.

American Psychiatric Association. (2000). *Diagnostic and statistical manual of mental disorders* (4th ed., text rev.). Washington, DC: Author.

Baker, R (1999, Fall). Codes of ethics: Some history. *Perspectives on the Professions, 19*(1). Retrieved June 18, 2007, from http://ethics.iit.edu/perspective/pers19_1fall99_2.html

Beauchamp, T. L., & Childress, J. F. (1979). *Principles of biomedical ethics.* New York: Oxford University Press.

Beauchamp, T. L., & Childress, J. F. (2001). *Principles of biomedical ethics* (5th ed.). New York: Oxford University Press.

Bruff v. North Mississippi Health Services, Inc., 244 F. 3d 495 (5th Cir. 2001).

Cashwell, C. S., & Young, J. S. (Eds.). (2005). *Integrating spirituality and religion into counseling.* Alexandria, VA: American Counseling Association.

Foltin, R., & Standish, J. (2004, Summer). Reconciling faith and livelihood: Religion in the workplace and Title VII (The 1964 Civil Rights Act: Forty Years and Counting). *Human Rights, 31,* 19.

Griffith, E. E. H., & Young, J. L. (2004). Clergy counselors and confidentiality: A case for scrutiny. *Journal of the American Academy of Psychiatry and the Law, 32,* 43–50.

Hagedorn, W. B. (2005). Counselor self-awareness and self-exploration of religious and spiritual beliefs: Know thyself. In C. S. Cashwell & E. J. Young (Eds.), *Integrating spirituality and religion into counseling* (pp. 63–84). Alexandria, VA: American Counseling Association.

Haldeman, D. C. (2004). When sexual and religious orientation collide: Considerations in working with conflicted same-sex attracted male clients. *Counseling Psychologist, 32,* 691–715.

Hathaway, W. L. (2005, August). *Preliminary practice guidelines for religious/spiritual issues.* Paper presented at the 113th Annual Convention of the American Psychological Association, Washington, DC.

Hathaway, W. L. (2006, August). *A meta-ethical prolegomena for professional ethics: Values or principles.* Paper presented at the 114th Annual Convention of the American Psychological Association, New Orleans, LA.

Hathaway, W. L. (2007). *Preliminary practice guidelines for religious/spiritual issues.* Manuscript submitted for publication.

Hawkins, I., & Bullock, S. (1995). Informed consent and religious values: A neglected area of diversity. *Psychotherapy: Theory, Research, Practice, Training, 32,* 293–300.

Hebert, R. S., Dang, Q., & Schulz, R. (2007). Religious beliefs and practices are associated with better mental health in family caregivers of patients with dementia: Findings from the REACH study. *American Journal of Geriatric Psychiatry, 15,* 292–300.

Hermann, M. A., & Herlihy, B. R. (2006). Legal and ethical implications of refusing to counsel homosexual clients. *Journal of Counseling and Development, 84,* 414–418.

Huyler, S. P. (1999). *Meeting God: Elements of Hindu devotion.* New Haven, CT: Yale University Press.

Institute of Medicine. (2001). *Crossing the quality chasm: A new health system for the 21st century.* Washington, DC: Author.

Johnson, W. B. (2001). To dispute or not to dispute: Ethical REBT with religious clients. *Cognitive and Behavioral Practice, 8,* 39–47.

Johnson, W. B., Ridley, C. R., & Nielsen, S. L. (2000). Religiously sensitive rational emotive behavior therapy: Elegant solutions and ethical risks. *Professional Psychology: Research and Practice, 31,* 14–20.

Jonsen, A., & Toulmin, S. (1990). *The abuse of casuistry: A history of moral reasoning.* Berkeley: University of California Press.

Josephson, A. M., & Peteet, J. R. (Eds.). (2004). *Handbook of spirituality and worldview in clinical practice.* Washington, DC: American Psychiatric Association.

Lomax, J. W., II, Karff, S., & McKenny, G. P. (2002). Ethical considerations in the integration of religion and psychotherapy: Three perspectives. *Psychiatric Clinics of North America, 25,* 547–559.

Lukoff, D. (1998). From spiritual emergency to spiritual problem: The transpersonal roots of the new *DSM–IV* category. *Journal of Humanistic Psychology, 38,* 21–50.

McClemore, C., & Court, J. (1977). Religion and psychotherapy—Ethics, civil liberties, and clinical savvy: A critique. *Journal of Consulting and Clinical Psychology, 45,* 1172–1175.

McMinn, M., & Dominguez, A. (Eds.). (2005). *Psychology and the church.* New York: Nova Science.

Miller, G. (2003). *Incorporating spirituality in counseling and psychotherapy: Theory and technique.* New York: Wiley.

Pargament, K. I. (1997). *The psychology of religion and coping.* New York: Guilford Press.

Percival, T. (1803). *Medical ethics: A code of institutes and precepts adapted to the professional conduct of physicians and surgeons.* Manchester, England: Johnson & Bickerstaff.

Richards, P. S., & Bergin, A. E. (2005). *A spiritual strategy for counseling and psychotherapy* (2nd ed.). Washington, DC: American Psychological Association.

Shafranske, E. P. (Ed.). (1996). *Religion and the clinical practice of psychology.* Washington, DC: American Psychological Association.

Sperry, L. (2007). *The ethical and professional practice of counseling and psychotherapy.* Upper Saddle River, NJ: Pearson Education.

Sperry, L., & Shafranske, E. P. (Eds.). (2005). *Spiritually oriented psychotherapy.* Washington, DC: American Psychological Association

Stratton, J. S., & Smith, R. D. (2006). Supervision of couples cases. *Psychotherapy: Theory, Research, Practice, Training, 43,* 337–348.

Tan, S. Y. (1994). Ethical considerations in religious psychotherapy: Potential pitfalls and unique resources. *Journal of Psychology and Theology, 22,* 389–394.

Tan, S. Y. (2003). Integrating spiritual direction into psychotherapy: Ethical issues and guidelines. *Journal of Psychology and Theology, 31,* 14–23.

Tan, S. Y., & Johnson, W. B. (2005). Spiritually oriented cognitive–behavioral therapy. In L. Sperry & E. Shafranske's (Eds.), *Spiritually oriented psychotherapy* (pp. 77–103). Washington, DC: American Psychological Association.

Tjeltveit, A. C. (1999). *Ethics and values in psychotherapy*. New York: Routledge.

West, W. (2000). *Psychotherapy and spirituality: Crossing the line between therapy and religion*. Thousand Oaks, CA: Sage.

Worthington, E. L., Jr., & Sandage, S. J. (2001). Religion and spirituality. *Psychotherapy, 38,* 473–478.

Worthington, E. L., Jr., & Sandage, S. J. (2002). Religion and spirituality. In J. C. Norcross (Ed.), *Psychotherapy relationships that work* (pp. 371–387). New York: Oxford University Press.

Yarhouse, M. A. (1998). When clients seek treatment for same-sex attraction: Ethical issues in the "right to choose" debate. *Psychotherapy, 35,* 248–259.

Yarhouse, M. A., & VanOrman, B. T. (1999). When psychologists work with religious clients: Applications of the general principles of ethical conduct. *Professional Psychology: Research and Practice, 30,* 557–562.

Zinnbauer, B. J., Pargament, K. I., & Scott, A. B. (1999). The emerging meanings of religiousness and spirituality: Problems and prospects. *Journal of Personality, 67,* 889–919.

3

THERAPIST SELF-AWARENESS OF SPIRITUALITY

MARSHA I. WIGGINS

> I want to beg you as much as I can . . . to be patient toward all that is
> unsolved in your heart and to try to love the questions themselves. . . .
> Do not now seek answers which cannot be given you because you would
> not be able to live them. And the point is to live everything. Live the
> questions now. Perhaps you will then gradually, without noticing it, live
> along some distant day into the answer.
>
> —Rainer Maria Rilke

In a multicultural and pluralistic world, therapists have the opportunity to work with clients from myriad backgrounds. Many of those clients have significant spiritual or religious components in their self-understanding and expect therapists to respect, if not directly address, those concerns. Therapists, too, bring their cultural perspectives and personal history of spirituality and religion into the therapeutic setting. The more they are aware of their stance vis-à-vis spirituality and religion, including both positive and negative associations, the better prepared therapists will be in serving clients for whom these issues are paramount. The purpose of this chapter is to help therapists to discover the impediments to working with clients' spiritual and religious issues and to become aware of their worldviews and their values toward and experiences of spirituality and religion.

COMMON IMPEDIMENTS TO WORKING WITH CLIENTS' SPIRITUAL AND RELIGIOUS ISSUES

Even after acknowledging one's spiritual and religious heritage and how it impinges on present professional practice, therapists may encounter potential barriers to working effectively with clients for whom spirituality and religion are critical constructs. Some of these impediments include (a) lack of training in regard to the interface between religion, spirituality, and psychotherapy; (b) minimizing the significance of spirituality and religion in clients' lives; (c) pathologizing spirituality and religion (see chap. 1, this volume); and (d) varieties of countertransference reactions.

Despite the legacy of negative attitudes toward spirituality and religion that some therapists inherit, there are several steps they can take to avoid common impediments to working with clients' spirituality and religious issues. First, therapists can assess the level of importance clients ascribe to spirituality or religion in their daily lives. Knowing how significant these constructs are for client functioning can help therapists take them more seriously. Second, therapists can learn more about the most prevalent forms of spirituality and religion in their geographical regions. Becoming familiar with the belief systems of local culture enables therapists to think about spirituality and religion as cultural artifacts and to give them a place in the therapeutic milieu. Third, therapists can rethink the way they categorize spirituality and religion. Instead of considering these client characteristics as ancillary or tangential to the therapeutic process, therapists can centralize them and place them alongside other important client factors such as gender, age, ethnicity, sexual orientation, and relationship status. Fourth, therapists work on their own issues and history with spirituality and religion. Fifth, therapists can consult professional research on the positive relationship between spirituality and religion and physical and mental health. For instance, Koenig (2004) estimated that, between 1980 and 2000, 500 studies had confirmed a positive association between spirituality and better mental health, improved well-being, and reduced substance abuse. Last, therapists can explore a variety of means for cultivating a sense of transcendence and wonder in their own lives. That is not to say therapists should become religious. Instead, it is to suggest a way of being in the world that invites the luminous and the mysterious to sit next to the cognitive and the scientific in one's construction of reality. Making these small changes in practice can assist therapists in becoming more successful in their work with clients for whom spirituality or religion is deemed paramount. Still, countertransference issues pose additional challenges unique to the therapeutic process.

THE ILL EFFECTS OF COUNTERTRANSFERENCE

A plethora of experiences may shape therapists' countertransference reactions and responses to clients' spiritual and religious issues. For example, therapists who grew up in families in which religion was considered unimportant, unscientific, or irrational may feel disloyal to their families of origin if they focus on their clients' spiritual or religious issues (Frame, 2003). They may get involved in arguments or other conflicts with dogmatic clients that may result in cementing clients' rigid beliefs rather than opening for them new opportunities. Or, conversely, therapists of all backgrounds may be unaware of how significantly religion influences their clients and thus not attend to it in ways that would be helpful (Benningfield, 1998). In either case, one remedy for this type of countertransference is for therapists to examine the motives behind their struggles with dogmatic clients. When therapists acknowledge that the source of the struggle is part of family-of-origin issues or personal theological perspectives, then it is easier to lay it aside. Therapists may also explore other examples of rigidity in these clients, thus unhooking themselves from the content related to spirituality and religion.

Some therapists may have been raised in orthodox religious homes and disassociated themselves with their family's religion during adolescence or young adulthood. It is developmentally typical for young people to question their religious or spiritual beliefs (Fowler & Keen, 1978). However, some people continue to wrestle with unresolved theological questions that make them anxious when religious or spiritual topics arise. When such anxiety strikes therapists, they may (consciously or unconsciously) redirect a therapy session toward another topic. This shift is often accomplished to avoid addressing the religious or spiritual concerns that create discomfort. Therapists who find themselves in this type of countertransference dilemma can seek consultation with an expert on their particular brand of religion and begin to address their own theological struggles. They may engage in self-awareness practices described later in this chapter, such as the spiritual genogram, autobiography, or journal. Increasing their self-knowledge can reduce defensiveness and increase objectivity in the face of spiritual or religious clients.

Some therapists may work with clients who are exploring their spiritual or religious beliefs and considering moving away from long-held fundamentalism to more open theological positions. A possible countertransference reaction may occur when therapists who are disturbed by such dogmatic religion are too eager to move clients beyond their inflexible views (Genia, 2000). As a result of therapists' critical reaction to clients' fixed religious worldviews, clients may feel unbalanced in their faith. Separating one's own wishes for the client from the pacing that best serves the client is a means of dealing with the kind of countertransference described earlier. Recognizing as well as underscoring client–therapist boundaries enables therapists to detach themselves from their clients' developmental and theological journeys. It frees therapists to concentrate on assisting clients' growth in relation to clients' comfort.

Other therapists who have experienced significant losses and trauma, such as school shootings or the tragic death of loved ones, may feel angry with a God they believed failed to prevent such disasters. These personal crises may also create crises of faith for people who previously thought they had made peace with their Higher Power and reconciled with their spirituality or religion (Frame, 2003). Consequently, when clients raise spiritual or religious issues, therapists may feel unprepared to deal with the powerful emotions these topics unleash. They may also feel incapable of responding effectively to their clients' distress and thus may attempt to minimize or avoid it. Getting supervision and possibly therapy for these troubling issues is a helpful way for therapists to address countertransference of this type.

Other therapists may have experienced higher consciousness, unity with others and the universe, and a palpable sense of self-transcendence. Despite the positive effect of these encounters, some therapists may not have a suitable spiritual, religious, or philosophical frame for integrating transpersonal experiences into their lives. They may feel at once excited and worried about these deeply moving occurrences. When they find themselves in this situation, their countertransference reaction may cause them to overidentify with clients who present similar situations (Frame, 2003). Again, separating one's own experience from that of one's clients is a helpful strategy for managing countertransference triggered by deeply moving transcendent or transpersonal experiences. Acknowledging the difference between the self and the client will assist therapists in keeping the focus on clients' goals for change.

Another possibility is that therapists' transpersonal revelations may be so intense and unresolved that they avoid the spiritual and religious domain altogether. Or therapists may seek help from clients to assimilate their transpersonal experiences. In such a case, counselors who rely on their clients would be placing their personal needs above the needs of their clients, an act that is clearly unethical (American Association for Marriage and Family Therapy, 2001; American Counseling Association, 2005; American Psychological Association, 2002; National Association of Social Workers, 1999). Getting appropriate clinical supervision is an effective antidote to both types of countertransference.

Similarly, another type of unresolved issue for therapists may be the conflict they feel when their clients hold social and political positions, buttressed by a particular spiritual or religious perspective, that are diametrically opposed to their own. For example, clients may be hostile and denigrating toward gay and lesbian persons and may lean on sacred texts for authoritative justification of their views. Or perhaps clients are against abortion because of the doctrine of their church or their beliefs regarding the right to life. Therapists who hold opposing views may find themselves in an adversarial position with their clients. These practitioners may assume their aversive responses are triggered by the spiritual or religious dogma undergirding their clients' beliefs. Thus, clinicians may be tempted to minimize clients' issues, to address only the social or political issue without its accompanying religious context, or to focus on freeing the clients from what they perceive as unsound religious or spiritual beliefs (Frame, 2003). All of these detrimental possibilities are derived from clinicians' lingering internal conflicts. They are best addressed by a combination of personal therapy and clinical supervision.

Benningfield (1998) raised other issues that potentially trigger countertransference. He suggested that some therapists might fail to set appropriate boundaries with clients. One example of unclear limit setting may involve therapists who focus on spirituality and religion to the neglect of important psychological issues. In their efforts for clients to have positive associations with spirituality and religion, the therapists may avoid needed confrontation. As a result, therapists who are unable to balance supportive interventions with confrontational ones may unknowingly keep clients from addressing important problems.

An illustration of positive countertransference occurs when spiritual or religious therapists do not probe clients about their spiritual or religious beliefs and practices (Benningfield, 1998). Because they themselves consider religious ideology sacred, they may be reluctant to address it as evenhandedly as they do other issues.

Finally, some therapists may hold strong religious opinions that make them vulnerable to imposing them on their clients (Frame, 2003). Even if they feel some desire to persuade others to adopt their spiritual perspective or religious practice, to do so in the therapy room is a violation of professional ethics. The challenge of being open to clients' diverse worldviews and beliefs is more difficult when clients ascribe special power to their therapists or see them as healers possessing unique knowledge (Guggenbuhl-Craig, 1982). It is critical that therapists with strong spiritual beliefs or religious traditions refrain from abusing the power of their role by attempting to convince their clients to adopt their beliefs and practices. Keeping focused on the purpose of therapy and the needs and goals of clients should minimize this countertransference reaction. There are several options therapists have to address countertransference triggered by clients' spiritual or religious disclosures. Countertransference that interferes with therapist effectiveness signals the need for supervision, personal counseling, and perhaps client referral (Frame, 2003).

Case Study 1: An Example of Countertransference

Jacob is a Jewish mental health professional working in a group practice.[1] He was raised in a conservative Jewish home in which religious ritual was practiced and his family was active in the local synagogue. During his late adolescence, Jacob began dating Nicole, a fundamentalist Christian, who took him to revivals and made every effort to convert him to Christianity. Jacob's parents

---

[1]For the cases presented in this chapter, pseudonyms are used, and identifying details have been altered for confidentiality.

were unsupportive of his relationship with Nicole and put pressure on him to end it. Jacob experienced considerable inner turmoil as a result of being torn by his love for Nicole, his struggle with her religious beliefs, and his conflictual relationship with his parents and extended family members. During a week-long mission trip to Central America, Jacob had an emotionally intense spiritual experience and decided to be baptized as a Christian. On learning of their son's conversion to Christianity, Jacob's parents withdrew their emotional and financial support, and he was left on his own. In his late 20s, after ending his tumultuous relationship with Nicole and struggling to make sense of his place within Christianity, Jacob renounced religion altogether.

One of Jacob's clients, Catherine, is a fundamentalist Christian. Jacob finds he becomes irritated when Catherine brings up her questions about how to manage her guilt at having had an abortion when she had been raised to believe abortion is a sin. Whenever she speaks of God and God's will for her life, Jacob redirects her and politely informs her that a psychotherapist's office is not the place to discuss her religious beliefs. Jacob makes an effort to reframe Catherine's religious concerns as psychological ones and tells her she should talk with her pastor about her spiritual dilemmas. After several sessions, he is aware he is avoiding spirituality and religion, perhaps to the detriment of his client.

In peer supervision, Jacob presents his struggle with Catherine and her unrelenting requests for him to help her untangle her religious beliefs and reconcile them with her behavior. Jacob's peers suggest that he might be having countertransference reactions to Catherine, and they begin asking him about his religious background and experiences. When Jacob shares his personal history with religion, he is acutely aware that he has many unresolved religious issues he must address before he is able to work effectively with Catherine and other clients similar to her.

As mentioned before, countertransference can be positive. For example, when therapists find themselves sharing a similar spiritual or religious orientation or practice with their clients, therapists may be more motivated to assist clients with whom they have a genuine and personally meaningful connection. Also, therapists may experience positive countertransference with clients who disclose personal stories of faith and inspiration. These countertransference reactions may increase therapists' respect and admiration for their clients, resulting in therapists' expectations of positive therapeutic outcomes.

Although some of the material in the preceding pages of this chapter focuses on the negative aspects of therapists' interactions with clients related to spirituality and religion, there are significant positive aspects as well. Therapists who take seriously clients' spiritual and religious convictions and practices and create space in the therapeutic milieu for exploration of these issues may make major headway in helping clients address their psychological distress. The fact that a therapist has honored a client's spiritual worldview may increase the client's trust and strengthen the therapeutic alliance. Moreover, therapists who invite spirituality and religion into their work with clients may gain a greater understanding of how clients make meaning in their lives and what types of interventions might be effective in addressing their concerns.

BECOMING AWARE OF ONE'S WORLDVIEW

Becoming aware of one's worldview, values, belief system, and cultural context is an important aspect of being a skilled therapist (Liddle, 1982; Whitaker & Keith, 1981). Taking seriously one's personal history as it affects the therapeutic process means addressing what Aponte and Winter (1987) called person-of-the-therapist issues. Failure to be aware of ways one's worldview affects and shapes therapy makes therapists vulnerable to clinical triggers (Guerin & Hubbard, 1987). For example, suppose clients present in therapy with a rigid, ultra-religious belief system. Therapists who were raised in but rejected similar belief systems could be "triggered" by these clients' dogmatism. Rather than being able to focus on intervening to help such clients, therapists could displace anger at their parents onto unsuspecting clients. Thus, unknowingly, therapists' issues and those of their clients may collide in such a manner that therapists are caught in the web of their clients' systems (Kramer, 1985), which may result in ineffective psychotherapy.

There are several strategies therapists may use to assist them in their quest for self-knowledge. The *spiritual genogram* and related self-addressed questions are tools that enable therapists to examine their families of origin and understand the ways transgenerational values, assumptions, roles, rules, rituals, traditions, and practices shape and influence their worldview. Writing a *spiritual autobiography* helps therapists come to terms with how they have or have not engaged with spirituality and religion across the life cycle. Participating in a spiritual and religious self-assessment regarding beliefs about spirituality and religion can clarify a personal stance toward common theological premises. As a result of this process, therapists' self-knowledge increases, and they become more cognizant of boundaries around their beliefs, how their affirmations are similar and different from those held in their family of origin, and where they may be likely to find themselves triggered by their clients' issues and perspectives.

The Spiritual Genogram

The genogram, a multigenerational family map, is a classic tool used to gather family information across generations. Bowenian family theory guided the process at the outset (Carter & Orfandis, 1976; Guerin & Pendagast, 1976; Orfandis, 1976; Pendagast & Sherman, 1977); however, now the genogram is used by therapists with diverse theoretical perspectives who work with a variety of populations (Carter & McGoldrick, 1998; Doherty & Baird, 1983; Garcia Preto, 1996; Hardy & Laszloffy, 1995; Kuehl, 1995, 1996;

Magnuson, Norem, & Skinner, 1995; McGoldrick, Gerson, & Shellenberger, 1996; Wachtel, 1982).

Using symbols to represent family composition and other demographics (McGoldrick et al., 1996), the genogram reveals the transmission of family patterns across generations. The spiritual genogram (Frame, 2000) provides clinicians with a means for approaching an aspect of life often ignored in therapy. It enables users to gain insight on how their spiritual or religious legacy continues to influence their current beliefs and practices.

Although the genogram has been used primarily with clients, therapists have much to gain by creating their own spiritual genograms. First, they draw a three-generational genogram. Then, they note significant events and dates, such as births, marriages, divorces, remarriages, and deaths, and as much data as possible about their family members, using the symbols offered by McGoldrick et al. (1996). The gender of each person is depicted, as is adoption, stillbirth, abortion, twins, unmarried couples, family members' sexual orientation, and family relationship quality.

The basic genogram may be color coded (Lewis, 1989) to indicate religious and spiritual traditions. For example, Jews may be illustrated with blue, Muslims with black, Buddhists with yellow, personal spirituality with green, and atheists or agnostics with pink. For various types of Christians, additional colors may be used. Roman Catholics may be colored red and Protestants orange. More specificity in terms of denomination or affiliation may be drawn, using additional colors and creating a legend on the genogram. No color is added when religious or spiritual background is unknown (Frame, 2000).

The color coding on the spiritual genogram reveals the multiplicity of spiritual and religious backgrounds present in an extended family. When one's spiritual and religious history is illustrated in full color on the genogram, religious conflict previously outside individuals' awareness may become clear. One also discovers the sources of beliefs, morals, values, and attitudes that persist and have an impact on the provision of psychotherapy.

Important events occurring in the family's spiritual or religious life should also be reported on the genogram. For example, baptisms, first communions, confirmations, bar and bat mitzvahs, and other rituals and rites of passage may be included. Significant events in the spiritual or religious community can be depicted when families have been extremely involved in them. Relevant events include, for example, a congregational relocation; sexual misconduct of a clergy member leading to dismissal; closing of a church, synagogue, mosque, or other religious center; death of a well-loved priest; building projects; or changing racial, ethnic, or class composition in the congregation (Frame, 2000).

Brackets ("[ ]") are placed around persons who have left particular religious communities. Converting to other religions or joining other types of religious or spiritual organizations involves adding another layer of color around the family member's symbol, indicating the type of change. Dates for leaving and joining religious communities should be indicated. This aspect of the genogram reveals the stability or fluidity of religious or spiritual affiliation (Frame, 2000). The arrow symbol ("→") depicts family members' spiritual or religious closeness (Frame, 2000). For example, a large extended Mormon family could be portrayed by this symbol. For this family, religion provides a bond that connects family members across generations. A family whose beliefs are more focused on moral behavior without a specifically identified religion or spiritual practice but who are united in this outlook may also be represented by the arrow symbol.

Family conflict with spiritual or religious roots is denoted by the symbol ("~"). Perhaps there is such conflict between a father and daughter that occurred when the daughter married someone from a different religion. Or perhaps a son and his partner have disagreements about how to raise their child because of differing traditions around this religious practice. Genogram constructors write on their genograms about overt conflict as well as different beliefs or moral stands. Then they reflect on the extent to which these conflicts are being perpetuated in their current couple or family relationships.

When the standard genogram has been constructed, therapists may wish to write their responses to the following questions to better understand how spiritual or religious beliefs, experiences, rituals, and practices are connected to their sense of themselves as clinicians:

1. What role, if any, did spirituality/religion play in your family of origin?
2. What role does spirituality/religion play now?
3. What specific spiritual/religious beliefs are most important for you now? How are they a source of connection or conflict between you and other family members?
4. How is gender viewed in your religious/spiritual tradition? Ethnicity? Sexual orientation? How have these beliefs affected you and your extended family?
5. What patterns emerge for you as you study your genogram? How are you currently maintaining or diverting from those patterns?
6. How does your spiritual/religious history connect with your current distress or with the problem you presented for counseling?
7. What new insights or solutions may occur to you based on the discoveries made through the spiritual genogram? (Frame, 2003, p. 107)

Therapists constructing their spiritual genograms may wish to contact extended family members when more information is needed. The following questions may be helpful under these circumstances:

1. How important do you think spirituality/religion was in our family?

2. How do you think your experience of the spiritual/religious atmosphere was similar to or different from mine?
3. Which members of our extended family seem to have had the most power when it came to spirituality/religion? Which ones had the least? How do you think the use of power in terms of spirituality/religion affected our family and our relationships with one another?
4. How difficult do you think it has been or would be for family members to seek a different spiritual or religious path than the one with which we were raised? Who in our family would be supportive and why? Who would not be supportive and why?
5. How do you think spirituality/religion has been a source of strength and coping for our family? How do you think it has interfered in our family's relationships? (Frame, 2003, p. 108)

Case Study 2: Using a Spiritual Genogram

Elizabeth is a Caucasian mental health professional in private practice. Her parents were both professors at Ivy League universities in the northeastern United States. She was raised to believe spirituality and religion were "crutches" for those who lacked either the intelligence or ego strength to face life's challenges. Her disdain for any life dimension that did not have scientific evidence was palpable. When she relocated to the southeastern United States, she found her clients to be exceptionally religious, most espousing some form of Christianity.

Elizabeth realized she had developed a habit of dismissing her clients' spiritual and religious concerns and judging such clients as uninformed and neurotic. In the course of peer supervision, Elizabeth disclosed her frustration with her religious clientele and sought help in confronting her bias against them. One of her peers, Mohammed, suggested Elizabeth examine the root of her mistrust of spirituality and religion and cautioned that her prejudicial posture could be interfering with her clinical effectiveness.

From her genogram (see Figure 3.1), Elizabeth discovered she belonged to a long line of atheists and agnostics who eschewed spirituality and religion of any kind. They were proud of their heritage as intellectuals and instilled this pride in their children. Moreover, after speaking with her siblings and cousins, Elizabeth learned that they, too, had been prevented from socializing with religious peers and from learning about the practice of religion in any form. Elizabeth then began to understand that her relationship to spirituality and religion was largely unexamined, and she vowed to challenge herself in this area. She became committed to taking the stance of "not knowing" (Anderson & Goolishian, 1992) in order to be receptive to her clients' diverse worldviews.

The elder Scott generation practiced no formal religion. Richard was an atheist and Laura was an agnostic.

1931–2006

(75)
Laura Anne Scott

1956
(51)
Sarah Jolene Powell

1951
[55]
Michael Francis Powell

1948
(59)
Lucinda Renee Powell

1946
[61]
Alexander Russell Powell

1927–2001

[74]
Richard Murray Powell

Elizabeth, the therapist, has little knowledge of or experience with spirituality or religion. She carries with her transgenerational patterns of intellectualism. She has been taught that religion is a crutch for the simple minded.

Suzanne [Singleton] Abernathy was a Quaker but gave up her religion when she married Albert.

(77)
Suzanne Elizabeth Singleton

1954
(52)
Sandra Kay Abernathy

1952
(55)
Carolyn Patricia Abernathy

1950
[56]
Robert Wilson Abernathy

1929–2000

[70]
Albert John Abernathy

1977
(30)
Elizabeth Jane Abernathy

1974
[33]
William Edward Abernathy

1972
[34]
Aaron Jay Abernathy

Elizabeth's parents are intellectuals. They eschew all types of religion.

Elizabeth's siblings are agnostic. They have no interest in organized religion and reported no spiritual practices.

Figure 3.1. Elizabeth's spiritual genogram. Circles represent female and squares represent male; numbers inside the circles represent ages.

Writing a Spiritual Autobiography

Writing a spiritual autobiography is another approach to addressing one's personal spiritual and religious story. This process provides therapists the opportunity to survey their lives from the vantage point of spirituality and religion to gain perspective on the unique journeys they have taken.

When writing a spiritual autobiography, therapists are encouraged to begin the autobiography with the earliest memories of spirituality or religion in their homes and families of origin. Following suggestions made by Faiver, Ingersoll, O'Brien, and McNally (2001), therapists may wish to use the categories listed subsequently to organize their autobiographies.

1. *Introductory statements:* In this section, writers are encouraged to use free association to think about their relationship with spirituality and religion. They consider how they describe themselves vis-à-vis spirituality and religion.
2. *Spiritual themes:* In this category, writers consider topics, subjects, Jungian archetypes, or metaphors that capture the spiritual themes that give tone and texture to their lives.
3. *Spiritual influences:* Here writers note people who have influenced and mentored them. They write about who has affirmed them, challenged them, and been dependable sources of care, comfort, and nurture.
4. *Life's lessons:* In this section, writers review what they have learned thus far in their life journey and consider what lessons they want to pass on to subsequent generations and how they want to transmit these lessons to others.
5. *Personal conclusions:* In the final section of the autobiography, writers discern their thoughts and feelings about the overall effect of spirituality in their lives.

Therapists writing their spiritual autobiographies may integrate their responses to a series of questions into the categories discussed previously so that they become aware of their spiritual and religious roots as they examine the themes that emerge when they analyze their formative experiences. The following questions may be used as a guide:

1. What kinds of experiences did you have with spirituality and religion through childhood, adolescence, young adulthood, and beyond? (Frame, 2003)
2. When were your religious or spiritual beliefs and values challenged or changed? (Frame, 2003)
3. What role do religion and spirituality play at this time in your life? (Frame, 2003)
4. What future directions would you like to take in this aspect of your life? (Frame, 2003)

5. What were sources of authority, values, and power? (Fukuyama & Sevig, 1999, p. 9)
6. What is your experience of transcendence? (Fukuyama & Sevig, 1999, p. 9)
7. What resistance or barriers exist that prevent you from connecting with sources of spirituality? (Fukuyama & Sevig, 1999, p. 9)
8. What are the implications of your discoveries for your mental health practice?

Another approach to the spiritual autobiography is the exceptional human experience (EHE) model (Palmer, 1999). Using the EHE model, therapists review and possibly integrate psychic, death-related, mystical, and other transcendent experiences into their larger life stories.

Case Study 3: Using a Spiritual Autobiography

Malcolm is an African American mental health professional working in a large community mental health facility. He is one of 4 children and the only son of parents who were both postal workers. Malcolm chose to write his spiritual autobiography not long after his mother died. It was then he became aware of how significant spirituality and religion had been in his family of origin. Malcolm wrote,

> I think I was born in a church. As early as I can remember, my family spent all day Sunday at church and every Wednesday night at prayer meeting. I went to Sunday school and sang in the choir and believed everything Brother Johnson said about God and Jesus. When I went to college, I quit church—not because I quit believing, but because it just wasn't cool anymore. I've never really thought about my religion much. I certainly haven't questioned it. Now that I'm an adult with a young son, I want to figure out what I believe now and what I want to teach my children about faith. I never really thought about religion playing much of a role in psychotherapy.

Malcolm is an example of a person whose past had been steeped in a religious tradition and who has managed to keep it quite separate from his work as a mental health professional. Through the process of writing his autobiography, Malcolm discovered an important but unexamined aspect of his life he wished to explore. He was interested in the intersection of religion and culture and the effects of these contextual factors on his clients' well-being and their experience in therapy.

Guided Journaling

Another approach to self-knowledge regarding one's spiritual and religious values and beliefs is through the use of guided journaling. A personal journal is a book in which one keeps a personal record of events in one's life, of one's different relationships, of one's response to things, of one's feelings about things—in essence, of one's search to find out who one is and what the meaning of one's life might be. It is a book in which one carries out the greatest of life's adventures, the discovery of oneself (Cargas & Radley, 1981).

Krug (1982) listed topics that lend themselves well to a spiritual journal. They include personal life events and one's reaction to them as well as significant and meaningful conversations and their effects. Another important facet of keeping a spiritual journal is to record life's questions and how one is wrestling with them in day-to-day life. Memories, quotations, or passages from books; insights about one's experiences; one's joys and sorrows; and one's achievements and failures are appropriate to be included in a spiritual journal.

Some guidelines for successful journal keeping include making time for writing, being honest, addressing feelings, being open to experimenting with the format, and refusing to make the journal an obsession (Krug, 1982). The spiritual journal is a tool to assist people in coming to terms with their lives and their place in the universe.

Therapists should consider keeping a journal to reflect on difficult life questions to which spirituality and religion provide responses. It is helpful for therapists to remember clients may be grappling with these same issues, which is why it is important for therapists to gain clarity on where they stand on these matters. Therapists can use the questions listed next to structure their thinking and writing, or they can use these questions as the focus of small-group discussions:

1. How do you view human nature? Are people good, evil, or neutral?
2. What about free will? Do people have the human agency to make their own choices, or are their thoughts, feelings, and actions determined by some other force such as instincts, reinforcements, or God?
3. How would you respond to the question, "Why do bad things happen to good people?" Is God responsible for evil? Is there an evil spirit that struggles against a good spirit? Is God powerless to contain evil? Do bad things happen because people make poor choices? Do bad things happen to good people because the "good people" aren't really as good as they think they are? Do bad things happen randomly?
4. What happens to people after they die? Is there some form of afterlife? If so, what does it look like? Who decides what happens to whom?
5. Do you believe in a Higher Power? What are the qualities of the Supreme Being if you believe in one? Why do you believe in a Higher Power or God? If you do not believe in a Higher Power or God, what are the reasons for your disbelief?

6. What is your understanding of spirituality? How have you experienced it in your life?
7. Which of the person-of-the-therapist issues seem to fit best for you? In which areas do you believe yourself to be most vulnerable to countertransference when clients raise religious or spiritual issues? What experiences have you had that lead you to believe that you are particularly vulnerable to clinical triggers?
8. Which types of clients or client problems involving religion or spirituality would be the most challenging for you? Why? Which ones would be the most engaging? Why? (Frame, 2003, p. 32)
9. What are your experiences with other faith groups? What is your level of comfort working with clients from other faith groups?

Case Study 4: Using Guided Journaling

Maria Elena is a Latina mental health professional working in a health care environment. She was raised a Roman Catholic but has not been to Mass in many years. Despite her absence from church, Maria Elena has visceral reactions to some of her clients' spiritual and religious beliefs and attitudes. She reported to her supervisor she disliked clients who "talked about God's will too much." Maria Elena suspected her responses to her clients had the potential to interfere with her effectiveness as a practitioner. She decided it was time to undertake an in-depth exploration of her spiritual and religious assumptions. She began with the questions noted earlier. The following is an excerpt from her journal:

> I believe in God, but I don't know if He (I'm not even sure God is a "He") has any influence on what actually happens in my life or in world affairs. I think some Intelligent Being created the universe, but not in six days like the Bible says. I believe there is a Power for good in the world and one for evil, but I don't know how to describe those forces. I believe people are basically good but make poor choices sometimes that result in tragedy. I also think some bad things happen for a reason and others happen for no reason. Whoever God is, I believe God is more merciful to us than we are to others. I'm fairly certain being a Catholic is not the ticket to heaven as I have been told. A really loving God would welcome anyone. My spiritual life is a big question mark right now. I want to go deeper, learn more, become more open.

Maria Elena's journal writing was the catalyst that helped her deal with her negative reactions to some clients and to explore her spirituality in the present. She was motivated to learn more about where her beliefs came from, to assess these beliefs in terms of how they fit with her other life philosophies, and to craft a spiritual worldview that was consistent with her mental health training and practice.

As an alternative to cognitive-based strategies, another vehicle for increasing self-awareness is through the practice of *mindfulness* (Hagedorn, 2005; Ott, Longobucco-Hynes, & Hynes, 2002; Walsh, 1999). Essentially, mindfulness involves being fully present in the moment. Tacon, McComb, Caldera, and Randolph (2003) defined mindfulness in this way: "Mindfulness encourages detached, non-judging observation or witnessing of thoughts, perceptions, sensations, and emotions, which provides a means of self-monitoring and regulating one's arousal with detached awareness" (p. 27). Mindfulness can take many forms, including relaxation exercises, breath work, body work, meditation, or introspection.

One of the most developed practices incorporating mindfulness is the *experiential focusing method* developed by Gendlin (1978) and expanded by Hinterkopf (1994). The method is a means of focusing on bodily reactions related to one's experiences. This approach has the capacity to help therapists process negative spiritual or religious experiences and integrate the positive aspects. This mindfulness practice has many benefits. Improved focus, concentration, and precision, as well as improved communications and relationships, may issue from mindfulness (Levey & Levey, 2006). In addition, mindfulness practice may deepen insight and intuitive wisdom, awaken more authenticity and caring, increase resilience in the face of change, and strengthen faith and self-confidence (Levey & Levey, 2006). These benefits can help therapists stay focused and centered to minimize the possible negative effects of their clients' spiritual and religious disclosures. Also, therapists who practice mindfulness may tune in to their own inner voice and be more able to trust their intuition when working with their clients' positive and negative spiritual experiences.

In addition to assisting therapists to process spiritual experiences, the experiential focusing method can help solidify a current spiritual orientation (Hinterkopf, 1994). In brief, the method involves deep breathing to achieve a relaxed stated followed by six steps: (a) *clearing a space*, (b) *getting a sense*, (c) *finding a handle*, (d) *resonating*, (e) *asking*, and (f) *receiving* (Gendlin, 1978). Each step involves an action and process questions that may be answered in a journal. Clearing a space involves examining a religious or spiritual problem and tuning into related bodily sensations. Getting a sense means allowing oneself to experience the feelings associated with the issue that emerged in the first step. Finding a handle involves asking oneself a series of questions about the issues and waiting for answers to come in words or images rather than cognitively constructing them. Resonating is a process in which one allows the words and images that emerged in the previous step to connect to a current feeling. It is less about organizing one's experience and more about letting it happen until there is a clear match between words, images, feelings, and bodily reactions. Asking involves putting direct questions to the self in regard to the felt sense emerging from the issues at hand. For example, one might ask, "Do these words accurately describe this feeling?" "What is the worst thing about this for me?" or "What does this whole thing need from me?" (Hagedorn, 2005, p. 79). Again, this step does not involve active seeking of answers but rather waiting for answers to appear that create a "felt shift" (Hagedorn, 2005, p. 79). This felt shift is "a physiological change that brings a feeling of liberation, with an accompanying increase of life energy" (Hagedorn, 2005, p. 79). The final step, receiving, includes assimilating the felt shift and sharing it with others if one feels comfortable doing so.

Case Study 5: Implementing a Mindfulness Practice

Anthony is a gay Caucasian mental health professional who works in a hospice program. For years he has struggled with negative messages he received in his youth from his fundamentalist church about his sexuality. Anthony spent much of his young adulthood being frightened that he would "burn in hell" because of his homosexuality. As a result, he abandoned his church and dismissed religion from his life. Now, as he works with dying patients, many of whom have AIDS, he is faced again with ultimate questions about life after death.

Anthony chose to use the experiential focusing method (Gendlin, 1978) in an effort to come to terms with the inner spiritual turmoil triggered by his unresolved religious issues in conjunction with his sexual orientation. In clearing a space, Anthony noted he experienced heart palpitations and sweaty palms when he began to reflect on the negative messages he had received in church about being gay. Then, in the process of getting a felt sense of the issue, Anthony was aware of the terror he had felt as a young person believing he would be eternally separated from those he loved. In his mind's eye he saw images of hell: fire, the devil, burning, suffering, and being rejected by God. Anthony was gripped by anxiety and fear. In addition, he found himself weeping with sadness for the losses he would have as a result of his eternal damnation. He also felt deep shame about not measuring up to what his family and church had expected of him. In finding a handle, Anthony stayed with the feelings, waiting for words and images to appear. Some of the words that emerged were "lost," "angry," "forsaken," "guilty," "powerless," "empty," "parched," and "alone." The most striking image for Anthony was being alone, lost in the desert, dying of thirst, trying to find his way. In resonating, Anthony sat with the feelings and words and waited for a connection. Anthony was struck by the feelings of terror and of being lost and abandoned by his loved ones only to die in the desert. When engaging in the fifth step, asking, Anthony put forth the questions, "What does this thing need from me?" "What should happen here?" After waiting in silence for nearly an hour, in a moment of shining insight, Anthony realized he had been passively awaiting his "spiritual death" and had done nothing to attempt to avoid his disastrous future. He was acutely aware he needed to try to rescue himself from his feelings of powerlessness, loneliness, and shame. In receiving, Anthony noticed he had new energy for coming to terms with his religious background and for seeking a way to develop a spirituality that was life giving rather than life threatening.

Therapists have the opportunity and responsibility to know themselves and to be aware of the potential for clinical triggers that may compromise the quality of the services they provide. By being attuned to their own spiritual and religious worldview, and by addressing person-of-the-therapist issues in personal therapy, supervision, or both, therapists increase the likelihood of being able to work effectively with clients' spiritual and religious concerns.

CONCLUSION

Being an ethical and competent therapist requires one to undergo a process of self-exploration with the goal of becoming self-aware (Hagedorn, 2005). In the domain of spirituality and religion, it is especially important for therapists to come to terms with their personal history, their unresolved issues, and their responses to critical life questions such as "Who am I?" "What is my purpose?" "How do I make sense of the universe?" "What is my belief about a Higher Power?" and "What are my experiences with transcendence?" because these are questions clients often wrestle with as well. In addition, therapists can benefit from exploring their notions about tragedy, forgiveness, faith, the after-life, altruism, materialism, and the sacred (Weinstein, Parker, & Archer, 2002).

Making a commitment to an ongoing process of self-knowledge can be accomplished through specific strategies and practices, such as constructing a spiritual genogram, writing a spiritual autobiography, keeping a spiritual journal, and practicing mindfulness. Therapists also can take advantage of acquiring more training so their knowledge and skills enhance their personal development. In this way, therapists can work effectively with clients who seek to integrate spiritual and religious orientations into their lives with the goal of becoming healthy individuals.

REFERENCES

American Association for Marriage and Family Therapy. (2001). AAMFT code of ethics. Alexandria, VA: Author.

American Counseling Association. (2005). Code of ethics and standards of practice. Alexandria, VA: Author.

American Psychological Association. (2002). Ethical principles of psychologists and code of conduct. American Psychologist, 57, 1060–1073.

Anderson, H., & Goolishian, H. (1992). The client is the expert: A not-knowing approach to therapy. In S. McNamee & I. J. Gergen (Eds.), *Therapy as social construction* (pp. 25–39). London: Sage.

Aponte, H. J., & Winter, J. E. (1987). The person and practice of the therapist: Treatment and training. *Journal of Psychotherapy and the Family, 3,* 85–111.

Benningfield, M. F. (1998). Addressing spiritual/religious issues in therapy: Potential problems and complications. In D. S. Becvar (Ed.), *The family, spirituality and social work* (pp. 25–42). New York: Haworth Press.

Cargas, H. J., & Radley, R. J. (1981). *Keeping a spiritual journal.* Garden City, NY: Doubleday.

Carter, E. A., & McGoldrick, M. (Eds.). (1998). *The expanded family life cycle* (3rd ed.). New York: Gardner.

Carter, E. A., & Orfandis, M. (1976). Family therapy with only one person and the therapist's own family. In P. Guerin (Ed.), *Family therapy* (pp. 197–199). New York: Gardner.

Doherty, W. J., & Baird, M. A. (1983). *Family therapy and family medicine.* New York: Guilford Press.

Faiver, C., Ingersoll, R., O'Brien, E., & McNally, C. (2001). *Explorations of counseling and spirituality: Philosophical, practical, and personal reflections.* Pacific Grove, CA: Brooks/Cole.

Fowler, J. W., & Keen, S. (1978). *Life maps: Conversations on the journey of faith.* Waco, TX: Word Books.

Frame, M. W. (2000). The spiritual genogram in family therapy. *Journal of Marital and Family Therapy, 26,* 211–216.

Frame, M. W. (2003). *Integrating spirituality and religion into counseling: A comprehensive approach.* Pacific Grove, CA: Brooks/Cole.

Fukuyama, M. A., & Sevig, T. D. (1999). *Integrating spirituality into multicultural counseling.* Thousand Oaks, CA: Sage.

Garcia Preto, N. (1996). Puerto Rican families. In M. McGoldrick, J. Giordano, & J. K. Pearce (Eds.), *Ethnicity and family therapy* (2nd ed., pp. 164–186). New York: Guilford Press.

Gendlin, E. T. (1978). *Focusing.* New York: Everest House.

Genia, V. (2000). Religious issues in secularly based psychotherapy. *Counseling and Values, 44,* 213–221.

Guerin, P. J., & Hubbard, I. M. (1987). Impact of therapists' personal family system on clinical work. *Journal of Psychotherapy and the Family, 3,* 47–60.

Guerin, P. J., & Pendagast, E. G. (1976). Evaluation of family system and genogram. In P. J. Guerin (Ed.), *Family therapy* (pp. 450–464). New York: Gardner.

Guggenbuhl-Craig, A. (1982). *Power in the helping professions.* Dallas, TX: Spring.

Hagedorn, W. B. (2005). Counselor self-awareness and self-exploration of spiritual and religious beliefs: Know thyself. In C. S. Cashwell & J. S. Young (Eds.), *Integrating spirituality and religion into counseling* (pp. 63–84). Alexandria, VA: American Counseling Association.

Hardy, K. V., & Laszloffy, T. A. (1995). The cultural genogram: Key to training culturally competent family therapists. *Journal of Marital and Family Therapy, 21,* 227–237.

Hinterkopf, E. (1994). Integrating spiritual experiences in counseling. *Counseling and Values, 38,* 165–175.

Koenig, H. G. (2004). Religion, spirituality, and medicine: Research findings and implications for clinical practice. *Southern Medical Journal, 97,* 1194–1200.

Kramer, J. R. (1985). *Family interfaces: Transgenerational patterns.* New York: Bruner/ Mazel.

Krug, R. (1982). *How to keep a spiritual journal.* Nashville, TN: Thomas Nelson.

Kuehl, B. P. (1995). The solution-oriented genogram: A collaborative approach. *Journal of Marital and Family Therapy, 21,* 239–250.

Kuehl, B. P. (1996). The use of genograms with solution-based and narrative therapies. *The Family Journal: Counseling and Therapy for Couples and Families, 4,* 5–11.

Levey, J., & Levey, M. (2006). *The luminous mind.* San Francisco: Conari Press.

Lewis, K. G. (1989). The use of color-coded genograms in family therapy. *Journal of Marital and Family Therapy, 15,* 169–176.

Liddle, H. A. (1982). Family therapy training: Current issues, future trends. *International Journal of Family Therapy, 4,* 81–97.

Magnuson, S., Norem, K., & Skinner, C. H. (1995). Constructing genograms with lesbian clients. *The Family Journal: Counseling and Therapy for Couples and Families, 3,* 110–115.

McGoldrick, M., Gerson, R., & Shellenberger, S. (1996). *Genograms in family assessment* (2nd ed.). New York: Norton.

National Association of Social Workers. (1999). *Code of ethics.* Washington, DC: Author.

Orfandis, M. M. (1979). Problems with family genograms. *American Journal of Family Therapy, 7,* 74–76.

Ott, M. J., Longobucco-Hynes, S., & Hynes, V. A. (2002). Mindfulness meditation in pediatric clinical practice. *Pediatric Nursing, 29,* 487–491.

Palmer, G. T. (1999). Disclosure and assimilation of exceptional human experience: Meaningful, transformative, and spiritual aspects. *Dissertation Abstracts International, 60*(5), 2358B.

Pendagast, E. G., & Sherman, C. O. (1977). A guide to the genogram. *The Family, 5,* 3–14.

Tacon, A. M., McComb, J., Caldera, Y., & Randolph, P. (2003). Mindfulness meditation, anxiety reduction, and heart disease: A pilot study. *Family and Community Health, 26,* 25–33.

Wachtel, E. F. (1982). The family psyche over three generations: The genogram revisited. *Journal of Marital and Family Therapy, 8,* 335–343.

Walsh, F. (Ed.). (1999). *Spiritual resources in family therapy*. New York: Guilford Press.

Weinstein, C. M., Parker, J., & Archer, J. (2002). College counselor attitudes toward spiritual and religious issues and practices in counseling. *Journal of College Counseling, 5*, 164–174.

Whitaker, C. A., & Keith, D. V. (1981). Symbolic–experiential family therapy. In A. S. Gurman & D. P. Kniskern (Eds.), *Handbook of family therapy* (pp. 187–225). New York: Bruner/Mazel.

4

NOTING THE IMPORTANCE OF SPIRITUALITY DURING THE CLINICAL INTAKE

MARK M. LEACH, JAMIE D. ATEN, NATHANIEL G. WADE, AND BARBARA COUDEN HERNANDEZ

[T]o a great extent, it is the therapist who determines how the concerns and questions of religion and spirituality will be approached and examined, and indeed, whether they will be approached at all.

—J. T. Chirban

The clinical intake can play a pivotal role in setting the course for therapeutic exchange between therapists and clients, especially around issues related to client spirituality and spiritual experiences. However, there is little empirical and nonempirical guidance from the literature that informs readers of means to include spirituality during the intake portion of treatment, the primary purpose of this chapter. This chapter offers a glimpse into ideas and strategies for addressing spirituality and overcoming barriers to including spirituality during the clinical intake and interview, on the basis of the current literature available as well as our own clinical experiences. Specifically, we discuss how therapists can integrate spirituality into the clinical intake through (a) facilitation of spiritual acceptance, (b) agency climate, (c) intake forms, (d) referral sources, and (e) the clinical interview.

THE CLINICAL INTAKE

The clinical intake is usually the first exposure clients have to the counseling process, and this exposure often determines whether clients will return for additional sessions. In Sue, McKinney, and Allen's (1976) well-referenced study, which examines over 13,000 client files, they found that ethnicity predicted early termination from counseling after the first session. In other words, clients of color were less likely to return after an intake session than Caucasian clients. The same holds true today. Though multiple reasons were noted, one particular reason (central to the purpose of this chapter) was that some clients may not feel initially comfortable, understood, or accepted by the counselor and therefore will not return. The same can be said for the clients hesitant or unsure of the role of spirituality in therapy (e.g., Erickson, Hecker, Kirkpatrick, Killmer, & James, 2002). Clinical intakes and interviews create the atmosphere for the rest of therapy and can often dictate whether clients will return for subsequent appointments. Other than information gathering and initial discussion of client issues, clinical intakes and interviews are intended to create a positive therapeutic alliance, either with an individual or the agency. They also set the foundation for client conceptualization, as some clients will benefit from subsequent spiritual interventions or at least acknowledge and discuss the role of spirituality during treatment. Therapists and intake workers should relay to clients that they or the agency are willing and open to discuss spiritual and religious issues in therapy, even if they are not eventually used in clients' therapy.

One major purpose of the intake interview is to conduct an initial client assessment. Essentially, the intake should answer questions that address whether the client warrants further counseling, case conceptualization, the type of treatment most beneficial, and the projected length of treatment. Through an intake interview, therapists should be assessing therapy goals based on client concerns, client interpersonal style and skills, a personal history, and the extent to which clients' current concerns are affecting their lives (Sommers-Flanagan & Sommers-Flanagan, 2002). By the end of the intake session, depending on agency type and format, it may be possible to develop a conceptualization of the client that includes diagnoses, treatment plans, and expected outcomes (see chap. 6, this volume). Often overlooked during intake sessions is the inclusion and introduction of spirituality. However, at intake, therapists can begin to initiate discussion about the inclusion of spirituality to set the therapeutic tone for the remaining sessions. The purpose of introducing the topic is to develop a spiritually safe and receptive therapeutic alliance (see chap. 8, this volume). It is a means of informing the client that, if desired, spiritual issues are acceptable areas for discussion.

Because of the history of animosity between psychology and religion, many clients arrive for an initial session believing that the two areas should be kept separate. In fact, we have had multiple clients overtly state that they wished for spiritual topics to remain the sole domain of their spiritual leader. However, for clients unsure of therapy but also willing to discuss spirituality, the intake process can initially create an atmosphere of spiritual trust and acceptance. For some clients wanting to maintain the separation of their treatment and spiritual and religious issues, briefly including spirituality during the intake can offer a change of mind during the course of treatment. Of course, many clients may not be receptive or the clients' concerns may not be conducive to spiritual inclusion, although a few initial questions can assist therapists in determining whether further conversation can occur. Still, other clients present to therapy expecting that spirituality will be naturally incorporated into treatment and that time will be devoted to specifically exploring spiritual issues and engaging in spiritual interventions.

FACILITATING SPIRITUAL ACCEPTANCE

Introducing spiritual acceptance in an intake session can be a nuanced task, often filled with behavioral and verbal subtleties. Behaviorally, clients who mention spirituality may be assessing therapists' nonverbal behaviors to look for clues as to whether the topic is acceptable. Verbal responses to a client's spiritual comments, or therapists actually asking spiritually based questions, can help determine client acceptance. Spiritual issues are grounded in values, thus therapy discussions are value laden. How does a counselor minimize imposing spiritual values on clients? To create this atmosphere, Richards and Bergin (2005) promoted an explicit minimizing value approach when dealing with client values. This ethical approach highlights that the best way to minimize value imposition is to explicitly discuss values at appropriate times, such as early in the first hour of the initial session. Means to achieve this goal could be modeling these values, being explicit about your own values (which may result in a referral to a different agency therapist if there are incongruous values between counselor and client), and communicating that discussions involving spirituality can promote client coping and change (for a broader discussion, see Richards, Rector, & Tjeltveit, 1999).

Richards and Bergin (2005) also presented spiritual goals and dimensions relevant to some therapy interactions, although they noted that these five general goals are not appropriate for every client. These goals are presented within a theistic philosophy intimately tied to personality and therapeutic change. Although Richards and Bergin discussed the following goals in relation to the full spectrum of therapy, it is easy to see why creating a mindset of spiritual inclusion during the intake can offer richness not often included in less spiritual counseling. The five goals are as follows:

1. Help clients experience and affirm their eternal spiritual identity and live in harmony with the Spirit of Truth.
2. Help clients examine and better understand what if any effects their religious and spiritual beliefs have on their presenting problems and their lives in general.

3. Help clients identify and use the religious and spiritual resources in their lives to assist them in their efforts to cope, heal, and change.
4. Help clients examine and resolve religious and spiritual concerns that are pertinent to their disorders and make choices about what role religion and spirituality will play in their lives.
5. Help clients examine how they feel about their spiritual growth and well-being and, if they desire, help them determine how they can continue their quest for spiritual growth and well-being. (pp. 116–118)

AGENCY CLIMATE

A number of issues influence the intake process, such as the type of setting and the intake procedures themselves. Agencies differ with respect to the quantity of clients requesting services and available staff, both of which may affect the format of the intake. Smaller agencies and private practitioners are more likely to act as both intake worker and counselor, allowing for more fluidity between the intake and the rest of the therapeutic process. These types of intakes allow for much greater incorporation of initial spiritual assessment. However, some high-volume agencies such as community mental health centers and hospitals are likely to have specialized intake workers or case managers who conduct the intake interview. Although these personnel are trained to conduct intakes, they primarily gather specific information from agency intake forms and rarely delve into deeper clinical issues; the goal is to simply obtain enough information to begin the treatment process. It is equivalent to a medical intake procedure and is essentially a fact-finding mission and may not exude the warmth, openness, and personal client responsibility hoped for in a therapeutic environment.

Agency climate and personal therapist preferences often dictate the degree to which an agency or individual is open to spirituality during the therapeutic process, including the intake interview. We are not advocating that spirituality must always be pursued in treatment, or even during the intake process if the intake worker deems it inappropriate at that time, but that the door could be opened for clients who want spirituality included. There are many good reasons for clients not to discuss spirituality, especially during the intake, and these must be respected (e.g., intake worker is not the eventual counselor or emergent crisis issues). However, the intake interview can be a time to gently begin discussion about the inclusion of spirituality in treatment. The purpose of opening the door for spiritual inclusion is to determine the extent to which (a) clients are spiritual, (b) spirituality is an appropriate topic given the therapeutic issue, and (c) clients are willing to discuss spirituality should it be relevant.

However, there is the potential for resistance not only from clients but also from agencies and therapists. First, the agency may not allow for spiritual exploration through its intake procedures, such as asking perfunctory spiritual questions similar to the ones listed earlier. Second, individual therapists may be unwilling to examine spiritual issues in therapy for a number of reasons. For example, Leach and Aten (2007) found that counseling students in training often have concerns that preclude them from initiating discussions about spiritual issues. They reported apprehension surrounding a lack of knowledge about clients' faith groups, their own faith discomfort, fear of offending clients, fear of being unable to respond to spiritual issues from clients should they elaborate, and the lack of theory to guide them. Each issue requires a slightly different intervention with the student but nonetheless shows anxiety about including spirituality in the therapeutic process. Other studies with mental health professionals continue to find that spirituality is not frequently included across the therapeutic or research realms (e.g., Bergin & Jensen, 1990; Schlosser, Foley, Holmwood, & Poltrock, in press; Smith & Orlinsky, 2004). Third, intake workers are not trained in spirituality, and myths about the non-inclusion of spiritual and religious issues abound (Leach & Aten, 2007). For example, many mental health professionals erroneously believe that initiating discussion on spiritual or religious issues is equated with engaging in a religious discussion, although these two topics are not consistent.

INTAKE FORMS

According to Corey, Corey, and Callanan (1998), "One of the best ways to protect the rights of clients is to develop procedures to help them make informed choices" (p. 112). Informed consent is a contract agreement between the mental health professional and the client that details what treatment options are available along with the potential benefits and risks. In most instances the informed consent is a part of the clinical intake and clinical interview process and is typically presented to the client in writing and verbally discussed, after which formal written consent is obtained. Not only does the informed consent serve as an ethical and legal contract to help protect the client, but it also helps educate the client about the therapeutic process (Sommers-Flanagan & Sommers Flanagan, 2002). Furthermore, the informed consent may be the client's first exposure to learning how mental health professionals conceptualize treatment and what is valued and appropriate to discuss in this process (e.g., Is it appropriate to discuss spiritual matters?).

We recommend that therapists who are interested in integrating spirituality into the therapeutic process address spirituality in the informed consent. How exactly this is done will vary depending on therapists' work setting, personal values and worldview, and theoretical orientation (Somberg, Stone, &

Claiborn, 1993). A spiritually sensitive mental health professional working at a spiritually oriented treatment facility that primarily serves spiritually committed clients should be more explicit about the role of spirituality in treatment during the informed consent (see Exhibit 4.1) compared with professionals working in a secular, state, or government facility, for example. Thus, spirituality could be directly mentioned throughout each section of the informed consent form in more explicit spiritual settings (e.g., agency mission, about the staff, process of therapy) or could be couched among a number of other important cultural constructs that are addressed in less explicit spiritual settings (e.g., race, gender, sexual orientation). Chappelle (2000) suggested that specific informed consent should be obtained from client and supervisor before using explicit spiritually oriented interventions (e.g., referencing sacred writings; see Exhibit 4.2). Professional disclosure statements (see Exhibit 4.3) have also been used as part of the clinical intake stage during informed consent to further orient potential clients to mental health professionals' qualifications, view of the therapeutic process, and philosophy associated with therapy (e.g., Haslam & Harris, 2004). In line with these practices some schools of thought suggest that the first session should be considered a time in which therapists discuss their value system surrounding healthy functioning, various interventions, and so on. This information can be given verbally or on the consent form (Jensen & Bergin, 1988). The purpose is for the client to make an informed decision regarding treatment. It is during the intake session that mental health professionals can begin discussion of their basic values and glean information from the client about his or her values, including spiritual values. Of course, therapists should use good clinical judgment when considering a discussion of values, especially during the initial session that can both help and hinder future sessions.

EXHIBIT 4.1
Sample Informed Agency Consent Addressing Spirituality

It is our belief that spirituality and/or religion are important elements of many people's lives. We believe that religion and/or spirituality can have a significant effect on the types of problems for which many people seek therapy. These effects might be positive (e.g., religious beliefs helping someone to cope with their concerns) or negative (e.g., disconnection from a religious community that makes other problems more severe). As a result, we seek to include a client's spiritual or religious commitments in the therapy process whenever appropriate. You can expect some questions about your spiritual/religious beliefs and practices in the initial assessment phase of your therapy. If spirituality and/or religion are important elements in your life or appear to have a role in your presenting concerns, with your consent, your therapist will integrate these issues into your treatment. However, if at any time you are not comfortable discussing spiritual or religious issues with your therapist, you may decline to answer or otherwise share your discomfort with your therapist. Your therapist will also be able to help you by providing a referral, in addition to our services, to appropriate spiritual leaders or clergy within your faith tradition.

EXHIBIT 4.2
Informed Consent for Using Spiritual or Religious Components in Therapy

Our therapists are trained to provide mental health counseling services. Many are also capable of integrating specific spiritual or religious practices with typical counseling practice. Your therapist may ask if you would like to integrate specific spiritual or religious practices into your treatment. These include, but are not limited to, praying with or for you, teaching and guiding you in meditation, assigning readings from scripture or sacred writings, encouraging you to practice specific religious or spiritual rituals, and helping you to access the resources of your spiritual or religious community. In all cases, the therapist will strive to provide you with interventions that are congruent with your spiritual or religious perspective and that fit within your faith tradition. You are free to decline these interventions at any time and request that your therapist refrain from including the spiritual or religious in therapy, if it makes you feel uncomfortable.

Intake forms from smaller agencies and private practitioners are often shorter, are more flexible, and allow for more therapist–client time during intake. Some range from including virtually no information about spirituality to including multiple questions, with the intent being follow-up. Intake forms at high-volume agencies may include a question or two in reference to clients' spiritual or religious preferences and influences, such as "Do you have any spiritual or cultural beliefs that may influence your treatment?" This important question may attempt to set the tone that it is appropriate to discuss religious beliefs, although the question itself is inadequate. Clients often arrive unaware that their spiritual and religious beliefs can actually influence their treatment.

EXHIBIT 4.3
Professional Self-Disclosure of View on Spirituality

I specialize in helping individuals, couples, and families cope with the impact of illness, accidents, or other medical issues on their lives. My therapy work is characterized by holism and focuses on the ways people make meaning of their life circumstances. Holism means that I assess health and wellness in mental, emotional, social, physical, and spiritual facets of experience. People seem to benefit from therapy the most when thinking, feelings, behavior, and action are all included in the work. It is my belief that many individuals approach life with moral beliefs or spiritual practices that inform their decisions and perspectives of life. Few people examine how these beliefs and practices are related to emotional issues or life circumstances. Such transcendent beliefs can provide tremendous support and meaning for the issues clients face or may even be associated with unpleasant emotions or exchanges. I typically invite my clients to discuss their religious beliefs and faith practices as a way to think through the challenges they face and to acquaint me with their worldview. Such discussions are for the purpose of enriching our understanding of the issues at hand and are not for the purpose of proselytizing or debating the correctness of our ideas. I am comfortable including religious practices in therapy, such as prayer, meditation, or discussion about guiding religious documents, if these things are valuable to you. It is your prerogative to include or exclude these, or any aspects of your personal thoughts or feelings.

Additionally, many clients respond by stating their religious identification, such as Buddhist, Catholic, or Jewish. The question does not typically allow for further discussion of spiritual issues from clients, nor does it create a strong therapeutic alliance in which the client understands that spiritual issues are acceptable topics of discussion. Questions on these forms appear to be almost obligatory ways of tapping diversity issues with clients. What is important for therapists, as Spilka, Hood, Hunsberger, and Gorsuch (2003) stated, is not whether someone is religious but how they are religious. Under different agency structures the intake interview can be a place for more client expansion, but in larger, publicly funded agencies it is often not permissible or accepted. Some community agencies have only one or two perfunctory questions on the intake form referring to spiritual or cultural issues that may influence treatment. However, discussions with some of the agency's counselors indicate that they either do not follow up with the question or admit that they are unsure how to follow up.

REFERRAL SOURCE

When considering spiritual inclusion, therapists must also consider the referral source, whether self, partner, family, clergy, business, educational system, or legal system. Referrals from clergy are particularly salient given the historical separation between religion and mental health fields. As with any referral source, therapists should discuss issues pertaining to the client, with appropriate consent. Therapists can ask clergy members about the reason for referral, their thoughts on the issues, and what role faith has in treatment from their perspective.

Although clergy are discussed in the literature as a rich resource (McMinn & Dominguez, 2005), therapists rarely include clergy during therapy sessions, including the intake session. Clergy, especially as the referral source, can offer a wealth of information that can reduce the time needed in treatment. Often, clients who initially seek help from a spiritual community are hesitant about seeking help from the mental health community. Having the religious referral source arrive with the client can help ease the client's anxiety and bridge the relationship between the two professions. Therapists will differ in regard to their ease of having the clergy member sit in the intake session, although this simple act can be extremely beneficial. For example, while working at a hospital with a small psychological unit, the first author (Mark M. Leach) received a call from a Catholic nun who discussed an older adolescent female parishioner who had been sexually abused by a stepfather 2 years earlier. On arrival to this small town, word quickly spread that the author's specialty was treating individuals who had been sexually abused. As expected, the parishioner was hesitant to see a male therapist for treatment, although she trusted the nun implicitly. The author invited the nun to sit in on the initial session to allay the fears of the parishioner. The nun's participation also allowed the author to initiate spiritual discussions at greater depth than would be typically expected because she offered information at the client's request. Her presence alone introduced spiritual components to the session. Simple questions such as "Can you talk to me about how you see your faith being a part of treatment?" were often all that was needed for the client to feel more comfortable. In this case the client began talking about God as a coping mechanism, although at the time it was also clear that the nun's presence in this session acted as a hindrance to discussion of the client's more negative feelings toward God. These were addressed in later sessions and are not unusual for sexual abuse victims.

CLINICAL INTERVIEW

When it comes to the clinical interview itself, there are different ways that therapists can inquire about spirituality and assess the spiritual resources, problems, or complications that a client might bring to therapy. One way of conceptualizing these different approaches is to categorize the interviewing into explicit and implicit inquiry (for more detail, see chap. 5, this volume). The explicit–implicit categorization helps to frame the ways in which a therapist might inquire about a client's spirituality and helps to describe the different spiritual assessment models that have been recommended.

Explicit Inquiry

Explicit inquiry is any method of direct questioning about spirituality, such as "Is spirituality an important part of your life?" or "Do you have any religious or spiritual beliefs that may be important to discuss in counseling?" One extensive model of explicit inquiry is Hodge's (2001, 2005, 2006) spiritual assessment model that includes two frameworks. The first is an *initial narrative* framework wherein therapists guide clients in creating an autobiographical spiritual history. According to this approach, therapists work empathically with clients to validate client experiences and help them express the range of their spiritual beliefs, commitments, and perspectives. In the second framework, the *interpretive anthropological* framework, the goal is to understand ways that clients' spirituality might be a strength or resource for coping with their mental health concerns. This approach does not appear to be focused on assessing spiritual or religious problems per se but on assessing spirituality as a resource for helping clients cope with their mental health concerns. For instance, spiritual coping has been found to be a protective factor against many client concerns. Dervic, Grunebaum, Burke, Mann, and Oquendo (2006) confirmed earlier studies that suggested that spiritual coping acts as a protective factor for adults sexually abused as children.

However, certain religious or spiritual approaches to life might exacerbate mental health concerns or in some cases be difficult to distinguish from the psychological presenting problem (e.g., Hathaway, 2003). Unhealthy spirituality can be conceived as life-restricting practices, such as cognitive rigidity and authoritarianism (Hood, Hill, & Williamson, 2003). For example, Exline and Rose (2005) discussed religious and spiritual strain that includes discomfort as a result of not being at peace with a Higher Power. Because some clients present with such spiritual struggles, therapists have developed tools for uncovering spiritual and religious problems (e.g., Chirban, 2001). Using this approach, therapists might inquire explicitly into various spiritual domains, such as spiritual affiliation or spiritual development. Used alongside traditional clinical interview questions, this approach allows therapists to quickly assess potential spiritual problems or concerns.

Richards and Bergin (2005) developed an assessment model that incorporates both dimensions mentioned earlier: spirituality as a strength or resource and as a potential area for intervention. This model of spiritual and religious assessment is also explicit, although the depth of the assessment unfolds over two levels. At the first level, therapists are encouraged to conduct a brief global ecumenical assessment, meaning an assessment that would be appropriate for a client of any religious or spiritual persuasion. If this general assessment provides religious or spiritual information that might be relevant to therapy, Richards and Bergin suggested moving to the next level. At this second level, the assessment is more detailed and may either remain ecumenical (i.e., appropriate for people of any faith tradition) or become denominational (i.e., specific to the client's religious worldview). In both situations, Richards and Bergin argued that more detailed information about clients can help to provide guidance to the therapist for the course of therapy. The detailed assessments that they suggested include the clinical interview and even formal scales (e.g., religious orientation or commitment) that are guided by research and theory in the psychology of religion. Furthermore, Richards and Bergin took a broad perspective on the usefulness of spiritual and religious assessment, claiming that therapists may want to understand not only their clients' specific religious or spiritual concerns that might exacerbate their presenting problems but also the potential of religious or spiritual resources that might aid the therapy process and promote healing.

For therapists who may lack the availability of time or resources to conduct a multilevel explicit assessment, the FICA method (which stands for Faith and belief, Importance, Community, and Address in care) may prove helpful. Originally outlined in the medical literature by Puchalski and Romer (2000), the FICA is an assessment tool to be used in a clinical setting and in a brief period of time. It can also be used during intake interviews to allow for greater client responses and get a better conceptualization of the client. Although the assessment tool can contain multiple questions, many researchers and therapists (e.g., Hills, Paice, Cameron, & Shott, 2005) use brief modified versions that include four questions: Do you consider yourself spiritual or religious (Faith)? How important is spiritual or religious faith to you (Importance)? Are you a member of a spiritual or religious faith community (Community)? and How would you like me to address these issues during our time together (Address)? As the reader can surmise, these questions are relatively innocuous and can be modified further depending on the therapeutic situation.

Implicit Inquiry

The overt spiritual questions of an explicit inquiry are often a useful and direct way to gather information about the client during a clinical interview. However, implicit inquiry may also be used to begin spiritual discussions without necessarily mentioning spirituality. Implicit inquiries commonly explore topics related to spiritual themes, such as meaning making, coping, and social support. There are several ways that therapists might include an implicit inquiry into the clinical interview. Griffith and Griffith (2002) argued that one powerful implicit technique is simply listening to clients' use of spiritually laden words. They recommended paying close attention to specific client word choice and noticing emotional shifts during the course of the story. Words such as *presence* and *eternity* may stand out in clients' stories, or emotionally laden terms may appear to have meaning for clients. Following up with these specific words or highlighting the emotional shift can be all that is necessary to encourage clients to talk more about their spiritual lives.

Another method of implicit inquiry is to explore clients' worldview, personal philosophies, or other areas that might not necessarily lead to a spiritual or religious answer (e.g., one's basis for morality). Questions in this area might explore clients' typical coping strategies, their purpose or meaning in life, or how they make personal decisions about right and wrong. Some questions include the following:

1. How do you cope with the stress in your life?
2. How do you find comfort in times of stress?
3. What meaning does your life have currently?
4. What gives your life purpose?
5. For what are you grateful?
6. How easy is it to forgive yourself and others for past hurts?

Related to these questions of meaning, coping, and morality is exploring clients' current experiences of the congruence between their values or ideals and their lifestyle (Richards & Bergin, 2005). Many clients struggling with mental health concerns may be struggling with inconsistencies between these two aspects of their life. Inquiring into these potential conflicts can open the door for spirituality while still providing useful information when spirituality or religion is not relevant to the client.

Another strategy that therapists might use toward implicit inquiry is appropriate self-disclosure. This can begin prior to the first question of the clinical interview, when clients first encounter therapists' offices. The decorations, books, and layout of the therapy room convey important information to observant clients. Therapists who include spiritually or religiously themed material in their offices are self-disclosing, although implicitly and perhaps vaguely, their interest in and perhaps commitment to some form of spirituality or religion (Constantine & Kwan, 2003). Some therapists may even advertise their services with spiritual or religious symbols. Although less indirect, self-disclosure of therapists' experiences or expertise with spirituality or religion might also be appropriate. These self-disclosures can communicate to the spiritual client the therapist's openness to talking about spiritual or religious issues and may allow clients more freedom to initiate conversations that include the spiritual.

Implicit inquiry during the clinical intake can have several benefits. First, it can be an effective way to engage spiritually with clients who are more defended about their spiritual or religious lives. Clients who are uncertain about a therapist's openness to spirituality or who are ambivalent about their own spiritual journey may be reluctant to engage more direct questioning. Implicit inquiry allows these clients the freedom to choose when they are ready to divulge the more personal or troubling aspects of spirituality. Implicit inquiry might also be helpful for clients who may be unaware of the many different forms that spirituality can take. Clients who have a narrow version of spirituality (e.g., spirituality is expressed only in the confines of one of the major world religions) may not respond to direct, explicit questions about spirituality. However, through implicit inquiry that explores meaning, coping, worldviews, and other life aspects connected to spirituality broadly defined, the therapist may be able to uncover a vast and rich spiritual life that is simply not labeled "spiritual" by the client. This allows the therapist to marshal these resources for the client and access client strengths and uncover important conflicts that might be otherwise overlooked.

CASE STUDY: INTAKE AND INTERVIEW PROCESS

Following is a case study that examines how spirituality can be integrated into the clinical intake stage and interview process. This case highlights both implicit and explicit forms of inquiry that can be used by therapists to explore clients' spirituality. Likewise, this case provides an example of how therapists might incorporate a collaborative relationship with spiritual leaders from the onset of therapy as a client resource.

Thomas was a 39-year-old Caucasian man who presented for therapy asking for help with his feelings of worthlessness, hopelessness, and sadness.[1] He described a long history of vegetative symptoms, with onset during his teen years. "I just can't get ahold of this thing," he lamented. "I know I shouldn't feel this way, but I just can't shake it." Thomas's depression had lifted for short periods during his life, which included the weeks leading up to his marriage, a few weeks surrounding the time when he joined his church, and more recently, for 1 week during a church retreat.

He described a job and social pursuits in which he typically found some degree of pleasure. His relationships with his wife and children were strong. He frequently saw his siblings during family functions and described those events as decidedly positive. He had no significant medical history and denied history of abuse or neglect. He had never engaged in high-risk behaviors such as unauthorized use of controlled substances, violence, or self-harming acts. It sounded like a straightforward case of major depression.

Thomas had not remarked on the devotional books on my (Barbara Couden Hernandez [BCH]) shelf nor volunteered any significant information pertaining to his faith or spiritual practices. I did recall that when he called to schedule our appointment, he asked whether I was a Christian. When I replied in the affirmative, he responded positively. I was therefore interested why, after nearly half an hour of discussion about his depressive symptoms and relational history, he had not remarked on his spirituality.

My assessment began with the question, "Do you have any spiritual beliefs or life philosophy that influences how you view your situation?" Thomas was a member of a large conservative Christian congregation close to my office. He added that a deacon had provided the referral but remarked that he'd best pray rather than to visit a therapist. I was intrigued. (Thomas was telling me about his faith affiliation but not his spiritual practices or beliefs.) I asked him to help me understand what his interest had been in my faith affiliation when he called to set up our appointment. Our conversation proceeded to this effect:

Thomas: Oh, I wanted to make sure that you wouldn't try to undermine my faith.

BCH: Are you concerned that I might do that?

Thomas: Well, my church doesn't believe in therapists and especially not people who will talk you into taking drugs. So I wanted to know if you are a Christian because you won't talk me into taking drugs.

BCH: Hmmm. Can you say more about that?

---

[1]For the case presented in this chapter, a pseudonym is used, and identifying details have been altered for confidentiality.

Thomas: Well, I was on [an antidepressant] for awhile and I felt pretty good. But our pastor preached a sermon about faith and how important it is to our standing with God. He said that people just need to trust God rather than be anxious or depressed. If we really believe that God is taking care of us, we'd never be depressed or anxious. My meds went down the toilet after I heard that. I've wanted to die. But I belong to God and I would rather trust God and die with His approval rather than take pills with His disapproval.

This was critical information for me as a therapist. Thomas's expectation was that I would somehow help him to cope with his depression without medication use. This ran counter to my own religious beliefs and clinical judgment, and I was alarmed about his suicidality. A spiritual history might yield other important information as well as demonstrate my openness and validation of his faith experience before we addressed his suicidality directly.

Thomas had grown up in a home without any religious training, yet he had prayed from a young age that God would make his mother love him. This occurred after she had angrily told him that she wished he had never been born because he was an inconvenience to her. As an adult Thomas recognized that his mother was doubtless overwhelmed with the care of three small children since his father had died in a traffic accident. However, he embarked on a lifelong quest to feel wanted. When he was a young adult he was invited to join a church near his home. This was a negative experience because he did not feel a sense of warmth or inclusion there. Believing that it was important for him to be part of a congregation, he visited other faith groups until he was warmly welcomed to his present church. He has been a member there for 6 years, citing his membership as an organizing feature of his social and spiritual life.

Thomas's remissions coincided with the periods of time during which he felt the greatest sense of belonging: his courtship and marriage, when he joined his church, and a church retreat. His sense of belonging to God could easily be threatened by a standard referral for medication evaluation. I hypothesized that his sense of belonging to God and his relationship to his church friends were a significant source of strength to him. Daily prayer, meditation, and Bible reading were mentioned as helpful in improving his mood.

After performing a suicide assessment, I scheduled a return appointment for the next day. Once consent was obtained, Thomas enthusiastically welcomed my suggestion that he invite his pastor to join us for a discussion about the best course of treatment. I suggested that Thomas consider reading Psalm 103 several times before our appointment, referencing passages that describe the loving tenderness with which God deals with humankind. Thomas was delighted and asked whether he could offer prayer as we closed our session. This he did with considerable fervor and relief.

The following day Pastor James discussed the ideas in his sermon by talking about antidepressant overprescription. It was noted that neither he nor Thomas understood the action of antidepressants or the indications for their use. Nor did they understand the heritability of mood disorders. Using Doherty's (1999) model for addressing religious beliefs in therapy, I provided clinical information about chronic depression and its symptoms. We discussed the moral imperative for parents to care for their own mental health to provide a healthy atmosphere for their children. I invited Pastor James to discuss God's will for our lives in terms of satisfaction and emotional health. He then clarified his comments in his sermon to have applied to those with transient worries or sad mood but not those with serious mood disorders. He suggested that Thomas refill his antidepressant prescription and begin taking his medications immediately. After a general discussion about common medication management issues and giving consent to speak with his prescribing physician, Thomas expressed relief and the intent to resume his medications. The following week's session was spent anchoring this new information and setting goals for therapy.

An understanding of Thomas's spiritual journey and religious beliefs led to a course of therapy that would have been different had these issues not been considered. In addition to addressing medication compliance and self-management, we were able to address his yearning for belonging and other unresolved issues from his family of origin. Because therapy was predicated on the investigation of Thomas's spiritual needs, compliance and motivation were high throughout the course of treatment.

CONCLUSION

The purpose of this chapter was to provide insight into how therapists might go about integrating spirituality into the clinical intake and interview. Overall, a number of approaches that therapists can use to include and explore the spiritual during this important phase of therapy have been highlighted. As suggested throughout the chapter, a number of factors, such as agency climate and client preference, need to be considered when incorporating spirituality into the clinical intake. Thus, both explicit and implicit approaches were discussed so that therapists can tailor an approach congruent with their own practices, agency policies, and client needs. Still, as mentioned at the beginning of the chapter, more research and practice guidelines are needed to guide therapists during this initial stage of the therapeutic process. It is our hope that this chapter will help facilitate a more intentional and examined method for integrating spirituality into the clinical intake and interview by therapists.

REFERENCES

Bergin, A. E., & Jensen, J. P. (1990). Religiosity of psychotherapists: A national survey. *Psychotherapy: Theory, Research, Practice, Training, 27*, 3–7.

Chappelle, W. (2000). A series of progressive legal and ethical decision-making steps for using Christian spiritual interventions in psychotherapy. *Journal of Psychology and Theology, 28*, 43–53.

Chirban, J. T. (2001). Assessing religious and spiritual concerns in psychotherapy. In T. G. Plante & A. C. Sherman (Eds.), *Faith and health: Psychological perspectives* (pp. 265–290). New York: Guilford Press.

Constantine, M. G., & Kwan, K. K. (2003). Cross-cultural considerations of therapist self-disclosure. *Journal of Clinical Psychology, 59*, 581–588.

Corey, G., Corey, M. S., & Callanan, P. (1998). *Issues and ethics in the helping professions*. Pacific Grove, CA: Brooks/Cole.

Dervic, K., Grunebaum, M. F., Burke, A. K., Mann, J. J., & Oquendo, M. A. (2006). Protective factors against suicidal behavior in depressed adults reporting childhood abuse. *Journal of Nervous and Mental Disease, 194*, 971–974.

Doherty, W. J. (1999). Morality and spirituality in therapy. In F. Walsh (Ed.), *Spiritual resources in family therapy* (pp. 179–192). New York: Guilford Press.

Erickson, M. J., Hecker, L., Kirkpatrick, D., Killmer, M., & James, E. (2002). Clients' perceptions of marriage and family therapists addressing the religious and spiritual aspects of clients' lives: A pilot study. *Journal of Family Psychotherapy, 13*, 109–125.

Exline, J. J., & Rose, E. (2005). Religious and spiritual struggles. In R. F. Paloutzian & C. L. Park (Eds.), *Handbook of the psychology of religion and spirituality* (pp. 315–330). New York: Guilford Press.

Griffith, J. L., & Griffith, M. E. (2002). *Encountering the sacred in psychotherapy: How to talk with people about their spiritual lives*. New York: Guilford Press.

Haslam, D. R., & Harris, S. M. (2004). Informed consent documents of marriage and family therapists in private practice: A qualitative analysis. *American Journal of Family Therapy, 32*, 359–375.

Hathaway, W. L. (2003). Clinically significant religious impairment. *Mental Health, Religion and Culture, 6*, 113–129.

Hills, J., Paice, J. A., Cameron, J. R., & Shott, S. (2005). Spirituality and distress in palliative care consultation. *Journal of Palliative Medicine, 8*, 782–788.

Hood, R. W., Hill, P. C., & Williamson, P. W. (2005). *The psychology of religious fundamentalism*. New York: Guilford Press.

Hodge, D. R. (2001). Spiritual assessment: A review of major qualitative methods and a new framework for assessing spirituality. *Social Work, 46*, 203–214.

Hodge, D. R. (2005). Spiritual lifemaps: A client-centered pictorial instrument for spiritual assessment, planning, and intervention. *Social Work, 50*, 77–87.

Hodge, D. R. (2006). A template for spiritual assessment: A review of the JCAHO requirements and guidelines for implementation. *Social Work, 51*, 317–326.

Jensen, J. P., & Bergin, A. E. (1988). Mental health values of professional therapists: A national interdisciplinary survey. *Professional Psychology: Research and Practice, 19*, 290–297.

Leach, M. M., & Aten, J. D. (2007). *Reasons for students' resistance to incorporating spirituality into counseling.* Unpublished manuscript.

McMinn, M. R., & Dominguez, A. W. (2005). *Psychology and the church.* New York: Nova Science.

Puchalski, C. M., & Romer, A. L. (2000). Taking a spiritual history allows clinicians to understand patients more fully. *Journal of Palliative Medicine, 3*, 129–137.

Richards, P. S., & Bergin, A. E. (2005). *A spiritual strategy for counseling and psychotherapy* (2nd ed.). Washington, DC: American Psychological Association.

Richards, P. S., Rector, J. M., & Tjeltveit, A. C. (1999). Values, spirituality, and psychotherapy. In W. R. Miller (Ed.), *Integrating spirituality into treatment: Resources for practitioners* (pp. 133–160). Washington, DC: American Psychological Association.

Schlosser, L. Z., Foley, P. F., Holmwood, J. R., & Poltrock, E. S. (in press). Why does counseling psychology exclude religion? A content analysis and methodological critique. In J. G. Ponterotto, J. M. Casas, L. A. Suzuki, & C. M. Alexander (Eds.), *Handbook of multicultural counseling* (3rd ed.). Thousand Oaks, CA: Sage.

Smith, D. P., & Orlinsky, D. E. (2004). Religious and spiritual experience among psychotherapists. *Psychotherapy: Theory, Research, Practice, Training, 41*, 144–151.

Somberg, D. R., Stone, G. L., & Claiborn, C. D. (1993). Informed consent: Therapists' beliefs and practices. *Professional Psychology: Research and Practice, 24*, 153–159.

Sommers-Flanagan, J., & Sommers-Flanagan, R. (2002). *Clinical interviewing* (3rd ed.). New York: Wiley.

Spilka, B., Hood, R. W., Jr., Hunsberger, B., & Gorsuch, R. (2003). *The psychology of religion: An empirical approach* (3rd ed.). New York: Guilford Press.

Sue, S., McKinney, H., & Allen, D. (1976). Predictors of the duration of therapy for clients in the community mental health system. *Community Mental Health Journal, 12*, 365–375.

5

CLINICAL ASSESSMENT OF CLIENTS' SPIRITUALITY

KENNETH I. PARGAMENT AND ELIZABETH J. KRUMREI

The religious is elusive not because it lurks behind ordinary phenomena but because it is woven into the phenomena.

—D. E. Capps

Spiritual assessment is a process that evolves over the course of therapy to aid in the process of addressing the spiritual dimension in treatment. This chapter considers how to assess the role of spirituality in the lives of specific clients, including the role that spirituality plays in their problems, their resources, their critical life events, and their larger context. Such assessment occurs through a three-stage process: initial spiritual assessment, extensive spiritual assessment, and implicit spiritual assessment. Before delving into the methodology of spiritual assessment, we offer a conceptual framework for thinking about spirituality.

CONCEPTUAL FRAMEWORK OF SPIRITUALITY

Spiritual assessment should be grounded in a clear understanding of spirituality, including how it works, how it may be part of clients' problems, and how it may be part of their solutions. Without a roadmap of spiritual under-

Portions of this chapter are from *Spiritually Integrated Psychotherapy: Understanding and Addressing the Sacred*, by K. I. Pargament, 2007, New York: Guilford Press. Copyright 2007 by Guilford Press. Adapted with permission.

standing to guide assessment, therapists may get lost in the spiritual domain. Spiritually disoriented themselves, therapists may overlook important spiritual issues to get back to familiar territory or misdirect clients in the search for solutions. We now offer a brief summary of one way to understand and evaluate spirituality (see Pargament, 2007, for a more extensive review).

People are motivated to seek out a relationship with something sacred, just as they are motivated to attain physiological, psychological, and social goals (Pargament, 1997). Although social scientists have often attempted to reduce spirituality to presumably more basic motives, we believe that spirituality can be a motive in and of itself. Spirituality refers to the effort to discover the sacred, conserve a relationship with the sacred once it has been discovered, and transform that relationship when necessary. By sacred, we are referring not only to God, higher powers, and transcendent reality but to any aspect of life that takes on attributes of divinity. Thus, the sacred can encompass relationships, nature, art, institutions, the self, sports, war, politics, time, place, sexuality, and so on, if it is imbued with divine character and significance. In short, spirituality is a search for the sacred, which can involve any aspect of life that is perceived as sacred.

The search for the sacred is a dynamic process rather than a static set of beliefs and practices (see Figure 5.1). The search begins with the discovery of something sacred. The discovery may occur through socialization (e.g., through family, religious institutions, or the larger culture) or through a personal spiritual encounter (e.g., hearing the voice of God or sensing the leading of the Holy Spirit). Once they have discovered the sacred, individuals may take traditional and nontraditional spiritual paths to conserve and foster their relationship with the sacred. This can include the pathway of knowing (e.g., Bible study, scientific study), the pathway of acting (e.g., rituals, virtuous deeds), the pathway of relating (e.g., building religious communities, acts of loving kindness), and the pathway of experiencing (e.g., prayer, meditation, music).

At times, however, people's relationships with the sacred can be threatened or damaged as a result of internal or external changes. For instance, experiencing unexpected hardships, such as an illness or financial loss, may challenge a person's conception of a benevolent God. In response to such challenges, people can draw on spiritual coping methods (e.g., seeking spiritual support, engaging in purification rituals, reframing an event as having positive spiritual meaning) to preserve and protect the sacred. These methods are often successful in sustaining people's relationships with the sacred. However, some life stressors can lead individuals to experience tension and conflict with the divine (e.g., feeling angry at God for allowing divorce to break up a family; Mahoney, Krumrei, & Pargament, 2008), with a religious community, or within themselves (Pargament, Murray-Swank, Magyar, & Ano, 2005). Such spiritual struggles are often short-lived, but they can also represent turning points with more profound implications. For example, spiritual struggles can

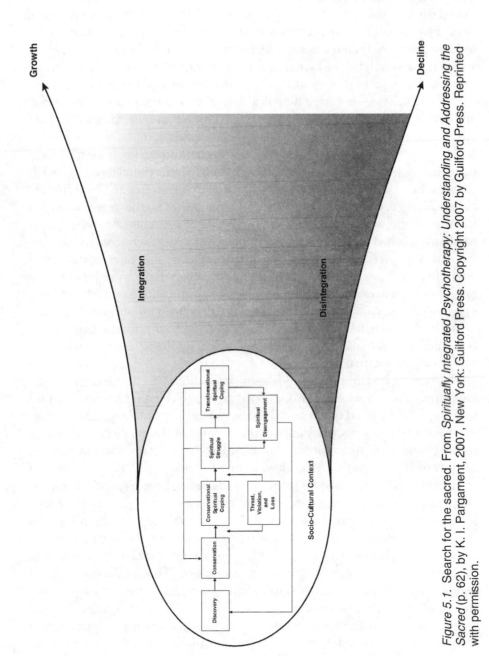

Figure 5.1. Search for the sacred. From *Spiritually Integrated Psychotherapy: Understanding and Addressing the Sacred* (p. 62), by K. I. Pargament, 2007, New York: Guilford Press. Copyright 2007 by Guilford Press. Reprinted with permission.

lead to temporary or permanent disengagement from the search for the sacred. They can also lead to efforts to fundamentally change the character of the sacred through transformational methods of spiritual coping (e.g., conversion, rites of passage). Once such a transformation takes place, people return to the task of conserving their relationships with the sacred. It is important to emphasize that the search for the sacred does not occur in a vacuum; it shapes and is shaped by a larger field of situational, social, cultural, and personal forces.

Spirituality as described here is a natural and normal part of life, a rich and diverse process that evolves over the course of an individual's life span. Although spirituality is often defined in positive terms, we believe that spirituality is not inherently good or healthy. Whether spirituality leads to growth or decline depends on the degree to which it is well integrated (see Figure 5.1; Pargament, 2007). A well-integrated spirituality is not defined by a specific belief, practice, experience, or relationship but rather by the degree to which the ingredients work together in synchrony with each other. At its best, spirituality is marked by pathways that are broad and deep, sensitive to life's situations, supported by the larger social context, capable of continuity and flexibility, and directed toward a sacred destination that can respond to the full range of human potential and provide the person with a powerful guiding vision. At its worst, spirituality is disintegrated, defined by pathways that lack breadth and depth, fail to meet the demands of life, clash with the larger social system, change too easily or not at all, and misdirect the person to pursue matters of limited spiritual value.

Drawing on this understanding of spirituality, we can identify several key topics and questions that orient therapists to spiritual assessment (see Exhibit 5.1). It should be stressed that these questions are designed to organize therapists' thinking. They are not questions that should be posed directly to the client. First, therapists should consider where clients stand in relation to spirituality. This involves understanding factors such as the centrality of spirituality and motivation for spirituality in clients' lives. Second, therapists should be aware that clients enter therapy at very different places in their spiritual journeys. For example, some people come to therapy in the midst of a spiritual struggle or transformation, whereas others enter therapy in a conservational mode with a spirituality that has been stable for much of their lives. Still others come to therapy spiritually disengaged. Third, therapists should examine the content of clients' spirituality. This involves getting a better picture of what the clients consider to be sacred, how they envision these sacred entities, and the pathways they take to the sacred. Fourth, therapists should gain a better understanding of how clients' spirituality is related to their social context. Fifth, therapists should be able to evaluate the efficacy of clients' spirituality by considering the various ways in which spirituality affects clients' lives. Finally, drawing on all of the information mentioned earlier, therapists should come away from the assessment process with a sense of how

EXHIBIT 5.1
Comprehensive Framework of Spiritual Assessment

1. Relation of clients to spirituality
   (a) Is spirituality central or peripheral to clients' lives and strivings?
   (b) Are clients aware or unaware of the place of spirituality in their lives?
   (c) Are clients' spiritual motivations internally based or externally based
       (e.g., guilt, social pressure)?
2. Location of clients in their spiritual journeys
   (a) Do clients have a long or short history of spiritual involvement?
   (b) Are clients spiritually engaged or disengaged?
   (c) Are clients in the midst of discovering their spirituality?
   (d) Are clients primarily focused on conserving their present spirituality?
   (e) Are clients in the midst of transforming their spirituality?
   (f) Are clients going through spiritual struggles?
   (g) Are clients working through or stuck in their spiritual struggles?
3. Content of clients' spirituality
   (a) What do clients hold sacred?
       (i) Are clients' representations of the sacred large enough to encompass the
           full range of life experiences, or are they constricted?
       (ii) Are clients' representations of the sacred benevolent or malevolent?
       (iii) Do clients recognize the limits in their understanding of the sacred?
       (iv) Do clients' various understandings of the sacred blend together, or do
            they clash with each other?
   (b) How do clients express their spirituality?
       (i) Are clients aware or unaware of how they experience and express
           spirituality?
       (ii) Which spiritual pathways do clients take? Do clients take some pathways
            to the exclusion of others?
       (iii) Do clients integrate their spirituality into their lives or do they compart-
             mentalize it?
       (iv) Are clients flexible or inflexible in selecting and following ways of
            expressing spirituality?
       (v) Are clients familiar with the variety of ways of expressing spirituality that
           are available to them?
       (vi) Are clients disciplined or undisciplined in pursuing spirituality?
       (vii) Are clients' relationships with the sacred secure or insecure (e.g., anxious,
             hostile, self-degrading)?
4. Context of clients' spirituality
   (a) How well do clients' spirituality fit with their social context?
   (b) Are clients' environments spiritually benevolent or malevolent?
   (c) Do clients experience spiritual support from or spiritual conflict with others?
   (d) Does clients' spirituality enhance or detract from the well-being of others?
5. Impact of spirituality on clients' lives
   (a) What kinds of emotions/affect are elicited by clients' spirituality?
       (i) Are clients satisfied with their spirituality?
       (ii) Do clients experience spiritual comfort or spiritual distress?
   (b) Does clients' spirituality lead to benefits and/or costs for them or those in their
       lives?
   (c) Does clients' spirituality increase or decrease their health and well-being?
6. Place of spirituality in treatment
   (a) In what ways are clients' spirituality well integrated or disintegrated?
   (b) Is spirituality a part of the solution or a part of the problem?
   (c) What spiritual resources can clients draw on in therapy?
   (d) What spiritual problems should clients address in therapy?
   (e) What spiritual obstacles are likely to arise in therapy?

spirituality should be addressed in treatment, on the basis of the ways in which clients' spirituality is well integrated or disintegrated and whether it is contributing to clients' problems or potential solutions.

This comprehensive framework can guide therapists in the assembly of a rich picture of clients' spirituality. Before we discuss the specific methods of clinical assessment, it is important to reflect on creating an atmosphere of open spiritual dialogue.

CREATING AN ATMOSPHERE FOR SPIRITUAL ASSESSMENT

Many clients enter therapy without an awareness of how spirituality is pertinent to their clinical situation. To open the door to spiritual dialogue in therapy, therapists can introduce spirituality as a topic for discussion and indicate how it could be relevant to the clinical problems or solutions. When spirituality is emerging as an important topic, therapists should inquire whether their clients are interested in talking about spiritual matters. It is vital that therapists respect clients' rights to control the nature and extent of spiritual conversation. Therapists must be judicious about when to move forward and when to retreat, all the while leaving the door open to future dialogues about spirituality.

Therapists should communicate an attitude of respect and interest when clients are willing to discuss spiritual matters in treatment. Clients may hesitate to raise spiritual issues in therapy because they expect their therapists to view spirituality as irrelevant at best, or silly, foolish, and maladaptive at worst. The antidote to these concerns is the therapist's expressed interest in learning more when clients bring up a topic related to spirituality. In essence, therapists convey openness to being taught by clients. Toward this end, therapists avoid making assumptions about clients' spirituality. For example, therapists should not assume that knowledge of a religious denomination is equivalent to understanding the clients' spiritual experiences, as there are diverse spiritual understandings within any denomination. Thus, even therapists and clients who share the same religious tradition cannot be assumed to share the same conception of spirituality. Furthermore, therapists should routinely ask for clarification before making interpretations of clients' spiritual language. Common spiritual terms such as *faith, spiritual experience, prayer, born again,* and *religious* have very different meanings to different people. The task for therapists is to understand the unique meanings that clients attach to such terms. In short, therapists respond to spiritual topics by expressing genuine interest in entering the spiritual world as clients see it.

In sum, creating an appropriate atmosphere for spiritual assessment involves obtaining consent from clients to address spirituality in therapy, expressing respect and interest concerning spiritual matters, and conveying a willingness to be taught by clients about their spirituality. This benevolent atmosphere sets the stage for an initial spiritual assessment. On the basis of clients' responses to initial questions about spirituality, therapists can decide whether to follow with an extensive spiritual assessment to gain a comprehensive picture of clients' spirituality or an implicit spiritual assessment that may reveal a deeper, spiritual dimension of clients' lives.

INITIAL SPIRITUAL ASSESSMENT

Time is at a premium during the intake session of therapy. Given the many areas of clients' lives that must be explored in the first session—presenting problems; risk factors; medical, psychological, and social histories; diagnostic questions; and treatment goals—there is little time for extensive interviewing about spirituality. Despite the time constraints, spirituality should not be overlooked in the initial intake (see chap. 4, this volume).

In the first session, questions can be raised about four important spiritually related areas: the importance of spirituality to clients, the religious affiliation of clients, the relevance of spirituality to the problems, and the relevance of spirituality to the solutions (see Exhibit 5.2). As previously noted, the assessment of spirituality is not a mechanical process. These questions must be tailored to the individual client. For example, if it becomes apparent that a client is not spiritually or religiously involved, then it is not necessary to pursue all four areas. Rather than separate the spiritual questions out from other assessment questions, they can be naturally integrated into the flow of conversation with clients.

The first question of the initial spiritual assessment is, "Do you see yourself as a spiritual or religious person? If so, in what way?" Responses to this question will provide insight into whether clients have a spiritual worldview. Information may be gained about the nature of clients' spirituality and the role it plays in various aspects of their lives. In addition, this is an opportunity to observe whether clients seem comfortable discussing spiritual issues in therapy.

EXHIBIT 5.2
Initial Spiritual Assessment Questions

1. The importance of spirituality to the client: "Do you see yourself as a spiritual or religious person? If so, in what way?"
2. Religious affiliation of the client: "Are you affiliated with a spiritual or religious denomination or community? If so, which one?"
3. The relevance of spirituality to the problem: "Has your problem affected you spiritually or religiously? If so, in what way?"
4. The relevance of spirituality to the solution: "Has your spirituality or religion been involved in the way you have coped with your problem? If so, in what way?"

This is followed by a question about clients' larger religious context: "Are you affiliated with a spiritual or religious denomination or community? If so, which one?" This will offer an indication of whether clients see their lives through the lens of a specific religious belief system. It is also important to listen for whether clients have rejected a particular religious community. These questions about religious affiliations and the importance of spirituality to clients can be interwoven with other questions about clients' identities, such as their occupations, roles in their families, and goals for the future.

Next, it is important to assess how spirituality relates to the presenting problems. Therapists may ask, "Has your problem affected you spiritually or religiously? If so, in what way?" This question fits well in the context of other questions about the effect of clients' problems on psychological, social, and physical functioning. Responses to this question will indicate whether clients conceptualize their problems in spiritual terms. One possibility is that clients experience their problems as spiritual struggles. They may feel abandoned by God or that the problems are a punishment from God. This could be associated with spiritual doubts or feelings of being judged by a religious community. Research has shown that people who voice spiritual struggles are at greater risk for psychological and physical problems (Fitchett, Rybarczyk, DeMarco, & Nicholas, 1999; Pargament, Koenig, & Perez, 2000; Pargament, Smith, Koenig, & Perez, 1998). However, more recent research has also highlighted the potential of spiritual struggles to elicit positive transformation and growth (e.g., Pargament et al., 2005).

The other side of the coin is to assess how spirituality relates to the solution. The final question of the initial spiritual assessment is, "Has your spirituality or religion been involved in the way you have dealt with your problem? If so, in what way?" This inquiry easily follows the more general question about ways in which clients have tried to deal with their problems. Responses to this question will provide insight into whether clients view their spirituality as a resource in the face of difficulties. Spirituality can be incorporated into the problem-solving process in many different ways. For example, clients have described looking to God for strength, turning to religious communities for help, relying on spiritual beliefs as a guide in making decisions, detaching from daily concerns through meditation or prayer, and engaging in spiritual activities and rituals to move past their problems. Thus, this question highlights the ways in which spirituality is helpful to clients in relation to their presenting problems. In addition, responses to this question may indicate whether clients are overlooking potential resources within spirituality.

These four questions launch the spiritual assessment in therapy. The clients' responses offer some initial glimpses into their spirituality. The initial assessment may indicate that spirituality is not relevant to certain clients. This can occur for various reasons and does not guarantee that spirituality will not emerge as a significant factor later in the therapeutic process. Implicit methods of assessment can be used in such cases to delve deeper into clients' experiences. However, it is also possible for the initial spiritual assessment to reveal directly the importance of spirituality to clients and their problems. In such cases, further details must be gained about the relevance of spirituality to the situation through a more extensive spiritual assessment.

EXTENSIVE SPIRITUAL ASSESSMENT

The purpose of an extensive spiritual assessment is to gain more detailed information about clients' spiritual beliefs, practices, and experiences and the role that each plays in their clinical problems or the solutions to them. The label *extensive spiritual assessment* may sound dry; however, it describes a rich, multidimensional process used to capture a phenomenon as multifaceted as spirituality. The extensive spiritual assessment should not be thought of as a rote, structured interview but as an opportunity to elicit clients' spiritual stories through the use of open-ended questions and clinical exercises. As clients' spiritual narratives unfold, therapists also focus on indirect cues, such as changes in facial expressions or patterns of speech. A robust picture of clients' spirituality is further bolstered through the use of quantitative measures and external sources of information.

Eliciting the Client's Spiritual Story

Spirituality can be a private and elusive phenomenon that is difficult to put into words. Many clients may not have had previous opportunities to describe their spiritual experiences. For these reasons, allowing clients to tell their spiritual story is the best method of gathering more extensive information about their spirituality. Rich information is gained when clients describe where they have been, currently find themselves, and are going spiritually. As mentioned before, spirituality is conceptualized as a dynamic process. A spiritual journey can encompass periods of discovering the sacred, periods of spiritual stability in which a variety of spiritual paths are taken to conserve and foster a relationship with the sacred, circumstances in which spirituality affects life for the better, periods of spiritual struggle in which the sacred is threatened or damaged, circumstances in which spirituality affects life for the worse, periods of spiritual change in which a variety of spiritual coping methods can be used to either preserve or transform the sacred, and periods of spiritual disengagement in which spirituality seems absent. Each type of spiritual experience can be embedded in clients' spiritual narratives. Telling a spiritual story allows clients to make use of images, symbols, and metaphors to communicate at a deeper level about a phenomenon as ineffable and mysterious as spirituality.

Using Open-Ended Questions

There is no formula for getting clients to share their spiritual narratives. Conducting a structured interview is likely to provide surface-level details about the clients' spiritual beliefs and practices. However, the goal of extensive spiritual assessment is to delve deeper into the experiences and circumstances of clients as spiritual beings. This is a process that must flow naturally from the conversations that occur in treatment. When appropriate opportunities arise, therapists can encourage clients to tell their spiritual story by posing spiritually relevant, open-ended questions. Exhibit 5.3 provides sample questions that can further the sharing of spiritual narratives. A case study, drawn from Pargament (2007), illustrates how such questions were adapted to a particular client and woven into the clinical conversation.

Case Study: Using Open-Ended Questions to Elicit a Client's Spiritual Story

Agnes, a 50-year-old woman, pursued treatment with me (Kenneth I. Pargament) after a stay in an inpatient psychiatric unit.[1] She had voluntarily committed herself after thinking of killing her husband or herself. We had been engaged in treatment for several weeks when an opportunity arose to explore some spiritual facets of her experiences.

"So, tell me," I asked Agnes, "How did you lose your soul?" Perhaps not the first question that comes to mind in conducting a spiritual assessment, but it seemed fitting for this client. Agnes was tall, thin, dressed in a severe black skirt and gray blouse, with her hair pulled back tightly off of her face. There was a tautness and brittleness about her.

I learned that Agnes spent much of her adult life living in the shadow of her husband. A charismatic businessman, active in charity work, Peter was well-known and respected in the community. Family and friends repeatedly reminded Agnes how fortunate she was to be married to him. Yet, she herself seemed invisible. Once, she and her husband had accompanied another couple to a restaurant only to learn that the couple had made the reservation for three people, forgetting to include Agnes in the tally.

Only Agnes knew that her husband was a terribly ineffectual businessman. Agnes was, in fact, keeping the business afloat, bringing in the lion's share of the business, and attending to its day-to-day operation. Even so, her accomplishments were hidden from others, and she herself took little pleasure from them. It was not what she wanted to be doing with her life. Her remark led to an exchange in which I began to elicit Agnes's spiritual story:

---

[1]For the cases presented in this chapter, pseudonyms are used, and identifying details have been altered for confidentiality.

EXHIBIT 5.3
Open-Ended Questions to Elicit the Client's Spiritual Story

1. Past spirituality
   (a) How was spirituality expressed in the environment you grew up in?[a]
   (b) When did you first discover the sacred?
   (c) How did you conceptualize the sacred when you were younger?
   (d) How did you express your spirituality?
   (e) What spiritual milestones have you experienced in your journey?
   (f) Have there been times that you felt the sacred was absent in your life?
2. Present spirituality
   (a) Conceptualizations of the sacred
       (i) What do you hold sacred in your life?
       (ii) How have your understandings and beliefs about the sacred changed?
       (iii) Why are you involved in spirituality?
       (iv) What do you feel God wants from you?
       (v) What do you imagine that God feels when he sees you going through this difficult time?[b]
       (vi) Do you ever experience a different side of the sacred than what you are experiencing now? What is that like?[b]
       (vii) Do you ever have mixed thoughts and feelings about the sacred? What are they like?
   (b) Expression and experience of spirituality
       (i) How would you describe your current spiritual orientation?[a]
       (ii) How do you experience the sacred in your life?
       (iii) What has helped nurture your spirituality?
       (iv) What has been damaging to your spirituality?
       (v) When/where do you feel most connected to the sacred?
       (vi) When/where do you feel the sacred is not present?
       (vii) What spiritual rituals or practices are important to you?
       (viii) What spiritual beliefs do you find especially meaningful?[a]
   (c) Spiritual efficacy
       (i) How has your spirituality changed your life for the better?
       (ii) How has your spirituality changed your life for the worse?
       (iii) To what degree has your spirituality given you pleasure? Meaning? A sense of connectedness to others? Hope for the future? Confidence in yourself? A feeling of being loved? Compassion for others?
       (iv) To what degree has your spirituality been a source of pain? Guilt? Anger? Confusion and doubt? Anxiety? Fear? Feelings of personal insignificance? Feelings of alienation from others?
       (v) In what ways has your spirituality helped you to understand or deal with your problems?
       (vi) In what ways has your spirituality been harmful in understanding or dealing with your problems?
   (d) Spiritual environment
       (i) Who supports you spiritually? How so?
       (ii) Who does not support you spiritually? How so?
3. Future spirituality
   (a) How do you see yourself changing spiritually in the future?
   (b) In what ways do you want to grow spiritually?
   (c) How does your spirituality relate to your life goals?

[a]Adapted from Hodge (2001). [b]Adapted from Griffith and Griffith (2002).

KIP: What is it that you would like to do?

CL: I just don't know. I can't get any traction. There's nothing to grab hold of inside of me. I feel such an emptiness in my core. I feel soulless.

KIP: So tell me, how did you lose your soul?

CL: I've often thought about that. I met Peter before I left for Europe to study the cello. Going to Europe was probably the most radical thing I had ever done. My parents discouraged me from going, telling me I could never support myself with music, and I had never been off on my own. But I won a scholarship to study music in Paris, and I had a wonderful time. I was going to stay another year, but over the summer, Peter proposed to me and said he wanted me to come home to be with him. I hesitated. My parents wanted me to return, too. On top of that, they were charmed by Peter and reminded me that I wasn't much in the looks department. Oh, and of course, I wasn't getting any younger. I left my music and came home to Peter.

KIP: You stopped playing the cello?

CL: Yes. [long pause and deep sigh] It's funny. Even though music was the heart and soul of my life, I didn't miss it at first. You have to understand that I adored Peter. He was utterly beguiling, and I was incredulous that this fascinating man would have any interest in me. I worshipped him.

KIP: How did you worship him?

CL: I just put everything else aside. My art, my music, and I devoted myself to him. Whatever Peter wanted, I supported. Wherever he went, I followed. I made allowances for him. I covered for him. I allowed him to live the life he wanted to live.

KIP: And what about you? Did you have other objects of devotion in your life?

CL: No, I gave everything to him. [pause]. And he took it all, without even a "thank you."

KIP: You feel like he took your soul?

CL: [pause] Maybe, but I was complicit in it. I was willing to give it up, to sacrifice even my soul for him.

KIP: We're talking about sacred matters here, and I hate to stop, but we're coming to the end of our time today. I'd like to leave you with a question to consider for our next session. You said that you feel soulless. Here's the question. Have you lost your soul or have you lost touch with your soul?

Our conversation continued in the next session:

CL: Well, I thought about your question. Actually, I thought about it quite a bit. My first reaction was that I've lost my soul completely, but I am wondering now whether there might be a little of me left inside. I used to think of my soul as a lantern, lighting my way in life, but for a long time I felt that the light had died out. Now I wonder whether there might be a little flicker of light left.

KIP: Are there times when you feel a bit of warmth from the light?

CL: Yes, I notice that there are times when I feel something stir inside of me.

KIP: When does that happen?

CL: Oh, when I listen to a piece of music, go to an art museum, or lose myself in poetry. I've never been beautiful on the outside, but something inside of me has always been receptive to beauty.

KIP: And that part of you is your soul?

CL: I think so. You see, God to me is all about creation and beauty. Those are the things that are truly immortal. I used to be able to create beautiful things. I don't do that anymore, but I can still appreciate beautiful things and that's the closest I can come to God.

Eliciting Agnes's spiritual story was not difficult. It flowed directly out of her larger life story. My questions were not intended to bracket spiritual matters from the dialogue of therapy but were tailored to incorporate spiritual conversation into the context of Agnes's problems, life history, social relationships, and vision of herself. Agnes's responses to my questions helped me to learn that she was suffering not only emotionally, in the form of a major depressive disorder, but spiritually as well. She had given up a spiritual pursuit, her love for the cello, to devote her life to the worship of her husband. As charming as he was, Peter was a poor substitute for the sacred. He was painfully human, unable to care for Agnes financially, emotionally, or spiritually. Family members were equally unsupportive of her expression of spirituality. Agnes was narrow and constricted in her spirituality. For years, she had sacrificed her own dreams to advance those of her husband. In the process, she had become a gaunt shadow figure, unknown to others, unknown to herself, unable to nourish herself spiritually. As Agnes became more aware of her poor choice of whom to worship and what it had cost her, she began to teeter on the edge of spiritual extremism. She came uncomfortably close to killing Peter, the idol who had accepted her sacrifices and failed to care for her in return. She also came uncomfortably close to killing herself to put an end to the emptiness she felt inside.

It is clear that spirituality was an important part of Agnes's problem, but there were signs that it might be part of the solution too. Agnes was spiritually flexible, open to exploring other sources of sacredness in her life. Perhaps she had not lost her soul but simply lost touch with it. She was able to identify a source of light and warmth within herself, her lantern. And she was beginning to broaden and deepen her approach to the sacred. Through her appreciation of creativity and beauty, she might turn up the light in the lantern from a flicker to flame. In my extensive spiritual assessment, I concluded that Agnes was emerging from a long period of deep spiritual struggle and entering a period of spiritual transformation. I saw her moving from a "false" god to a more authentic sense of her own spirituality and from self-derogation to more fulfilling ways to nurture her soul. She had little external support for the spiritual steps she was beginning to take, but I could offer some of that in therapy. Facilitating Agnes's transformation toward a more fully integrated and effective spirituality would become a central part of our work together in therapy.

Using Clinical Exercises

Clients who have difficulty conceptualizing or describing their spiritual journeys may benefit from exercises that provide a bit more structure. A host of activities can be done to help clients examine their spiritual pasts, presents, or futures. For example, clients who enjoy writing can be encouraged to author their own spiritual autobiographies. This provides clients the opportunity to reflect on the spiritual experiences, questions, ideas, beliefs, practices, relationships, and events that have been important in their spiritual journeys.

If writing a spiritual autobiography seems too daunting, clients can be encouraged to start with letter writing. Blanton (2006) described unique ways in which therapists can use the narrative elements of letter writing to enter the spiritual experiences of clients. Clients may benefit from writing spiritual letters of their own. Such letters can include any or all of the following components: descriptions of spiritual struggles, descriptions of spiritual goals and progress toward those goals, descriptions of recent encounters with the spiritual realm or the sacred, and questions that the client has about spiritual topics.

Clients who prefer to represent their spirituality in visual form can create a spiritual life map, a pictorial representation of the spiritual milestones that they have encountered in their lives. Hodge (2005), for example, wrote an article on the use of spiritual life maps in therapy. He provided a case study of a 42-year-old African American male whose spiritual life map illustrates how specific life experiences were tied to spiritual changes, such as crying out to God in desperation, being spiritually dead, and experiencing a spiritual awakening.

Exercises such as these can offer clients a more integrated perspective on their own spiritual experiences. Additionally, these exercises can shed light on the particular social forces that have affected clients spiritually. Family, friends, churches, communities, and culture play a large role in defining spiritual characteristics. For example, Miller and Kelley (2005) pointed out that in some communities, a person would be considered insane *not* to believe that the spirits of the dead actively influence people's lives. Similarly, another exercise that is particularly helpful for gaining information about clients' social contexts is the spiritual genogram (see chap. 3, this volume). An adaptation of the family genogram, the spiritual genogram depicts clients' spiritual heritages visually. It can include the spiritual dynamics of family (e.g., conflicts, closeness), inspirational models, antispiritual models, and key positive and negative spiritual events (Sperry, 2001). These exercises can be used in session or assigned as homework to help clients form more integrated understandings of their spirituality. These activities also provide useful tools for aiding clients in communicating their spiritual narratives to therapists.

Gathering Information Indirectly

It is important to attend not only to what clients say in their spiritual stories but also to how they convey the stories. Therefore, therapists attend to the type of information that clients do not verbalize and assess the level of fit between clients' words, feelings, and actions.

Important insights can be gained by reflecting on the topics and statements that are absent from clients' verbal communication. For example, clients may describe one spiritual pathway to the neglect of others, such as meditation without knowledge, belief without involvement in a community, or ritual without an emotional connection. Some clients may describe a spiritual life without talking about the meaning or satisfaction that they derive from it. Other clients may describe overarching spiritual beliefs without ever connecting them to their daily experiences. In such instances, the therapist can learn a lot about the client's spiritual beliefs and experiences by following up on the things that are not being said.

Furthermore, the level of congruence between clients' statements, emotions, and behaviors may reveal that there is more than meets the eye when it comes to their spirituality. A lack of fit in these areas may offer an indication of clients' spiritual authenticity. People may be spiritually involved for a host of reasons that are disconnected from the sacred. For example, a husband who is generally unconcerned with religious involvement or righteous living could coerce his wife to stay in the marriage on the grounds that the church does not sanction divorce. In this case, the discrepancy between the husband's avowed commitment to religious principles and his unloving attitude and behavior may reveal a spirituality that is less than authentic.

Gathering Information Quantitatively

Quantitative measures provide a secondary source of information that can be used as a check for potential biases and preconceptions of therapists in regard to clients' spirituality. Quantitative data can also be used to compare clients' spiritual functioning with that of a normative sample or to monitor changes in clients' spirituality over time.

The key for quantitative spiritual assessment is to select a measure that is appropriate for the individual client and provides an in-depth perspective of his or her spirituality. There is no shortage of measures of spirituality and religiousness (see Hill & Hood, 1999). However, many of the existing measures are inappropriate for clinical use because they are functionally disconnected from the life of the individual. Most measures of spirituality offer only superficial, descriptive information about an individual's basic spiritual beliefs and practices. Regrettably, this is not of much use for the therapeutic process, for which it is important to understand how spirituality expresses itself in the events and experiences of everyday life. In addition, most measures of spirituality have been developed and normed for Christians or similar theists. Therefore, the language and concepts of these measures are irrelevant, if not offensive, to those of other religious traditions.

Although scales of spirituality have traditionally been simple and limited in diversity, this is slowly changing. Fortunately, researchers and practitioners are beginning to develop measures that tap into the deeper and more elusive aspects of spirituality (see Table 5.1), such as an individual's spiritual pathways (e.g., Hall & Edwards, 1996; Hays, Meador, Branch, & George, 2001; Idler et al., 2003), spiritual strivings (e.g., Emmons, Cheung, & Tehrani, 1998; Mahoney et al., 2005), spiritual struggles (e.g., Exline, Yali, & Sanderson, 2000; Pargament et al., 2000, 2005; Yanni, 2003), spiritual changes (e.g., Cole, 2005), spiritual efficacy (e.g., Abramowitz, Huppert, Cohen, Tolin, & Cahill, 2002; Peterman, Fitchett, Brady, Hernandez, & Cella, 2002), spiritual flexibility (e.g., Batson & Schoenrade, 1991), and the role of spirituality in coping with problems (e.g., Pargament et al., 2000; Yanni, 2003). Measures are also being developed that have utility for non-Christians (e.g., Tarakeshwar, Pargament, & Mahoney, 2003). Using such sophisticated quantitative measures of spirituality will provide additional richness and accuracy to the extensive spiritual assessment.

Consulting External Sources of Information

Gathering information from those who are in relationship with clients, such as family members and significant others, may contribute to therapists' understanding of clients' spiritual contexts. This kind of information can be particularly helpful in situations when therapists are unsure whether their

TABLE 5.1
Instruments for Assessing Spirituality in Psychotherapy

Dimension	Scale and author	Scale description	Sample item
Spiritual pathways	NIA/Fetzer Short Form for the Measurement of Religiousness and Spirituality (Idler et al., 2003)	33 items assessing 10 spiritual pathways: public and private activity, congregation support, coping, intensity, forgiveness, daily spiritual experience, spiritual beliefs and values, commitment, and religious history.	"Because of my religious or spiritual beliefs, I have forgiven those who hurt me" (forgiveness).
	Spiritual History Scale (Hays et al., 2001)	23 items assessing degree to which religion has been source of support and conflict over the life span.	"For most of my life, my social life has revolved around the church/synagogue."
	Spiritual Assessment Inventory (Hall & Edwards, 1996)	36 items measuring 4 dimensions of individual's quality of relationship with God: instability, grandiosity, defensiveness/disappointment, realistic acceptance.	"God recognizes that I am more spiritual than most people" (grandiosity).
	Hindu Spiritual Pathways Scale (Tarakeshwar et al., 2003)	27 items assessing degree of involvement in 4 Hindu pathways: devotion, ethical action, knowledge, and restrain.	"How often do you perform *puja* in honor of your deity?" (path of devotion).
Spiritual strivings	Spiritual Strivings (Emmons et al., 1998)	Coded spiritual responses to list of 15 personal strivings ("An objective you are typically trying to obtain").	Sample spiritual strivings: "To approach life with mystery and awe," "To deepen my relation with God," "To achieve union with the totality of existence."
	Spiritual Strivings (Mahoney et al., 2005)	Ratings of degree to which each of 10 personal strivings is perceived as a manifestation of God or holding sacred qualities.	"This striving reflects what I think God wants for me" (manifestation of God).

(continues)

TABLE 5.1

Instruments for Assessing Spirituality in Psychotherapy *(Continued)*

Dimension	Scale and author	Scale description	Sample item
Spiritual struggles	Negative RCOPE (Pargament et al., 2000)	35 items assessing divine, interpersonal, and intrapsychic spiritual struggles.	In coping with my negative event, I "wondered whether God had abandoned me."
	Negative Religious Triangulation Scale (Yanni, 2003)	7 items measuring efforts to triangulate spirituality into familial conflicts.	When I differ with my mother/father/child, I "suggest that my mother/father/child is rejecting God's will."
Spiritual changes	Spiritual Transformation Scale (Cole, Hopkins, Tisak, Steel, & Carr, 2008)	50 items assessing spiritual changes and disengagement following a major trauma.	Since my trauma, "I more often see my own life as sacred."
Spiritual efficacy	Religious Comfort Scale (Exline et al., 2000)	13 items assessing experience of comfort through religion.	To what extent are you currently experiencing "feeling comforted by your faith"?
	Penn Inventory of Scrupolosity (Abramowitz et al., 2002)	19 items measuring religious obsessive–compulsive symptoms.	"I worry I must act morally at all times or I will be punished."
	FACIT-Spiritual Well-Being Scale (Peterman et al., 2002)	12 items assessing spiritual well-being following illness.	"I find strength in my faith or spiritual beliefs."
Spiritual flexibility	Quest Scale (Batson & Schoenrade, 1991)	12 items of open, changeable approach to religion.	"As I grow and change, I expect my religion to grow and change."
Spiritual coping (conservational)	Positive RCOPE (Pargament et al., 2000)	40 items assessing positive methods of spiritual coping (e.g., spiritual support, benevolent spiritual reappraisals, collaborative spiritual coping).	In coping with my negative event, I "looked to God for strength, support, and guidance."

Note. NIA = National Institute on Aging; RCOPE = Religious/Spiritual Coping Scale; FACIT = Functional Assessment of Chronic Illness Therapy.

clients' beliefs and behavior fall within or outside the normative boundaries of nontraditional religious or spiritual groups. Of course, therapists should pursue such contact only with clients' consent (and necessary releases of information). When appropriate, therapists may involve additional individuals in treatment. Clergy or members of clients' religious communities can provide unique knowledge that may be essential to making assessment and treatment decisions. Similarly, bringing a spouse or a whole family into the sessions may be helpful when clients are experiencing interpersonal spiritual conflicts or a lack of spiritual support.

Therapists can draw on a host of other resources to aid the spiritual assessment. Various texts can be referenced to increase understanding of specific religious traditions. Some articles and book chapters have been geared specifically toward clinical work, such as those that address working with religiously diverse clients (e.g., Lovinger, 1984; Richards & Bergin, 2000) or those that compare the philosophical assumptions underlying various theistic and nontheistic viewpoints of clients and therapists (e.g., Richards & Bergin, 2004). Studying clients' religious traditions or even visiting congregations within clients' denominations can further lead to valuable clinical insights. For example, therapists may discover unique ways in which the religious teachings or social climate of a client's religious tradition has the potential to aid or threaten the client's progress in treatment.

Thus far, this chapter has provided an overview of two stages of a spiritual assessment process. The process begins by including questions about spirituality in the intake session. This initial spiritual assessment may indicate that spirituality is clinically significant. In that case, a more extensive assessment is conducted to yield rich, detailed information about spirituality and the way it functions in clients' lives. Conversely, the initial assessment may not offer any indication that spirituality is relevant to the case. For some clients, spirituality will not be an important component of treatment. However, therapists should also consider whether underlying spiritual issues did not surface during the initial assessment because clients are unaware of the role of spirituality in their lives, are reluctant to discuss spirituality early in treatment, or do not identify with the therapist's explicitly spiritual language. One way to determine whether there are undetected spiritual issues that deserve consideration in treatment is to conduct an implicit spiritual assessment.

IMPLICIT SPIRITUAL ASSESSMENT

Sometimes spirituality emerges as an essential topic in treatment not as the result of direct questioning about spirituality and religion but through a more implicit process. Therapists should be aware of less direct ways in which they can uncover the deeper, spiritual dimensions of clients' lives. This form of spiritual assessment may be most appropriate for clients who are hesitant to discuss the topic of spirituality with a therapist or do not resonate with explicitly religious language. Assessing spirituality implicitly involves listening for implied spiritual content in clients' descriptions, asking clients questions that hint at the possibility of spiritual experiences, and attending to clients' emotions.

Listening for Implicitly Spiritual Language

The first component of an implicit spiritual assessment involves listening for implicitly spiritual language from clients. Just as clients may not connect to the explicitly religious language of therapists, therapists may not cue into the implicitly spiritual language of clients. Therefore, therapists must take care to listen for unique terms and phrases of clients that might open the door to further spiritual exploration. Three specific cues suggest that clients may be describing deeper spiritual issues: speaking in extremes, using major polarities, and making statements that parallel the spiritual.

First, clients who speak in extremes may be offering insight into their conceptions of the sacred. For example, clients may exalt the positive qualities of a person, activity, or thing. When clients speak of someone or something as all good, perfect, or never at fault, then they may be ascribing sacred qualities to this aspect of life. Similarly, clients may fixate on the negative qualities of someone or something in their lives. When clients can acknowledge only the negative, this may be a sign of "demonization" or the perception that they have been spiritually violated or desecrated. Understanding what clients have sanctified or demonized in their lives may provide specific directions for treatment. At times it may be necessary to help clients develop a more differentiated spiritual view of the person, object, experience, or activity at hand. For example, some clients will have the tendency to project sacred qualities onto the therapist (Pattison, 1982). If clients speak of their therapists in terms of being completely good and helpful, a lifeline, a miracle worker, or a savior, then it is essential to help them see the humanness of the therapist. This will prevent an inevitable "falling from grace" when the therapist proves unable to live up to the sacred qualities.

Second, clients may use extreme contrasts in their descriptions. Such major polarities may point to deep spiritual struggles (Nash, 1990). Examples are the contrast between brokenness and wholeness, curse and blessing, foolishness and wisdom, bondage and freedom, revenge and mercy, arrogance and humility, faithlessness and faithfulness. Therapists should be especially attuned to clients ascribing stark contrasts to themselves and their present or past experiences. Further exploration of such statements may open the door for conversations about clients' spiritual understandings that have been challenged or shaken (Park, 2005).

Third, therapists should be aware of statements that hint at spiritual processes in clients' lives. Clients may describe beliefs, practices, or experiences that initially do not seem overtly spiritual but that have an underlying spiritual nature. For instance, Schreurs (2002) noted,

> One may hear in other people's anger their disappointment about the general injustice of life, indicating that even though they do not believe in God, they deep down still relate to life itself as if it were a supreme judge who should administer justice but neglects to do so. (p. 121)

Listening for language that appears to parallel spiritual thoughts, feelings, or behaviors can lead to meaningful conversations about spirituality.

Using Psychospiritual Questions

An implicit spiritual assessment involves the use of questions that open the door for discussion about a broad range of spiritual experiences. These psychospiritual questions probe the possibilities of emotionally rich experiences of transcendent reality, connection to larger forces, or deeper meaning in life. These spiritual experiences may manifest themselves in a variety of different concepts, such as peace, courage, solace, sustenance, devotion, faith, hope, love, letting go, forgiveness, regret, despair, or suffering. Exhibit 5.4

EXHIBIT 5.4
Implicitly Spiritual Questions

1. Conceptualizations of the sacred
   (a) Who/what do you put your hope in?
   (b) Who/what do you rely on most in life?
   (c) To whom/what are you most devoted?[a]
   (d) To whom/what do you most freely express love?[a]
   (e) When have you felt most deeply and fully alive?
2. Spiritual goals
   (a) What are you striving for in your life?
   (b) Why is it important that you are here in this world?[a]
   (c) What legacy would you like to leave behind in your life?
3. Spirituality as a resource
   (a) What sustains you in the midst of your troubles?
   (b) From what sources do you draw the strength/courage to go on?[a]
   (c) When you are afraid/in pain, how do you find comfort/solace?[a]
   (d) Who truly understands your situation?[a]
   (e) For what are you deeply grateful?[a]
4. Spiritual struggles
   (a) What are the deepest questions your situation has raised for you?
   (b) What causes you the greatest despair/suffering?
   (c) How has this experience changed you at your deepest levels?
   (d) What have you discovered about yourself that you find most disturbing?
   (e) What has this experience taught you that you wish you had never known?
   (f) What are your deepest regrets?
   (g) What would you like to be able to let go of in your life?

[a]Adapted from Griffith and Griffith (2002).

provides examples of questions that can be used to indirectly assess the nature of clients' spirituality and its place in their lives.

Attending to Emotions

As every therapist knows, it is important to attend not only to what clients say and think but also to what they feel. This is particularly true for spiritual assessments because many people experience their spirituality primarily through feelings. Paying attention to the presence or absence of emotions may highlight something about clients' spiritual engagement. For example, clients might express that they do not believe in God, yet harbor anger and resentment at what a Higher Power has allowed to happen in their lives. In such cases, observing strong emotions may indicate that clients are in fact spiritually engaged in ways that they do not realize. The opposite could also occur. For example, clients could describe a high level of spiritual involvement, yet never display feelings about spiritual topics. A lack of emotion could suggest that even the most religious individuals are disengaged spiritually.

Spiritual experiences are particularly capable of eliciting strong emotions. These include both pleasant and unpleasant emotions, such as awe, peace, joy, inspiration, love, gratitude, excitement, sadness, anger, emptiness, shame, guilt, fear, and so on. The presence of particular positive emotions may indicate that a spiritually relevant topic has been broached.

Feelings such as gratitude, humility, love, and obligation are prevalent when people perceive God or sacredness in their lives (Pargament & Mahoney, 2005). Understanding what elicits excitement and joy in the lives of clients may provide important clues about their sources of sacredness. Therefore, watching for hints of emotion, such as a smile or a sparkle in the eye of a client who is depressed, may indicate that a sacred topic has been touched on. Similarly, observing that clients are exceptionally peaceful may indicate that they have accessed a powerful spiritual resource. Therapists should key into such cues and further explore the reason for changes in tone: Has the client identified a source of deeper meaning? Has the client experienced a connection with transcendent reality?

Past research has indicated that positive spiritual emotions far outnumber negative ones but that negative spiritual emotions have a stronger impact on people's lives and are predictive of declines in physical and mental health (e.g., Pargament, Koenig, Tarakeshwar, & Hahn, 2001). Therefore, it is important to include a screening for spiritual distress in the spiritual assessment. For example, extreme sadness or anger may indicate that clients are experiencing the loss or violation of something sacred in their lives. In such cases, it is important to assess whether clients are experiencing spiritual struggles, and if so, how they are handling the struggle and how it is affecting their lives.

In sum, when it comes to an implicit spiritual assessment, therapists should pursue topics that are accompanied by emotions that are especially strong or rare for their clients, including pleasure, solemnity, awe, profound sorrow, terrible fear, and gripping excitement. Such cues can lead to deeper conversations about clients' experiences of the sacred.

The process of implicit spiritual assessment, consisting of listening for clients' underlying spiritual language, asking clients implicitly spiritual questions, and attending to emotions, may reveal that spirituality is relevant to clients' lives and problems. A case example from Pargament (2007) described how implicit spiritual assessment can elicit a therapeutic breakthrough. In such instances, following up with an extensive spiritual assessment provides the opportunity to gather more detailed information about the nature of clients' spirituality and the degree to which it is well integrated or poorly integrated in clients' lives. However, an implicit spiritual assessment may not reveal that spirituality is relevant to a client's life or problems. In the end, the purpose of such an assessment is merely to offer clients a nonthreatening invitation to explore the spiritual domain in therapy.

Case Study: Conducting an Implicit Spiritual Assessment

A 39-year-old accountant, Joe was of average build, average appearance, and average disposition. In fact, everything about Joe seemed average. He had come to therapy a few months earlier complaining about depression. Although he had a stable job and marriage, he felt as if he were just going through the motions. There were no highs or lows in Joe's life. His days were marked by a sameness and a grayness that left him feeling as if he were living in a perpetual fog. Over the past 15 years, he had tried antidepressants, different forms of therapy, meditation, reading, and exercise, but nothing had altered the dreariness of his life.

I (Kenneth I. Pargament) went through a litany of therapeutic activities in an effort to help Joe generate a spark in his life, to no avail. Our sessions were mirroring his life. Trying to inject some enthusiasm in my voice, I would ask, "How did your week go, Joe?" "SOS, same old stuff," he would invariably reply in a monotonically average voice.

One day, feeling sleepy, ineffective, and rather desperate, I asked Joe, "Have you ever had a time in your life when you felt deeply and fully alive?" Joe paused to consider, and I awaited what I assumed would be another lifeless response. Instead, Joe said, "Well, there was the time in college when I flew jets." I almost jumped out of my skin. "You flew jets, Joe?" I shouted. "Well, tell me about it." Joe's parents had given him flying lessons for his 21st birthday. He loved the experience and spent his free time in his college years flying and qualifying for more and more technically sophisticated planes. "Joe," I said, "I never knew you were a pilot. What was it like to fly a jet?" "It was unbelievable," he said. "That sensation of power taking off. Never knowing quite what to expect. Feeling like I was testing myself. And the experience of flying—racing through the clouds, a speck in the vastness of the skies. Man, I was in Heaven, soaring with the angels. I told you I'm not a religious man, but if there's a God, well, that's the closest I've come to Him." This was not the Joe I knew. Eyes bright, voice animated, perched precariously on the edge of his seat, Joe had made a complete transformation.

"Have you ever had a time in your life when you felt deeply and fully alive?" My question had helped uncover a sacred spark in Joe that had been hidden for many years. Now the question was whether Joe could fan that spark into a flame. "Why did you stop flying?" I asked. "Oh, I moved away, got a job, things came up, you know," he responded. "But, Joe," I exclaimed, "When you talked about flying just now, you came to life. You took off in here." With a very unaverage, embarrassed grin, Joe admitted, "Yeah, it did feel good."

Flying became the focus of our subsequent sessions, not only flying airplanes but also flying in other areas of his life. Using this potent metaphor, we talked about ways Joe could take the skills and qualities of a pilot—mastery, planning, self-confidence, courage, an adventurous spirit—and apply them to his job, his relationships, and his life more generally. And Joe did take off. He began to fly airplanes once again, and he began to approach his life with a new enthusiasm.

Nothing in my initial assessment of Joe had suggested that spirituality would be a relevant part of this case. Like many others, Joe had never made the connection between his situations in life and his spirituality. Spirituality emerged as an important concern, not by hitting Joe over the head with questions about God, the church, or prayer, but by a more implicit, indirect effort to reveal a deeper, spiritual dimension to his life.

CONCLUSION

Spiritual assessment is designed to provide insight into the role of spirituality in clients' lives and how it might be a part of clients' problems or solutions. Effective assessment is a prerequisite to responsible treatment decisions. In this chapter, we have conceptualized spiritual assessment as a process that grows out of the relationship between client and therapist. Rich spiritual dialogue can develop only in an atmosphere of trust, respect, and openness. Effective assessment is also based on a clear conceptual framework for thinking about spirituality—what it is, how it works, how to distinguish spirituality at its best from spirituality at its worst.

Spiritual assessment is a multimethod, multilevel process. This chapter described three stages of assessment, beginning with a few questions about spirituality in the intake session. When appropriate, extensive spiritual assessment provides an opportunity for therapists to gather a more comprehensive picture of clients' spirituality. This involves using open-ended questions and clinical exercises to elicit clients' spiritual stories. As clients' spiritual narratives unfold, therapists also listen for what clients do not verbalize and consider the level of congruence in clients' spiritual experiences. In addition, therapists can draw on quantitative measures and external sources of information.

Some clients may not resonate to the explicitly spiritual language used in the initial and extensive spiritual assessments; others may be unaware of the role spirituality plays in their lives or hesitant to broach the topic. In the process of implicit spiritual assessment, therapists attend to indirect references to spirituality in the language of clients, make use of implicitly spiritual questions, and attend to clients' emotional tones to uncover a broader range of spiritual experiences. This provides clients with an invitation to enter into a spiritual conversation with their therapists, an invitation which may or may not lead to more extensive discussion of spiritual matters.

It would be inappropriate to end this chapter without emphasizing that assessment is not a simple process. People and problems are far too diverse and complicated for that to be the case. A spiritual assessment is more than the sum of its parts. Therapists must integrate information from each component of the assessment and draw on indirect means of learning about clients' spirituality. For this reason, clinical judgment is absolutely essential to the process of spiritual assessment. Therapists gather a plethora of information about many different variables from a variety of sources. The task is to weigh these variables in interaction with each other in hopes of garnering a broader contextual perspective. Real questions about real people are anything but simple. Therefore, sound clinical judgment is especially important in our efforts to understand and evaluate a process as rich, complex, and dynamic as spirituality.

REFERENCES

Abramowitz, J. S., Huppert, J. D., Cohen, A. B., Tolin, D. F., & Cahill, S. P. (2002). Religious obsessions and compulsions in a non-clinical sample: The Penn Inventory of Scupulosity (PIOS). *Behaviour Research and Therapy, 40,* 825–838.

Batson, C. D., & Schoenrade, P. (1991). Measuring religion as quest: 1. Validity concerns. *Journal for the Scientific Study of Religion, 30,* 416–429.

Blanton, P. G. (2006). Introducing letter writing into Christian psychotherapy. *Journal of Psychology and Christianity, 25,* 77–86.

Cole, B. S. (2005). Spiritually-focused psychotherapy for people diagnosed with cancer: A pilot outcome study. *Mental Health, Religion, & Culture, 8,* 217–226.

Cole, B. S., Hopkins, C., Tisak, J., Steel, J. S., & Carr, B. L. (2007). Assessing spiritual growth and spiritual decline following a diagnosis of cancer: Reliability and validity of the spiritual transformation scale. *Psycho-Oncology, 17,* 112–121.

Emmons, R. A., Cheung, C., & Tehrani, K. (1998). Assessing spirituality through personal goals: Implications for research on religion and subjective well-being. *Social Indicators Research, 45,* 391–422.

Exline, J. J., Yali, A. M., & Sanderson, W. C. (2000). Guilt, discord, and alienation: The role of religious strain in depression and suicidality. *Journal of Clinical Psychology, 56,* 1481–1496.

Fitchett, G., Rybarczyk, B. D., DeMarco, G. A., & Nicholas, J. J. (1999). The role of religion in medical rehabilitation outcomes: A longitudinal study. *Rehabilitation Psychology, 44,* 1–22.

Griffith, J. L., & Griffith, M. E. (2002). *Encountering the sacred in psychotherapy: How to talk with people about their spiritual lives.* New York: Guilford Press.

Hall, T. W., & Edwards, K. J. (1996). The initial development and factor analysis of the Spiritual Assessment Inventory. *Journal of Psychology and Theology, 24,* 233–246.

Hays, J. C., Meador, K. G., Branch, P. S., & George, L. K. (2001). The Spiritual History Scale in Four Dimensions (SHS-4): Validity and reliability. *The Gerontologist, 41,* 239–249.

Hill, P. C., & Hood, R. W., Jr. (Eds.). (1999). *Measures of religiosity.* Birmingham, AL: Religious Education Press.

Hodge, D. R. (2001). Spiritual assessment: A review of major qualitative methods and a new framework for assessing spirituality. *Social Work, 46,* 203–214.

Hodge, D. R. (2005). Spiritual lifemaps: A client-centered pictorial instrument for spiritual assessment, planning, and intervention. *Social Work, 50,* 77–87.

Idler, E. L., Musick, M. A., Ellison, C. G., George, L. K., Krause, N., Ory, M. G., et al. (2003). Measuring multiple dimensions of religion and spirituality for health research: Conceptual background and findings from the 1998 General Social Survey. *Research on Aging, 25,* 327–365.

Lovinger, R. J. (1984). *Working with religious issues in therapy.* Northvale, NJ: Jason Aronson.

Mahoney, A., Carels, R., Pargament, K. I., Wachholtz, A., Leeper, L. E., Kaplar, M., & Frutchey, R. (2005). The sanctification of the body and behavioral health patterns of college students. *International Journal for the Psychology of Religion, 15,* 221–238.

Mahoney, A., Krumrei, E. J., & Pargament, K. I. (2008). Broken vows: Divorce as a spiritual trauma and its implications for growth and decline. In S. Joseph & P. A. Linley (Eds.), *Trauma, recovery, and growth: Positive psychological perspectives on posttraumatic stress* (pp. 105–124). Hoboken, NJ: Wiley.

Miller, L., & Kelley, B. S. (2005). Relationships of religiosity and spirituality with mental health and psychopathology. In R. F. Paloutzian & C. L. Park (Eds.), *Handbook of the psychology of religion and spirituality* (pp. 460–478). New York: Guilford Press.

Nash, R. (1990). Life's major spiritual issues: An emerging framework for spiritual assessment and diagnosis. *The Caregiver Journal, 7,* 3–42.

Pargament, K. I. (1997). *The psychology of religion and coping: Theory, research, practice.* New York: Guilford Press.

Pargament, K. I. (2007). *Spiritually integrated psychotherapy: Understanding and addressing the sacred.* New York: Guilford Press.

Pargament, K. I., Koenig H. G., & Perez, L. (2000). The many methods of religious coping: Development and initial validation of the RCOPE. *Journal of Clinical Psychology, 56,* 519–543.

Pargament, K. I., Koenig, H. G., Tarakeshwar, N., & Hahn, J. (2001). Religious struggle as a predictor of mortality among medically ill elderly patients: A two-year longitudinal study. *Archives of Internal Medicine, 161,* 1881–1885.

Pargament, K. I., & Mahoney, A. M. (2005). Sacred matters: Sanctification as a phenomena of interest for the psychology of religion. *International Journal for the Psychology of Religion, 15,* 179–199.

Pargament, K. I., Murray-Swank, N., Magyar, G. M., & Ano, G. (2005). Spiritual struggle: A phenomenon of interest to psychology and religion. In W. R. Miller & H. Delaney (Eds.), *Judeo-Christian perspectives on psychology: Human nature, motivation, and change* (pp. 245–268). Washington, DC: American Psychological Association.

Pargament, K. I., Smith, B. W., Koenig, H. G., & Perez, L. (1998). Patterns of positive and negative religious coping with major life stressors. *Journal for the Scientific Study of Religion, 37,* 710–724.

Park, C. L. (2005). Religion and meaning. In R. F. Paloutzian & C. L. Park (Eds.), *Handbook of the psychology of religion and spirituality* (pp. 295–314). New York: Guilford Press.

Pattison, E. M. (1982). Management of religious issues in family therapy. *International Journal of Family Therapy, 4,* 140–163.

Peterman, A. H., Fitchett, G., Brady, M., Hernandez, L., & Cella, D. (2002). Measuring spiritual well-being in people with cancer: The Functional Assessment of Chronic Illness Therapy—Spiritual Well-Being Scale (FACIT–Sp). *Annals of Behavioral Medicine, 24,* 49–58.

Richards, P. S., & Bergin, A. E. (Eds.). (2000). *Handbook of psychotherapy and religious diversity.* Washington, DC: American Psychological Association.

Richards, P. S., & Bergin, A. E. (2004). A theistic spiritual strategy for psychotherapy. In P. S. Richards & A. E. Bergin (Eds.), *Casebook for a spiritual strategy in counseling and psychotherapy* (pp. 3–32). Washington, DC: American Psychological Association.

Schreurs, A. (2002). *Psychotherapy and spirituality: Integrating the spiritual dimension into therapeutic practice.* London: Jessica Kingsley.

Sperry, L. (2001). *Spirituality in clinical practice: Incorporating the spiritual dimension in psychotherapy and counseling.* Philadelphia: Brunner-Routledge.

Tarakeshwar, N., Pargament, K. I., & Mahoney, A (2003). Measures of Hindu pathways: Development and preliminary evidence of reliability and validity. *Cultural Diversity and Ethnic Minority Psychology, 34,* 377–394.

Yanni, G. M. (2003). *Religious and secular dyadic variables and their relation to parent–child relationships and college students' psychological adjustment.* Unpublished doctoral dissertation, Bowling Green State University.

6

INCLUDING SPIRITUALITY IN CASE CONCEPTUALIZATIONS: A MEANING-SYSTEMS APPROACH

CRYSTAL L. PARK AND JEANNE M. SLATTERY

> If you reject the food, ignore the customs, fear the religion and avoid the people, you might better stay home.
>
> —James Michener

The authors of this volume, along with many others (e.g., Hawkins & Bullock, 1995; Slattery, 2004), have argued that spirituality and religion—as well as other features of culture and context—are important aspects to which to attend in working with clients. Failing this, as Michener noted, we may as well "stay home." This chapter outlines a strategy for attending to clients' spirituality and religion and weaving this information into a coherent and effective case conceptualization. Because we see spirituality and religion as integral components of meaning systems, the strategy that we outline focuses directly on their roles in our clients' lives and also attends to how they influence other aspects of life (e.g., coping strategies or family life).

OUR APPROACH TO CONCEPTUALIZING CASES

Case conceptualizations are the end result of a systematic attempt to understand clients and their worldviews. Creating strong case conceptualizations helps therapists to understand clients and facilitate their change. Case conceptualizations view clients' behavior and symptoms from a perspective that is, ideally, broader and more contextualized than either clients or therapists could do on their own. Therapists gather numerous details of clients' lives, but more important, use these details to systematically develop productive hypotheses. This new view gives both therapists and clients greater freedom and more options in the counseling process.

A case conceptualization serves several important functions (Nelson & Hastie, 2005). First, this theory- and research-driven organization of clients' background, symptoms, problems, and strengths organizes disparate data in a systematic and coherent manner. Second, it helps therapists to develop useful hypotheses about the dynamics underlying clients' behavior. Finally, these hypotheses are used to formulate interventions, which in turn are used to test therapists' hypotheses. When these hypotheses are not supported, therapists should refine their case conceptualization and develop new hypotheses and interventions (see Figure 6.1).

Chapters 5 (assessment), 6 (case conceptualization), and 7 (treatment planning) of this volume are integrally related. Chapter 5 presents systematic

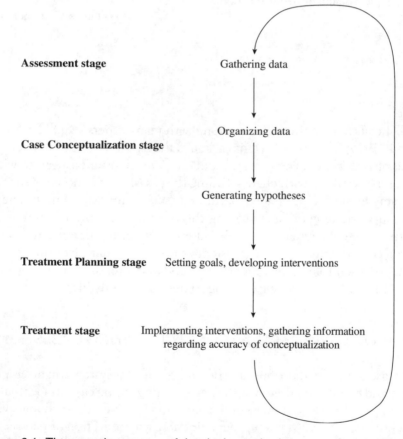

Figure 6.1. The recursive process of developing and using case conceptualizations.

approaches for gathering information about the roles that spirituality and religion play in a client's life. The present chapter focuses on the first two functions of a case conceptualization (i.e., organizing data and generating hypotheses). The third function of case conceptualizations (i.e., forming interventions) is discussed in chapter 7.

In this chapter, we describe a meaning-making approach to conceptualizing cases. According to this approach, there is nothing inherent in situations themselves that makes them stressful; rather, the meanings drawn from and the coping strategies chosen in response to situations create their effect (e.g., Lazarus & Folkman, 1984; Park, 2005). Spirituality and religion, among other cultural and contextual factors (e.g., race, ethnicity, family of origin, social class, and individual trauma history), are frequently a significant or even central source of individuals' meaning systems. The meaning-making framework is related to a broader cognitive perspective, focusing on a continuum of meanings we create, including positive and negative interpretations. In addition, this view focuses particularly on the discrepancies that exist among people's goals, their expectations about what should happen, and their beliefs about situations, as well as the distress generated by those discrepancies.

This theoretical perspective, only one of many possible, is further developed in the next sections. In the last section of this chapter, we present strategies for applying our approach to case conceptualization to other theoretical viewpoints.

THE NOTION OF MEANING SYSTEMS

To understand people, one must understand their unique ways of construing their worlds (Evans, 1993). The meaning-systems perspective proposes that every individual has a global meaning or orienting system and that this system has been significantly influenced by spirituality and religion along with other contextual factors. Meaning systems provide the general framework through which individuals structure their lives and assign meanings to specific situational encounters with their environment. This approach assumes that people's behavior, problems, and attempted solutions are understandable once their individually constructed meanings (global and situational) and given context are understood.

Global meaning consists of three aspects—beliefs, goals, and feelings (Park & Folkman, 1997)—and is central in determining behavior patterns in both everyday life and situations of adversity (Park, 2005; Silberman, 2005a; see Table 6.1). Global beliefs are widely encompassing assumptions about the world, such as beliefs in the benevolence and fairness of the world, as well as personal beliefs in control, luck, fairness, and vulnerability (Janoff-Bulman, 1992; Koltko-Rivera, 2004). Through these beliefs, people interpret their

TABLE 6.1
Relationships Between Aspects of Global and Situational Meaning and Their Presentations in Daily Life (Experiences of Congruent and Dissonant Events)

Measure	Global meaning — Ultimate/highest level of meaning	Situational meaning of a particular event — Event congruent with global meaning: receiving an award	Situational meaning of a particular event — Event dissonant with global meaning: being sexually assaulted
Beliefs	High-level beliefs, pattern, or style of approaching daily events (e.g., fairness, justice, self-esteem, controllability).	"Life is fair; I worked hard and deserve this recognition. I am good." Global beliefs are reinforced; person feels happy, positive emotions.	"I am a good person so this cannot be happening to me." Creating inconsistencies between perceived fairness or goodness and the meaning of the event. Generates a great deal of distress.
Goals	Highest aspirations, long-term projects, and ubergoals (e.g., developing a meaningful relationship with God; desiring to improve humankind's fate by studying science and curing a disease).	Reinforces aspirations and reduces discrepancies between current state of affairs and goals.	A basic goal, safety, was violated, generating intense distress and introducing questioning of deeply held spiritual goals.
Subjective sense	Sense of meaning and purpose in life, leading to satisfaction and well-being (e.g., "I have a worthwhile purpose and can understand the universe").	Increased life satisfaction and well-being, sense of being "on track" with life.	Drop in sense that life is meaningful, decreases in life satisfaction, well-being, and connectedness to God.

experiences of the world. Global goals are those high-level ideals, states, or objects toward which people work (Karoly, 1999), commonly reported as relationships and intimacy, religion, and achievement (Emmons, 2005). Ideally, people set and meet a series of short-term, concrete goals that lead to the achievement of their higher level goals; however, their behavior is often discrepant with their expressed goals (Baumeister, 1991; Emmons, 2005; Park, 2005). The emotional or feeling aspect of global meaning refers to experiencing a sense of "meaningfulness," a sense of meaning or purpose in life, as having plans and intentions (Klinger, 1977; Reker & Wong, 1988). This sense of meaningfulness comes from seeing one's actions as oriented toward or making progress toward a desired future state or goal (Baumeister, 1991; McGregor & Little, 1998). It is often, but not always, experienced as a spiritual state.

Global meaning exerts powerful influences on people's thoughts, actions, and feelings and gets translated into their daily lives through their interpretations of daily occurrences as well as major life events, their personal projects (smaller, more concrete goals that people pursue on a daily basis), and their general sense of well-being and life satisfaction (e.g., Emmons, 1999). According to a meaning-systems perspective, people constantly assign meaning to their daily lives, their own behaviors, and the situations that they encounter. Thus, situational meaning refers to the particular understanding or significance that an individual assigns to particular objects, relationships, or events. In the course of therapy, especially, these are often particularly challenging (e.g., bereavement, relationship endings or discord, violence or trauma).

Consistency among various aspects of individuals' situational and global meaning creates a sense of contentment and harmony. Discord among aspects of meaning can create great stress and distress; individuals typically work to reduce such discrepancies and create consistency in dysfunctional ways. Discrepancies occur when situations are interpreted as violating one's global beliefs (e.g., that the world is fair or that one has control) or one's goals (e.g., failing to be accepted for graduate school or losing a loved one). They can also arise when global beliefs or goals are in conflict with one another (e.g., one desires to fully express one's sexuality but is also afraid of displeasing God; Exline, 2002). Discrepancies can also be created when real events are appraised as differing from personal ideals (Alexander & Higgins, 1993; Avants, Margolin, & Singer, 1994; Higgins, 1987) or developmental, cultural, or community norms (Lansford et al., 2005).

When situational meaning does not fit with global meaning, people typically attempt to change or distort their views of their world and life events to incorporate them into their global meaning (assimilation). When the discrepancy is too great, people may change their global meaning to accommodate new life events. This issue of consistency or discord among meanings is central to the meaning-systems approach to case conceptualization.

A MEANING-MAKING APPROACH
TO CASE CONCEPTUALIZATION

The case conceptualization process uses sound theoretical frameworks and research findings to organize disparate client data (e.g., interviews, observations, objective and projective measures) to generate hypotheses explaining the underlying dynamics of the presenting problem (Nelson & Hastie, 2005). An understanding of the forces that has led to and that maintains the complaint leads to useful and effective treatment implications and appropriate interventions.

It is worth noting that case conceptualizations generally use a systematic approach to understanding the problem. Taking a systematic approach prevents therapists from overlooking variables that may be important to the problem. Just as the reliability of interviews is higher for structured interviews than for unstructured interviews (Campion, Campion, & Hudson, 1994), we predict that systematic case conceptualizations will also be more reliable than unsystematic ones.

The Roles of Spirituality and Religiosity in Case Conceptualizations

Although many therapists consciously and deliberately assess cultural worldviews related to race, ethnicity, and gender, the importance of spirituality and religiosity to understanding clients' worldviews and choices has been relatively ignored. However, because of the high levels of spirituality and religiousness in the general population (in the United States), therapists ignore them at their own peril—and to the detriment of those they are attempting to help. In fact, although its importance varies among individuals, spirituality and religiousness are central to the meaning systems or orienting systems of most clients (Bergin, 1991).

Spirituality and religion are closely tied to concepts of meaning and serve as a primary lens through which most people perceive and interpret their world (McIntosh, 1995; Ozorak, 2005). Similar to other systems of meaning, spirituality and religion influence beliefs, goals, and emotions (Silberman, 2005a) but are unique in centering on what individuals hold to be sacred (Pargament, Magyar-Russell, & Murray-Swank, 2005). This sacred content is often reflected in beliefs, goals, and emotions that are not explicitly spiritual or religious (e.g., marriage and parenting).

Spirituality and religion can provide stability and control in a world that otherwise often feels unpredictable and uncontrollable, providing comprehensive and integrated frameworks of meaning that are able to explain events in highly satisfactory ways (Spilka, Hood, Hunsberger, & Gorsuch, 2003). These frameworks of meaning are particularly important in interpreting and responding to the most challenging aspects of life, such as suffering, death, tragedy, and injustice (e.g., Pargament, 1997), but the frameworks also provide a way of understanding more mundane occurrences (e.g., Geyer & Baumeister, 2005; Spilka et al., 2003).

In addition to explicitly spiritual or religious beliefs such as the existence of God and the possibility of an afterlife, spirituality and religion can inform and influence other global beliefs that are less explicitly religious, such as beliefs in fairness, control, coherence, benevolence of the world and other people, and vulnerability (Pargament, 1997). The influence of spirituality and religion on global beliefs is far reaching. When spirituality and religion are incorporated into people's global meaning systems, their understanding of God or of the divine (e.g., loving and benevolent, wrathful) is connected to beliefs about the nature of people (e.g., inherent goodness, made in God's image, sinful human nature), of the self (e.g., as unworthy of God, as chosen), and of this world (e.g., the coming apocalypse, the illusory nature of reality) as well as, perhaps, the next (e.g., heaven, reincarnation; McIntosh, 1995; Silberman, 2005a).

Spirituality and religion are central to the life purposes of many people, providing their ultimate motivation and primary goals for living, as well as prescriptions and guidelines for achieving those goals (e.g., Baumeister, 1991; Pargament, 1997). Increasing knowledge of concern about one's ongoing relationship with God or a Higher Power are examples of this sort of ultimate motivation. Other goals can be derived from these superordinate ones, including having peace of mind, working for peace and justice in the world, devoting oneself to one's family or vocation, or finding deep intimacy with others. Of course, it must be noted, people also often embrace negative goals in the name of religion, including supremacy and destruction (see Silberman, 2005b). Although some goals are explicitly spiritual or religious, any goal can take on spiritual value if the individual ties it to his or her conceptualization of the sacred (Pargament et al., 2005). Secular pursuits that are often sanctified include marriage, parenthood, and vocation.

Spirituality and religion are extremely potent sources of values for individuals as well as for entire cultures (Baumeister, 1991). They often define what is right and good and to be sought after and what is wrong and bad and to be avoided. Predominant religions within a culture are in an unusually powerful position to determine or establish criteria of right and wrong and good and bad, even for people who are not overtly religious.

Spiritual and religious aspects of global beliefs can be central to how one experiences life on a daily basis. For example, beliefs in salvation can influence an individual's understanding of his or her life, provide guidance regarding which goals to pursue and which decisions to make, and infuse life with a deep sense of purpose. Furthermore, people may find great and ongoing comfort in notions of salvation for the just and ultimate punishment (i.e., the deprivation of eternal life) for the unjust (Hall & Johnson, 2001).

In sum, to understand clients and to work effectively with them, therapists need to understand their global meaning (beliefs, goals, and sense of life meaning) in view of their current circumstances, events, and self. Violations or discrepancies within global meaning or between global and situational meanings suggest hypotheses to explore further and guide the formulation of interventions. Rather than viewing global meaning, which is typically based on spiritual and religious meanings, as separate from other parts of clients' lives and contexts, this approach systematically ties global meaning to the rest of their lived experience.

This approach is useful for highly religious clients, whose religious and spiritual meanings are integral to their global and situational meanings. As our examples demonstrate, however, people draw meaning in response to all sorts of situations, large and small. In addition, even clients who are not overtly religious, such as those discussed in the following sections, can be better understood by keeping their spiritual and religious contexts in mind.

A Strategy for Developing Case Conceptualizations

A case conceptualization should begin with a framework that encourages a broad view of the person. The framework described in Exhibit 6.1 (Slattery, 2004) is one such possibility and is used in the balance of this discussion. Data from interviews and assessment measures, as well as population- and practice-specific information, should flesh out or modify these categories. For example, in a neurological rehabilitation setting, one might choose to focus to a greater degree on neurological functioning and medical issues. As just discussed, however, in any setting, spiritual and religious issues should be examined as a central source of clients' meanings.

A broad range of background information can help therapists develop a strong sense of their clients in terms of how their spirituality and religion inform their global meanings as well as their understanding of current problems. The categories in Exhibit 6.1 are the broad net for gathering details that lead to hypotheses about clients' meanings. In particular, a psychosocial history and other information gathered during assessments can be organized to identify (a) spiritual and secular meanings that clients ascribe to precipitating and associated events, as well as to their cognitive, affective, and physical symptoms; (b) places where life events are assimilated into global meaning, noting the distortions required to do so; (c) places where life events violate global meaning and necessitate changes in it; (d) discrepancies among different aspects of global meaning; and (e) discrepancies among real events, attitudes, beliefs, values, or behavior and cultural, spiritual, or developmental norms and expectations. Obviously, to meet the goals outlined in (a) through (e), we need to understand cultural and religious norms, developmental norms and benchmarks, and values and functions of events, for example, that belonging to a religion generally provides a sense of community, meaning, and hope.

EXHIBIT 6.1
Questions to Guide Organization and Hypothesis Generation
During the Case Conceptualization Process

The Problem

Current Problem or Symptoms

What symptoms does the client report? How severe are they? How chronic? When did they begin? How much are they interfering with functioning? Are they specific to certain situations, or do they occur across situations? What are his or her beliefs about what is wrong? About the appropriate treatment for his or her symptoms? Does he or she expect to get better?

Because clients often have difficulty reporting "bad" symptoms, be careful to assess major concerns, especially about suicide, rather than expecting clients to freely disclose them. Ask, "What else?"

Precipitating Event and Other Recent Events

Why is the client having problems now? Why is he or she entering treatment now? What negative or positive events have occurred recently at home, work, school, and in important relationships? What ongoing stressors? Are reactions proportional or disproportional to the stressor?

Personal and Family History of Psychological Disorders

Has the client or family experienced either similar symptoms or different ones at some time in the past? How were problems handled? Specifically assess whether suicide was used to cope with problems. What was helpful?

If either the client or family received formal treatment in the past, how might this affect current treatments? Were previous therapists respectful? Hopeful? Effective? Empowering? Is current therapy an extension of previous work or, from the client's viewpoint, working on the same old issues or totally new and unrelated ones?

Current Context

Physical Condition

How is the client's physical health? Can any medical conditions account for the symptoms reported? Have these been ruled out? In what health-promoting (or health-interfering) practices has the person been or is currently using?

Drug and Alcohol Use

Is the client taking any drugs (medicinal or recreational) that could cause symptoms? Is he or she taking any street drugs that could interact with medications prescribed to treat symptoms? Has the client been compliant with medications and treatment in the past?

Intellectual and Cognitive Functioning

What are his or her intellectual strengths and deficits? Could symptoms be caused by cognitive deficits?

Coping Style

Is he or she engaging in generally adaptive or maladaptive coping strategies? When is he or she most successful in coping with the problem? What works? Are coping strategies generally short-term or long-term solutions? How do these coping strategies fit with spiritual and religious goals?

Self-Concept

What are his or her beliefs about him- or herself (e.g., "I'm helpless with regard to the winds of fate")? What beliefs about self or problems in the past are particularly helpful? Does he or she have a generally strong or weak sense of self-efficacy?

(continues)

Sociocultural Background

In what culture was the client raised? If an immigrant, how long has he or she been in this country? Why did he or she come to this country? What are his or her connections to his or her homeland? What is his or her level of acculturation? What other group identifications (e.g., race, affectional orientation, gender, age, physical abilities) are most important?

How does his or her culture or group influence reactions to symptoms? How does cultural background influence symptoms? Could the behavior be "normal" in his or her culture and not in the therapist's (or vice versa)? Could differences in group identification influence the nature and quality of your relationship?

Spirituality and Religion

What (if any) religious affiliation does he or she report? Is religion important to the client? In what ways? How do spiritual and religious beliefs, values, goals, behaviors, and resources influence current functioning? Do they provide a supportive network? Are the client's beliefs typical or atypical of his or her culture? How does the nature of the client's beliefs influence his or her feelings of support and acceptance in the community?

Resources and Barriers

Individual Resources

What does he or she do particularly well or feel good about? How can these attributes (e.g., persistence, loyalty, optimism, intelligence) be resources for treatment? How might they undermine it?

Relational Style

What relational style characterizes most of the client's relationships? Open? Trusting? Suspicious? Manipulative? What are the client's general views of others? What is the therapeutic relationship like? Can the client be honest about symptoms, actions, side effects, and concerns? Can he or she honestly disclose the level of compliance with recommendations? Does he or she feel comfortable correcting any misassumptions made in the course of treatment?

Mentors and Models

What real, historical, or metaphorical figures serve as pillars of support or spiritual guides? How have they handled similar problems? It is important to note that some models may be primarily negative in tone. What are the positive aspects of these "negative" models?

Sense and Sources of Meaning

What sense of meaning does the client have and from where? Is life meaningful? Chaotic? Unpredictable? What is his or her worldview? From where is meaning drawn? Does the client have a strong sense of purpose or mission in life? A strong sense of direction? How "on track" does the client perceive his or her life to be regarding ultimate sources of meaning and purpose?

Social Resources (Friends, Family, School, Work)

How supportive are the client's family, friends, and colleagues? Are they sufficient in both quantity and quality to meet the client's needs? Do they increase or decrease the client's stress levels? Do they empower or undermine him or her?

EXHIBIT 6.1
Questions to Guide Organization and Hypothesis Generation
During the Case Conceptualization Process   *(Continued)*

Community Resources
   What agencies (if any) are involved? How supportive are they? How well do they work together? Are they at loggerheads, undermining each other's recommendations, or do they generally share information in an open and collaborative manner?

Community Contributions
   How does the client contribute to the community? Does this feel useful and meaningful to him or her? Are contributions acknowledged by important people in his or her support system? Are they related to and do they feed spiritual goals?

Obstacles and Opportunities to Change Process
   What things might serve as potential obstacles or aids to the change process? These can be financial, educational, social, intellectual, spiritual, and so forth. What does the client believe will (or might) happen when change happens (e.g., marriage will dissolve, family will work together more effectively, will lose financial support, will be excommunicated from the church)?

Note. From *Counseling Diverse Clients: Bringing Context Into Therapy* (pp. 14–15), by J. M. Slattery, 2004, Belmont, CA: Wadsworth. Copyright 2004 by Wadsworth. Adapted with permission.

Case Study: Building a Framework for Case Conceptualization

Julia is a bright 17-year-old college freshman whose best friend recently died unexpectedly of a stroke.[1] As a result of this event in combination with her brother's near death from a car accident 2 years earlier and her recent departure for college, Julia was experiencing significant moodiness, depression, occasional suicidal ideation, and difficulties in her relationships with her parents. Significant life events, her global and situational meanings, and potential discrepancies among meanings are presented in Table 6.2.

Repeated themes seen in Julia's assessment and interview data are (a) feelings of alienation and being "different," (b) failing to recognize or acknowledge the gifts that she has, (c) wanting to make a difference yet feeling impotent in both her own life and her community, (d) seeing a conflict between the values shared with her friends and those held by her parents and the community in which they live, and (e) an increasing spiritual search guiding her growth. These issues seem to be made more salient by the recent death and near-death experiences of those close to Julia.

Despite the significant stressors precipitating Julia's current crisis, she has left home for college and started new friendships with people in her dormitory. Rather than backing away from college, learning, and friendships,

---

[1]All case material is disguised through the use of pseudonyms. Identifying material is changed, and some cases are composites of several people.

TABLE 6.2

Meaning-Based Case Conceptualization of Julia

Variable	Objective description	Client's global and situational meanings	Potential discrepancies among meanings[a]
The problem			
Presenting problem or symptoms	Depression, significant moodiness and irritability, and occasional suicidal ideation following friend's death. Probably dysthymic as a teenager.	Sees recent symptoms as normal response to abnormal situation. Sees dysthymia as a result of living in a materialistic culture and having changed to a larger school in a new community. Wants a deeper, more spiritual connection.	Friends take a somewhat cynical view of culture, supporting dysthymia.
Precipitating event and other recent events	Sudden death of best friend at 18 by a stroke caused by a congenital aneurysm. Brother had been nearly killed in car accident 2 years earlier. Less than 1 month after friend's death, she moved away to college.	Death is unfortunate chance event. Sees friend's death as opportunity to rethink how she is living life. Rather than blaming others for problems, she believes she should begin to take control over her own life.	Her newly emerging global meaning is more consistent with family ideal of internal locus of control. Friends tend to take external locus of responsibility, internal locus of control. Death of friend did, however, violate her goal of maintaining her friend in her life.
Personal and family history of psychological problems	Reports a history of dysthymia throughout much of life. Reports no significant family history of depression or other mental health problems.	Sees a pessimistic and cynical approach to life as "healthy" and "aware."	Friends are introspective and "dark," so Julia sees her moodiness, irritability, and dysthymia as normal and appropriate, although she is also aware that this is not how her family approaches life.
Current context			
Physical health	Near-sighted, but no other health problems. Walks and rides bike regularly, sometimes for weekend trips. Is in good physical condition.	Is grateful for health and opportunities it provides.	Note contrast between her health and that of friend's previously undiagnosed aneurysm, and brother's serious accident, both underlining the fragility of life.

Drug/alcohol use	Reports infrequent use of marijuana. No other recreational or prescription drugs.	Does not identify this as a problem.	Her drug use is normative for group, although parents are negative about any drug use.
Intellectual/ cognitive functioning	Bright, abstract thinker whose intellectual passions—books, art—were product of learning on own.	Sees self as "different" but neither "bright" nor especially well educated.	Friends and father, especially, are bright and well read, reinforcing sense of being "average."
Coping style	Reads. Talks with friends. Withdraws from family. Has attributed problems outward and beyond her control.	With friend's death, she is beginning to recognize places where she could and should exercise control over her future.	Mother, in particular, believes Julia reads too much. She tends to be matter-of-fact and expects that her daughter should respond that way, too.
Self-concept	Sees self as bright but "nothing special." Has seen herself as "flotsam on the stream of life," although less so now.	Struggles between self-control and external attributions of control, with friend's death forcing her to think about the direction of her life.	These struggles are typical of closest friends' concerns. All see themselves as bright and capable but appear to underestimate abilities.
Sociocultural background	White, upper-middle class, professional background. Current community is wealthy, achievement oriented.	Sees community as self-absorbed, superficial, and materialistic.	Friends also reject the materialism of community, although they accept its intellectual strivings.
Religious background	Catholic with 9 years of Catholic school. Continues to attend church, although neither church nor religious upbringing was described as important. Recently has become less involved with formal religions but more spiritual.	Sees Catholic Church as rigid and "off-track" with issues like abortion and marriage of priests and nuns. "If God exists, He would not micromanage events, deciding who would live and who would die." Sees spiritual ideals more broadly, altruistically, not in a rule-bound manner.	Consistent with friends', although her parents want her to be more overtly religious. No violation in global beliefs was caused by friend's death, as she sees life as capricious rather than reflecting relationship with God.

(continues)

TABLE 6.2
Meaning-Based Case Conceptualization of Julia   (Continued)

Variable	Objective description	Client's global and situational meanings	Potential discrepancies among meanings[a]
Resources and barriers			
Individual resources	Bright, hard-working (but unfocused), and in honors classes. Loves to read. Compassionate, although has weak social skills.	Sees self as slightly above average in intelligence, below average in skills and achievements.	Community is achievement oriented and father is at top of field. These may contribute to her underestimates of her abilities.
Relational style	Appears to be reserved but willing to be open. More reserved and even oppositional with adults.	Does not expect to find easy intimacy. This seems to be changing, though, as she begins to accept responsibility for the nature of her relationships.	Mother pushes her to relate well to adults and derogates her when she is unsuccessful or uninterested.
Mentors and models	When pressed, she reported that JFK, the Berrigans, and Martin Luther King were models. No mentor was identified.	Wants to be passionate, make a difference, and take difficult moral stands.	Approach is consistent with friends' values; sees this as inconsistent with parental values, although this may be an inaccurate view of their viewpoint.
Sense— and sources— of meaning in life	Sees meaning as coming from her relationships and actively changing world to make it a better place.	Is active in community but does not make the impact that she believes she should. Has begun recognizing the ways that she has backed away from relationships and life, rather than making it what she wants.	Underestimates her individual control. Has vague notions of her purpose in life but is searching for ways to advance those ubergoals.
Social resources (family and friends)	Small, strong community of close friends both in high school and at college. Family is supportive, although relationships with parents are often oppositional and	Does not feel like she has many friends or social supports.	Perceived problems in social support may reflect that her high school, college, and community are large and often feel anonymous.

	argumentative. She had been close to her younger brother before his accident, although now sees him as "obnoxious."		
Work/school	B student in honors classes in high school; doing just enough to get by. In self-directed school program as a senior. Has recently begun college with an undeclared major. She sees college as affirming on a personal level as well as an intellectual one. She has become more successful in her college classes.	Saw her work in high school as "barely adequate." Attributes her increasing acceptance of control over her future to involvement in self-directed school.	Others see her as an "under-achiever" and worry about her future. She seems to be struggling between her own previously low goals and expectations and an awakening awareness of her desire to do something special with her life.
Community resources	Relationships with high school teachers and community were not particularly close, although with college faculty are closer. Several strong spiritual guides, although no ongoing relationship with them. No other agencies involved.	Adds to her sense of alienation from mainstream community.	Relationships are probably normative or better; her assessment may reflect desire for more support.
Community contributions	Although not currently volunteering in college (other than donating blood), has volunteered consistently throughout high school in a range of health and educational settings.	Feels good about her contributions to the community. Feels like she makes a difference.	Volunteers more than average and recognizes this.

[a]Includes own meanings and those of culture, family, friends, or own ideals.

Julia seems to have approached this new stage of her life with an unanticipated excitement. This transition, though, has been rocky, hence her request for counseling.

Although Julia denied being negatively affected by the age-atypical nature of her friend's death, together with her brother's near death (again, age-atypical), it does seem to have jarred her global meaning. Although she has backed away from the Catholic Church, perhaps because her friend's death did not fit her previous religious framework, she seems to have begun an existential and spiritual search for increased meaning, purpose, and intimacy in her life. Providing a framework for exploring and creating more effective spiritual and secular meanings, as well as helping her act on these new meanings, may then be a useful direction for intervention.

Despite the time apparently being ripe for change, Julia's oppositional style with adults should be considered. Rather than pushing her to commit to change or allowing her parents to push her to change, consider allowing her to choose frequency of meetings, goals, and even whether she wants to be in therapy at this point.

The ideas generated in a case conceptualization are hypotheses but can frame strategies for looking at the issues that clients bring to treatment. With this framework comes an increased empathy for the client and, generally, a strengthened therapeutic alliance (Slattery, 2004). The framework also highlights places to intervene.

Illustration of the Spirituality/Meaning-Systems Approach

To further illustrate the use of a spirituality/meaning-systems approach to conceptualize a case, we present the following case study, walking the reader through the steps of this approach. The first step in this process is to pull together a wide range of apparently unrelated observations about different realms of functioning (e.g., social, occupational, spiritual), as well as about the client's beliefs and expectations about life. The framework in Exhibit 6.1 can guide this data collection.

Case Study: Using the Spirituality/Meaning-Systems Approach

Ira Goldberg (age 52) was seriously depressed when he first entered treatment, although he denied current suicidal ideation. He reported significant periods of depression and anxiety throughout his life, but he had recently stopped doing the things that he used to enjoy. He was extremely lonely and felt isolated and "an outsider" among his acquaintances, while simultaneously being irritated by their "superficial" topics of conversation and narrow interests. He reported no close friendships, although he enjoyed the company of his girlfriend of 3 years. He seemed to have little sense of meaning or purpose to his life and believed that his physical health and life were on an inevitable decline. He is well educated and a leading businessman in his small urban community.

Mr. Goldberg was raised in a Jewish family in a primarily Christian community. His mother had a history of recurrent depressive episodes. He described his parents as "distant," although he did not see this as a problem. He married an Episcopalian woman, whom he described as "engaging" and "popular" and who seemed to be his primary source of friendships and social connections. After her untimely death 5 years ago, he dated several women, none of whom were Jewish. He made large donations each year to his synagogue but had not attended services recently; his current girlfriend resists his request to accompany him to services. He chose a non-Jewish therapist although a Jewish one was available (they would not have had a dual relationship).

Case conceptualizations are organized, but their usefulness comes from their ability to generate a cohesive set of hypotheses about the client. Our goal is not only to gather data but also to interpret them in a meaningful and useful way in light of both theory and research on the issue. A range of possible hypotheses should initially be brainstormed and considered, although these may later be narrowed to a much smaller set of working hypotheses. As with other forms of hypothesis testing, rather than using only a single observation or a single category of observations, conclusions are more reliable when disparate and converging pieces of information lead to and support conclusions.

In the case of Mr. Goldberg, a number of discrepancies can be noted. Losing his wife, a primary source of social connection and meaning, was vastly discrepant from his global meaning system, leading to a loss of companionship, social connection, security and safety, and a sense of life as coherent and meaningful. Her untimely death may also have violated his sense of fairness, justice, and predictability of the world. In addition, there were discrepancies from community norms (e.g., being Jewish in a Christian community) as well as developmental norms (e.g., being a young widower). All of these discrepancies would likely lead to problems in reconciling global and situational meanings (e.g., How can one proceed in a world that is chaotic and uncontrollable? How can one value self when one is very different from the community norm? How can one value self when one's strengths differ markedly from one's adopted community?). These ideas are outlined subsequently.

Hypotheses

Although Mr. Goldberg has a family history of depression, which suggests that his depression may have a biological component, being raised and living as a Jew among Christians seems to have been a significant contributing factor. Being Jewish appears to contribute both to his sense of isolation and feelings of inferiority and, paradoxically, also to his "arrogance" and "elitist attitudes." Rather than pursuing his previously broad and idiosyncratic interests, he had taken to following his girlfriend's interests and those of her friends. He looked to his Christian friends for companionship but had chosen friends who were less intelligent and ambitious than him. He seemed to believe that, as a Jew, he did not deserve better, although he admired the easy acceptance that they seemed to expect and what he saw as their relative lightheartedness.

As he had stopped doing the things that he had previously enjoyed and thought much of what he did was meaningless and trivial, he also lost his sense of meaning and purpose. This seems to be related both to his wife's death and to his ambivalence about his intellectual and professional goals, which were apparently not valued by his girlfriend and her friends.

Finally, case conceptualizations should lead to systematic rather than haphazard treatment interventions. As discussed further in chapter 7 (this volume), intervention strategies should derive directly from hypotheses generated in the course of the case conceptualization, should be acceptable to client and therapist, and should be useful. When possible, interventions should build on client strengths, while addressing client weaknesses, and reduce factors maintaining symptoms.

Interventions

Mr. Goldberg refused a referral to a psychiatrist, although he was willing to see one if initial psychosocial interventions were unsuccessful. Because he was very isolated, initial work focused on increasing his activity levels, exercise, and opportunities for meaningful interactions with intellectual and religious peers.

Once he became more stable, Mr. Goldberg contracted with his therapist to explore the meanings of violations in global meaning created by his wife's death and by being an outsider in his community. He agreed to examine his life choices and their meanings for him as well as to consider ways of renewing a sense of meaning and purpose. In particular, he agreed to think about ways to build a supportive and intellectually stimulating community and, perhaps, explore the meanings that being Jewish held for him at this point in his life.

During this period he repeatedly discussed the prejudice and discrimination he perceived in his day-to-day interactions (e.g., having an acquaintance talk about "money-hungry, dirty Jews"). Feeling powerless, despite being professionally, financially, and intellectually powerful, he left one such exchange both accepting the slight and feeling badly that he had not "stood up like a man." During this period therapy focused on ways that he could reduce the discrepancies between his real and ideal selves.

His wife's death continued to be a sore spot. With her death he lost someone who understood him, who bridged the Jewish and Gentile communities, and who was his intellectual equal but who was also playful and socially graceful. This period of treatment focused on integrating these apparent discrepancies and allowing him to meet needs that had gone unmet since her death, especially those involving feeling connected, understood, and accepted.

Use of This Approach to Inform Other Theoretical Case Conceptualizations

What is included in a case conceptualization varies widely across theoretical viewpoints. From our perspective, what is most important in doing a case conceptualization is not the specific details but the systematic generation of hypotheses. The categories listed in Exhibit 6.1 compose only one approach (see Ingram, 2006, for an integration of theoretical approaches to case conceptualization). Although we have been describing the roles of spirituality and religiousness in case formulation from a meaning-making viewpoint, the fundamental ideas are compatible with and can enrich case conceptualizations from many theoretical viewpoints.

We have already discussed the significant points of commonality with cognitive–behavioral case formulations, which explicitly emphasize cognitive representations. Similarly, the meaning-systems approach is obviously consistent with the client-centered approach, which explicitly focuses on discrepancies among aspects of self (e.g., real vs. ideal) or between self and others (Higgins, 1987). However, the meaning-systems approach is compatible with many other approaches as well. For example, the psychoanalytic case conceptualization focuses on both structural and dynamic features of personality, along with developmental issues and resources (Messer & Wolitzky, 1997). The structural features concern the *form* of functioning of the ego (reality testing) as well as affects, drives, and defenses (characteristic ways of experiencing impulses and feelings and containing them), object relations (basic modes of relating to others, including internal representations of self, other, and links between self and other), and self (coherence, stability, and evaluation of the self, identity, ideals, and goals). It is clear that the meaning-systems approach is highly relevant in understanding the particular meanings that individuals assign to these aspects of their personality. Dynamic features concern the content of functioning, especially the clashes or discrepancies between aspects of structure, such as major areas of conflict among elements of personality such as wishes, fears, impulses, and needs, which, according to psychoanalytic views, are often of a sexual, dependent, or aggressive nature. It is important to note that many of the discrepancies in meaning (beliefs and goals) may be beneath the level of a client's awareness, consistent with the psychoanalytic perspective.

CONCLUSION

In this chapter, we have attempted to provide therapists with an overview of the meaning-systems approach to conceptualization, highlighting the central role that spirituality and religiousness play in the meaning systems of the majority of clients. As noted earlier, although our approach focuses on gathering a broad range of details about clients, these details are important only in their ability to help us generate productive hypotheses. These hypotheses facilitate our ability to take a broad perspective of clients, leading to the establishment of deeper levels of sensitivity, understanding, and empathy in our work with them.

REFERENCES

Alexander, M. J., & Higgins, E. T. (1993). Emotional trade-offs of becoming a parent: How social roles influence self-discrepancy effects. *Journal of Personality and Social Psychology, 65*, 1259–1269.

Avants, S. K., Margolin, A., & Singer, J. L. (1994). Self-reevaluation therapy: A cognitive intervention for the chemically dependent patient. *Psychology of Addictive Behaviors, 8*, 214–222.

Baumeister, R. F. (1991). *Meanings of life.* New York: Guilford Press.

Bergin, A. E. (1991). Values and religious issues in psychotherapy and mental health. *American Psychologist, 46*, 394–403.

Campion, M. A., Campion, J. E., & Hudson, J. P. (1994). Structured interviewing: A note on incremental validity and alternative question types. *Journal of Applied Psychology, 79*, 998–1102.

Emmons, R. A. (1999). *The psychology of ultimate concerns.* New York: Guilford Press.

Emmons, R. A. (2005). Emotion and religion. In R. F. Paloutzian & C. L. Park (Eds.), *Handbook of the psychology of religion and spirituality* (pp. 235–252). New York: Guilford Press.

Evans, I. M. (1993). Constructional perspectives in clinical assessment. *Psychological Assessment, 5*, 264–272.

Exline, J. J. (2002). Stumbling blocks on the religious road: Fractured relationships, nagging vices, and the inner struggle to believe. *Psychological Inquiry, 13*, 182–189.

Geyer, A. L., & Baumeister, R. F. (2005). Religion, morality, and self-control: Values, virtues, and vices. In R. F. Paloutzian & C. L. Park (Eds.), *Handbook of the psychology of religion and spirituality* (pp. 412–432). New York: Guilford Press.

Hall, M. E. L., & Johnson, E. L. (2001). Theodicy and therapy: Philosophical/ ethological contributions to the problem of suffering. *Journal of Psychology and Christianity, 20*, 5–17.

Hawkins, I. L., & Bullock, S. L. (1995). Informed consent and religious values: A neglected area of diversity. *Psychotherapy, 32*, 293–300.

Higgins, E. T. (1987). Self-discrepancy: A theory relating self and affect. *Psychological Review, 94*, 319–340.

Ingram, B. L. (2006). *Clinical case formulations*. New York: Wiley.

Janoff-Bulman, R. (1992). *Shattered assumptions*. New York: Free Press.

Karoly, P. (1999). A goal systems-self-regulatory perspective on personality, psychopathology, and change. *Review of General Psychology, 3*, 264–291.

Klinger, E. (1977). *Meaning and void*. Minneapolis: University of Minnesota Press.

Koltko-Rivera, M. E. (2004). The psychology of worldviews. *Review of General Psychology, 8*, 3–58.

Lansford, J. E., Chang, L., Dodge, K. A., Malone, P. S., Oburu, P., Palmérus, K., et al. (2005). Physical discipline and children's adjustment: Cultural normativeness as a moderator. *Child Development, 76*, 1234–1246.

Lazarus, R. S., & Folkman, S. (1984). *Stress, coping, and appraisal*. New York: Springer Publishing Company.

McGregor, I., & Little, B. R. (1998). Personal projects, happiness, and meaning: On doing well and being yourself. *Journal of Personality and Social Psychology, 74*, 494–512.

McIntosh, D. N. (1995). Religion-as-schema, with implications for the relation between religion and coping. *International Journal for the Psychology of Religion, 5*, 1–16.

Messer, S. B., & Wolitzky, D. L. (1997). The traditional psychoanalytic approach to case formulation. In T. D. Eells (Ed.), *Handbook of psychotherapy case formulation* (pp. 26–57). New York: Guilford Press.

Nelson, A., & Hastie, M. (2005). *Teaching the art of case conceptualization*. Austin, TX: Austin Child Guidance Center. Retrieved December 1, 2006, from http://www.austinchildguidance.org/pro.jsp?pageId=2161392210281123098047139

Ozorak, E. W. (2005). Emotion and religion. In R. F. Paloutzian & C. L. Park (Eds.), *Handbook of the psychology of religion and spirituality* (pp. 216–234). New York: Guilford Press.

Pargament, K. I. (1997). *The psychology of religion and coping*. New York: Guilford Press.

Pargament, K. I., Magyar-Russell, G. M., & Murray-Swank, N. A. (2005). The sacred and the search for significance: Religion as a unique process. *Journal of Social Issues, 61*, 665–687.

Park, C. L. (2005). Religion as a meaning-making framework in coping with life stress. *Journal of Social Issues, 61*, 707–730.

Park, C. L., & Folkman, S. (1997). Meaning in the context of stress and coping. *General Review of Psychology, 1*, 115–144.

Reker, G. T., & Wong, P. T. P. (1988). Aging as an individual process: Toward a theory of personal meaning. In J. E. Birren & V. L. Bengston (Eds.), *Emergent theories of aging* (pp. 214–246). New York: Springer Publishing Company.

Silberman, I. (2005a). Religion as a meaning system: Implications for the new millennium. *Journal of Social Issues, 61*, 641–663.

Silberman, I. (2005b). Religious violence, terrorism, and peace. In R. F. Paloutzian & C. L. Park (Eds.), *Handbook of the psychology of religion and spirituality* (pp. 529–549). New York: Guilford Press.

Slattery, J. M. (2004). *Counseling diverse clients: Bringing context into therapy*. Belmont, CA: Brooks/Cole.

Spilka, B., Hood, R. W., Jr., Hunsberger, B., & Gorsuch, R. (2003). *The psychology of religion: An empirical approach* (3rd ed.). New York: Guilford Press.

7

INTEGRATING SPIRITUALITY WITH CLINICAL PRACTICE THROUGH TREATMENT PLANNING

BRIAN J. ZINNBAUER AND JOHN J. BARRETT

Successful treatments rarely occur by chance.
—S. R. Woody, J. Detweiler-Bedell, B. A. Teachman, and T. O'Hearn

Even with the best of intentions, therapists can damage the therapeutic relationship with certain clients or even doom the process of therapy if they lack awareness of spiritual and religious concerns or skill at working with these issues. Such dire outcomes need not occur, however. The choice of theoretical framework and the process of explicitly negotiating treatment goals may increase a therapist's chances of providing spiritually sensitive and effective care. Thus, the purpose of this chapter is to propose a model that integrates spirituality into treatment planning and is grounded within a multicultural framework. Case examples and sample treatment plans are used to illustrate this approach.[1] We begin with an actual case that provides one example of how not to address spiritual and religious issues in mental health care.

---

[1]For the cases presented in this chapter, pseudonyms are used, and identifying details have been altered for confidentiality.

CASE STUDY: HOW NOT TO ADDRESS SPIRITUAL
AND RELIGIOUS ISSUES IN MENTAL HEALTH CARE

After years of struggling to cope with a series of health problems and "blue moods," Edward sought help from the community mental health agency near his home. His heart attack and stroke 6 years before had left him unable to work. Partial facial paralysis and an unsteady gait often drew him too much attention in public, so he spent most of his time in his house by himself. He felt despondent and feared going outside during the daytime. All of his grocery shopping was done in the middle of the night at the local 24-hour market.

At his initial appointment, his assigned therapist, Jill, seemed friendly and asked him many different questions. After the intake interview was complete, they scheduled a first therapy session for the following week. Jill's intake summary was unremarkable: "47-year-old, divorced Caucasian man with dysthymia and increasing problems with social phobia. Recommend individual psychotherapy with possible referral to psychiatry."

The first several therapy sessions were helpful to Edward. He did not know exactly what therapy was about, but he was able to tell his story and talk with someone about his life for the first time in many years. He even told his sister on the phone one night that his therapist "really understood him." Edward wanted to ask Jill what was wrong with him but thought that a direct question like that would be impolite. He also worried a little that he did not know what he should do during his therapy sessions; therapy on TV was about "talking out your problems," and so Edward assumed that talking was the right thing to do. He further interpreted Jill's smiles and attentive listening as signs that he was a good client.

After a dozen more therapy sessions Edward began to wonder how long therapy was supposed to take. His therapist remained warm and supportive, but he noticed that the good feelings he experienced when talking with her dissipated soon after he left the mental health center. He had already discussed most of his life and the events surrounding both his stroke and heart attack. His anxiety about being in public was still a problem, but he recognized how his fears of other people's reactions were probably more "mind reading" than accurate.

During the next session his therapist brought up the topic of spirituality. Edward was quiet and more reserved than normal in his answers. He told her that he was raised Baptist but had "fallen away" from the church. After his long pause, Jill suggested that there may be a helpful spiritual perspective on his current problems. When Edward was quiet again, she suggested that his health problems may be due to karma and that spirituality may reveal the "silver lining" to his "dark cloud." Later, Jill told Edward, "You might even think about your change in health as a 'spiritual test.' " She ended the session by saying, "God bless you." Edward left quickly at the end of the 50 minutes, a change from previous sessions in which he and Jill had walked back to the waiting room together.

At home, Edward was upset. He did not like that his therapist was talking like a minister. They never discussed religion before—why now? As he thought more about it, the whole conversation evoked uncomfortable memories of being forced to attend church as a child and being disciplined by his mother with threats that he was "going to hell." Over the next several days he began to worry that his therapist might try to convert him to another faith. He did not know what "karma" was, but it sounded foreign. The day before his next session Edward canceled his appointment and never returned.

SPIRITUALITY

It is a welcome sign of progress that therapists no longer argue whether mental health treatment ought to include attention to the spiritual and religious lives of clients (Richards & Bergin, 2004). With the easy question aside, more difficult questions remain. What exactly is spirituality? How is spirituality related to client problems and strengths? And how do we effectively include spirituality in treatment planning?

Research that investigates the broad links between spirituality and health is abundant, but a thorough review is beyond the scope of this chapter (see chap. 1, this volume; also see summaries by Koenig, 2005; Oman & Thoresen, 2005; Pargament 1997). For the present purposes, we suggest that spiritual difficulties and strengths may be relevant to mental health work at several levels of analysis, including the individual, social, cultural, and global levels (see also Zinnbauer & Pargament, 2005). For example, a given client may find herself in conflict with her faith community over social or political issues (social level problem) but also draw strength and guidance in living from her spiritual beliefs (individual level strength). Another client may have recently immigrated from a culture that oppresses members of his faith (cultural level problem) but find current inspiration and the strength to overcome from his spirituality (individual level strength) and support from a new faith community (social level strength). A third client may feel condemned by God for a past mistake and experience extreme guilt (individual level problem) and also hold contradictory beliefs about his own faith that contribute to his distress (individual level problem). Additional examples are offered in Table 7.1.

These illustrations are by no means exhaustive, but they touch on relevant topics for treatment planning addressed in the mental health and multicultural literatures, such as the adequacy of spiritual and religious coping efforts (Butter & Pargament, 2003; Pargament, 1997), assessment of cognitive distortions in spiritual views and beliefs (Neilson, Johnson, & Ellis, 2001), developmental models of spirituality (e.g., Fowler, 1981; Wilber, 2006), spirituality in positive psychology (Peterson & Seligman, 2004), the effects of psychopathology on religious functioning (Hathaway, 2003), and the effects of social and political forces on individual functioning (Sue & Sue, 2003).

TABLE 7.1

Spiritual Strengths and Problems as a Function of Level of Analysis

Level	Potential problem	Potential strength
Individual	Irrational faith or beliefs.	Adaptive sacred beliefs.
	Incoherent or contradictory belief system.	Integrated spiritual worldview.
	Sacred prescriptions or goals mismatched to current problems.	Flexible sacred rituals or adaptive guidelines for living.
	Spiritually driven emotional distress (e.g., excessive guilt).	Spiritually inspired perseverance.
	Barrier to integrated personal identity or growth (e.g., spiritually justified self-hatred).	Sacred source of integrated identity or growth.
Social	Conflict with faith community.	Harmony with faith community.
	Conflict with family over faith.	Faith as unifying force in family.
	Promotes religious intolerance.	Promotes tolerance as virtue.
Cultural	Creates cultural/national violence.	Promotes peace.
	Culture oppresses certain faiths.	Culture respects/promotes spiritual diversity.
Global	World events cause loss of faith.	World events prompt renewal of faith and opportunities to display virtue.
	Divisive faiths can promote global competition or enmity.	Common virtues across faiths can promote global community.

The critical issue for treatment planning is that a therapist must accurately assess the various dimensions of spirituality in and across therapeutic encounters and determine their salience to mental health treatment (see chap. 5, this volume). This process clearly requires a great deal of interpretation and judgment. The dangers of imposing personal or cultural beliefs are very real for the therapist who is ignorant or inexperienced with spiritual concepts and beliefs (Arthur & Stewart, 2001). In addition, research has demonstrated that mental health professionals commonly make cognitive errors in clinical judgment because of mental shortcuts such as the *availability heuristic, representativeness heuristic,* and *confirmatory bias* (Dunning, 2005; Falvey, 2001; Falvey, Bray, & Hebert, 2005; Westin & Weinberger, 2004). When this judgment process is extended to complex areas such as spirituality or culture, the opportunities for errors increase.

To avoid these pitfalls, therapists are advised to take cognitive precautions (see Dunning, 2005; Falvey, 2001; Falvey et al., 2005; Westin & Weinberger, 2004; see also chap. 3, this volume). Therapists should actively consider alternative case conceptualizations and treatment plans during the course of clinical work (see chap. 6, this volume) and take into account both contextual and intrapsychic explanations for client behaviors. Also, reliance on memory and experience alone to guide decision making should be supplemented with formal decision aids, such as diagnostic criteria (e.g., Hathaway, Scott, & Garver, 2004; Scott, Garver, Richards, & Hathaway, 2004), data on base rates, and psychological testing. Given the documented limits to individuals' self-awareness (Dunning, 2005; Dunning, Heath, & Sols, 2004), peer consultation, training, and ongoing self-assessment are also suggested to implement these advisories.

It is also important to recognize that spirituality at times may be irrelevant to treatment and that spiritual functioning may be irrelevant to some individuals and groups. We must not assume or suggest a spiritual identity for the atheist, secular humanist, or agnostic who does not profess a belief in the sacred. To do so would amount to the same questionable imposition of values and worldview as the atheist therapist who pathologizes all faiths and sacred traditions.

Although necessary, accurate assessment and clinical judgment may not be sufficient to effectively integrate spirituality with therapy and treatment planning. A growing number of authors (e.g., Griffith & Griffith, 2003; Miller, 1999; Richards & Bergin, 1997, 2000, 2004; Shafranske, 1996; Sperry, 2001) have provided frameworks that integrate spiritual issues, strengths, and worldviews into mental health interventions, but no single approach has emerged as a standard for treatment. We believe that the most broadly applicable framework for this integration can be found within the multicultural literature. Spirituality is increasingly recognized by many advocates of multiculturalism as an element of culture and a vital area for mental health assessment and intervention (Fukuyama & Sevig, 1999; Hays, 2007; Sue & Sue, 2003). To conduct effective treatment planning, we suggest that therapists adopt a multicultural framework that emphasizes wise judgment based on self-knowledge, critical thinking, cultural knowledge, and a culturally sensitive stance.

MULTICULTURALISM

In response to the changing demographic within North America, the philosophical implications of postmodernism and contextualism (Blanter, 1997; Wilber, 2006), and a commitment to social justice and equity (Arthur & Stewart, 2001; Pedersen, 1997), there have been increasing calls within the field of mental health for therapists to work in ways that are sensitive to cultural differences. Ethical guidelines have been established by the American Psychological Association (2003), the American Counseling Association (2005), the U.S. Surgeon General (U.S. Department of Health and Human Services, 2001, cited in Hwang, 2006), the Canadian Psychological Association (1996), and the Canadian Counselling Association (2002) that stress the importance of respecting cultural diversity and avoiding discrimination in clinical practice. Numerous researchers and clinicians have also argued for multicultural competency as a professional necessity (Beiser, 2003; Lo & Fung, 2003), and some have gone further, suggesting that all mental health work is multicultural in nature (Pedersen, 2001; Sue & Sue, 2003). If this latter statement is true, then every new therapeutic encounter requires a bridge of cultures. Given the nature of the relationship, most of the responsibility lies with the therapist to ensure that an adequate bridge has been built and that it can support the flow of information and experiences that therapy will require.

Several authors have recognized spirituality as an element of culture (e.g., Fukuyama & Sevig, 1999; Hays, 2007; Russell & Yarhouse, 2006; Tarakeshwar, Stanton, & Pargament, 2003; Weinrach & Thomas, 2001), and guidelines generated in the multicultural literature are directly applicable to the realm of spiritual issues in therapy. For example, in her well-conceived and well-presented book on multicultural assessment and treatment, Hays (2007) offered the ADDRESSING framework for cultural assessment and a number of suggestions for culturally responsive practice. According to the ADDRESSING framework, a full accounting of culture must address multiple domains, including Age or generational influences, Developmental or acquired Disabilities, Religion and spiritual orientation, Ethnicity, Socioeconomic status, Sexual orientation, Indigenous heritage, National origin, and Gender. Hays summarized this information on "Axis VI," which is her addition to the multi-axial diagnostic system from the *Diagnostic and Statistical Manual of Mental Disorders, Fourth Edition, Text Revision* (*DSM–IV–TR*; American Psychiatric Association, 2000; see also Lo & Fung, 2003, for a different discussion of cultural analysis).

Hays (2007) further offered a number of suggestions to therapists to promote culturally responsive practice. These directives, modified here to specifically focus on the spiritual aspect of culture, are consistent with those from the research on clinical judgment. Hays (2007) suggested that therapists need to participate in ongoing self-assessment and use structured frameworks to assess the nature and relevance of spirituality to treatment. To avoid cognitive errors, she advised therapists to look for spiritual strengths as well as difficulties and to consider multiple sources of information (e.g., client, family, social environment, culture) in assessment and intervention. Finally, she promoted a central theme found in multicultural treatment: the importance of collaboration in mental health treatment.

Other scholars, such as Fukuyama and Sevig (1999); Kirmayer, Groleau, Guzder, Blake, and Jarvis (2003); and Stuart (2004), have also provided specific suggestions for multicultural mental health treatment that are applicable to spiritually sensitive therapy. Therapists should develop sensitivity to the timing and manner of introducing spiritual interventions into treatment, be cognizant of the dangers of assuming even the appearance of dual roles (e.g., cleric and therapist), and use thorough cultural and spiritual assessments. Theses authors also stress the importance of obtaining permission from clients to include spirituality as part of mental health work and collaborating with clients toward mutual understandings of culturally defined concepts and meanings. In addition to procedural suggestions, therapists are strongly encouraged to discuss and reflect on their own worldview and beliefs to reduce potential countertransference issues and misunderstandings.

Multicultural approaches thus suggest a middle way that balances individual and contextual assessment in treatment, acknowledges both spiritual strengths and deficits, emphasizes collaboration, and recognizes that the salience of spirituality within treatment is a variable that must be assessed rather than assumed. As such, these guidelines are not terribly controversial. However, advocacy for two additional issues relevant to multiculturalism, client–therapist matching and group-specific knowledge, is not as clear cut.

Some have questioned whether clients prefer therapists who match them on certain demographic variables (e.g., race, ethnicity, religion) and whether such matching leads to better outcomes. According to the affirmative version of this argument, the Baptist client would prefer and work best with a Baptist therapist, the Buddhist client would fare poorly with a Catholic counselor, and the Muslim client would invariably resist a referral to a Jewish psychiatrist. As summarized by Speight and Vera (1997), the research on client preference is mixed and the empirical results are often artifacts of the methodologies used in the studies (see also Patterson, 2001). These authors argued that there is a need for more research that documents the link between this matching process and clinical outcomes. Also needed are investigations that assess multiple client and therapist characteristics rather than single dimensions, as well as scholarship that advances theory development and testing (Speight & Vera, 1997).

Critics have noted a contradiction between exclusive demographic matching and multiculturalism. For example, some have suggested that insistence on this type of matching in clinical work and research (e.g., only Methodists can counsel Methodists, only Methodists can study Methodists) is counterproductive and contrary to the multicultural values of diversity and inclusiveness (Negy, 1999; Weinrach & Thomas, 2001). Daya (2001) argued that too much attention to external aspects of culture may obscure important ways in which culture is internalized and functions in people's lives.

Instead of simple demographic matching, Cardemil and Battle (2003), Daya (2001), Patterson (2001), and Yeh et al. (2005) emphasized cognitive matching and the nonspecific factors of mental health treatment. In other words, rather than a match on simple physical characteristics or ethnic membership, it may be more important that therapists are able to develop an effective therapeutic relationship, including the willingness to conduct open discussions about cultural differences and promote a shared perspective with their clients. It is clear that a cross-cultural match in which the therapist is accurately viewed as respectful, genuine, competent, caring, and effective is more likely to generate a positive alliance than a cultural or religious match lacking these elements. Whether the demographic characteristics predict better outcomes over and above cognitive matches and nonspecific factors is a question for additional research.

Another important issue is that of group-specific information (Pedersen, 2001). A universal recommendation is that therapists need more direct knowledge of and experience with the groups they serve. To this end, multiculturalists (e.g., Sue & Sue, 2003) and psychologists (e.g., Richards & Bergin, 2000) have generated publications with chapters focused on the specific characteristics of ethnic and religious groups. This approach may be necessary but not sufficient (Arthur & Stewart, 2001; Daya, 2001), however, to reach the goals of providing culturally or spiritually sensitive treatment. Given the wide within-group variance with regard to beliefs, acculturation, linguistic skills, exposure to discrimination, socioeconomic status, and other variables, it is not enough to memorize a list of group descriptions. If therapists stop there, such a superficial approach risks stereotyping and reducing individual uniqueness to cultural generalities (Daya, 2001). Again, we emphasize here that to provide effective treatment and produce useful treatment plans, therapists need to acquire accurate self-knowledge, knowledge of their clients' cultural and spiritual lives, and an appropriate framework that balances attention to individual, group, and spiritual diversity.

Therefore, equipped with a culturally sensitive framework, a caring stance, critically evaluated self-knowledge, a cultural and spiritual knowledge base, and solid interpersonal skills, the therapist is ready to address the practical ways in which to use this approach in actual clinical situations with spiritual clients. Given the potentially endless combinations of culture, faith, and other aspects of diversity, specific algorithms for assessment and intervention may never be possible (Patterson, 2001). Instead, we believe that it is more helpful to present a flexible method to guide treatment planning that can be applied across situations and types of clinical work but can also be tailored to individual therapeutic encounters.

TREATMENT PLANNING

As explained by Maruish (2002) and Jongsma and Peterson (1995), treatment planning as a distinct activity is a recent development in mental health care. This emphasis on clear treatment goals and specific interventions guided by a formal plan of care has been prompted by changes in reimbursement for mental health services, the rise of managed care, accreditation requirements by organizations such as the Joint Commission for the Accreditation of Healthcare Organizations, and increased concerns about legal liability and documentation. This emphasis has also come from therapists who work with structured interventions, such as cognitive and behavioral therapies, brief treatment models, integrated care models that align mental health care with primary care (e.g., O'Donohue, Byrd, Cummings, & Henderson, 2005), and manualized treatments (Mumma, 1998).

Woody, Detweiler-Bedell, Teachman, and O'Hearn (2003); Falvey (2001); and Jongsma and Peterson (1995) persuasively summarized the benefits and purposes of using formal treatment planning. These authors suggested that treatment planning provides clarity and focus to treatment, sets realistic expectations, establishes standards for measuring progress and completion, assists with quality improvement, facilitates communication with other professionals, improves clinical judgment, and provides protection from certain forms of litigation. Also, and in line with the suggestions of multicultural therapy, formal treatment planning helps ensure that the client and therapist work collaboratively (Chinman et al., 1999), that the content and general process of therapy are understandable to all participants (Yeh et al., 2005), and that clients have access to enough information to provide informed consent (Maruish, 2002).

As a brief aside, several authors (e.g., Harkness & Lilienfeld, 1997; Mumma, 1998; Woody et al., 2003) have argued for the use of empirically verified or supported treatments as part of the treatment planning process. Although we recognize the clear benefits of using such treatments, there are few such treatments designed and tested with the religious or spiritual client (see Pargament, Murray-Swank, & Tarakeshwar, 2005). Furthermore, there is an ongoing debate in the multicultural literature about whether to alter existing treatments to meet the needs of specific groups or to design novel treatments from within the worldview or culture of specific populations (see Hwang, 2006). We hope that ongoing research will explore these questions and provide culturally appropriate guidelines. Until then, case conceptualization and clinical theory guide practice (Mumma, 1998), and therapists working with spiritual clients must heed the suggestions of the multiculturalists and the researchers on clinical judgment presented earlier to provide accurate and culturally sensitive treatment.

The model that we present here is drawn from the excellent work of Hays (2007), Makover (1992), Maruish (2002), and Woody et al. (2003). The reader is referred to these works for additional explication of treatment planning methodology. Treatment planning in this proposal consists of seven steps: (a) identifying the presenting complaint, (b) using the initial ADDRESSING cultural assessment, (c) developing a problem list and a strengths list, (d) identifying the desired final outcome, (e) setting goals and resolving measurement issues, (f) selecting and implementing interventions, and (g) periodically reviewing progress. To illustrate these steps, we offer the following case example. For space reasons, some of the suggested elements for culturally sensitive treatment described earlier, such as generating rapport, adopting critical self-awareness, and negotiating cultural meanings, are assumed rather than described.

CASE STUDY: RELATIVELY SIMPLE

Jeanine Madison, a 38-year-old, married Caucasian mother of three young children, was referred to Dr. Donald Johnson by her family doctor for help with crying spells, irritability, and hypersomnia. Despite reporting marital conflict, the client requested individual therapy to address her difficulties. After an initial consultation, the following cultural assessment (Hays, 2007) was developed. The items were confirmed with the client to ensure accuracy.

Cultural Assessment

Age and generational influences: 38 years old; "Generation X, whatever that means."

Developmental or acquired disabilities: None reported

Religion or spiritual orientation: Raised Methodist; very active with church in youth and in college. Media reports of worldwide religious violence and terrorism have led her to question her identification with religion; currently identifies as "more spiritual than religious."

Ethnicity: Ancestry is European American; social network is largely European American; she denied that her ethnic background holds any particular salience for treatment. (The therapist, Don, is also European American.)

Socioeconomic status: Upper middle class; the client and her husband both have graduate degrees; the client is currently not working, having chosen to take 5 years away from career to start a family.

Sexual orientation: Heterosexual; married for 13 years

Indigenous heritage: None

National origin: United States

Gender: Female; middle child of three; has three children and views her self-identity as very connected to her status as mother and wife.

Problem List

The problem list contains those issues identified by the client, referral source, or therapist that cause clinically significant distress or impairment in functioning and can be addressed with mental health intervention. If possible, these entries should be phrased in concrete, specific, and potentially measurable terms. The inadequate list that follows is contrasted with a useful problem list based on the case information and negotiated between therapist and client.

The inadequate problem list included the following:

- bad marriage
- depression
- low self-esteem
- spiritual problems

The useful problem list included the following:

- daily conflicts with husband over finances and parenting
- crying spells average of three times per day
- nighttime sleep lasts 10 to 14 hours per day
- self-criticism related to parenting marital problems and mixed feelings about not working
- spiritual distress described as feelings of unworthiness and distance from God
- infrequent church attendance—once per month
- decrease in practice of prayer from daily use to once per month

Those items in the second list are specific and measurable. In contrast, those in the first list are too general and need to be broken down into more concrete and behavioral terms. If problems are too general or too vague, it becomes more difficult for therapists to design appropriate interventions or to measure the progress of treatment (Woody et al., 2003).

Strengths List

The list of strengths is a counterpoint to the problem list. Strengths may include positive traits or abilities relevant to the treatment, or favorable states and circumstances. The list developed for Jeanine included four entries proposed by Don: psychologically minded, intelligent, motivated, and socially supported by several friends and family members.

Final Outcome

The next step is to determine clients' overall objective or hopes for treatment (Makover, 1992) and to work with them to ensure that this overarching goal is clear, reasonable, and can be addressed in the given treatment setting. Here is another contrast, this time between problematic and useful versions of Jeanine's goal of therapy.

Problematic final outcomes: Make my husband agree with me and "see it my way." Force my schedule to allow full-time parenting, working, and volunteering.

Useful final outcome: Reduce symptoms of depression and resolve the ambivalence I feel about my role in the family and my choices in life.

The useful goal is clear and can be addressed in treatment. The other goals are potentially problematic. The first inadequate goal hinges success on the involvement of the husband, who may not be similarly invested in that outcome, and the second such goal may be impossible given the constraints of opportunity, energy, and the 24-hour day. After a brief and lightly humorous discussion, Jeanine admitted that changing her husband or bending space-time to accommodate too many daily activities was not realistic.

Setting Goals and Measuring Progress

This process connects the problem list with the desired final outcome. The client and therapist choose one to three problems from the problem list and then design interventions to address those goals. The means by which changes are to be measured and tracked are also identified. For those therapists who wish to use scales to measure aspects of spirituality during treatment, sources such as Hill and Hood's (1999) compendium can be helpful. However, the therapist must ensure that a given scale is appropriate for a given client and that issues of language, culture, and meaning are addressed. Furthermore, therapists are advised to consider the problem of arbitrary metrics that has been identified as a limitation of treatment efficacy studies (see Blanton & Jaccard, 2006; Kazdin, 2006).

Selecting and Implementing Interventions

In this case example, Jeanine decided that the chief barrier to resolving her internal conflicts about her work and home lay within her spiritual life. She stated that her childhood church upbringing stressed ritual, obedience, and a domestic homemaking role for women. Her current church appeared less prescriptive about gender roles and often focused on practical applications of scripture, but she remained conflicted about which was the "true" doctrine. Exposure to news stories describing religious violence and terrorism further clouded her beliefs in religion. Also, through conversations with several women in her social network, Jeanine became interested in Christian contemplative prayer and mysticism. At the end of the second treatment session, Jeanine prioritized her spiritual distress and depressive symptoms as the most important places to start. Exhibit 7.1 shows the initial treatment plan for Janine.

Review of Progress

At the end of 1 month, Jeanine was partially successful with the outlined treatment goals. She reported that she found the meetings with her pastor and

EXHIBIT 7.1
Treatment Plan 1 for Jeanine

Goal 1: Resolve spiritual distress; restore religious participation to once per week (with family)

Measurement:
1. Self-rated spiritual distress on a scale from 1 (*low*) to 7 (*high*); current rating: 6
2. Frequency of church attendance: currently once per month

Strategies:
1. Meet with pastor from church to discuss Christian doctrine and family role
2. Write expressive letter to God describing current conflicts
3. Use petitionary and contemplative prayer to seek spiritual strength and guidance
4. Attend Sunday services at church for 1 month

Review: 1 month

Goal 2: Reduce hypersomnia and crying spells by 50%

Measurement:
1. Hours of sleep each day
2. Frequency of crying spells

Strategies:
1. Structure sleep–wake schedule using handout on sleep hygiene
2. Eliminate daytime naps
3. Increase daily exercise to 20 minutes per day

Review: 1 month

---

her expressive letter exercise to be helpful in reducing her spiritual distress from a rating of 6 to 2 (out of 7). In addition, attending church again on a regular basis helped structure family time on the weekends when stress and chaos in the home were the highest. It also provided a source of social connection that she had been lacking. Jeanine was not as successful with the second goal and asked to put that goal on hold to focus more on her spiritual distress. After consulting together, Jeanine and Don decided to rewrite her treatment plan (see Exhibit 7.2).

At the end of the 2nd month, Jeanine reported significant improvements in spiritual satisfaction and success with her spiritual practices goal.

EXHIBIT 7.2
Treatment Plan 2 for Jeanine

Goal 1: Increase spiritual practice to 30 minutes per day

Measurement: Minutes of spiritual practice each day

Strategies:
1. Daily use of prayer, church attendance, and bibliotherapy related to Christianity and modern living; expressive letter writing; or meditation totaling 30 minutes minimum
2. Development of daily ritual to ensure spiritual participation
3. Invitation to husband to join spiritual pursuits

Review: 1 month

She further indicated that she used the structure of nightly prayer to assist with stress management and to maintain her sleep schedule. Her morning ritual of taking a walk while listening to spiritually oriented books on tape provided the added benefit of reducing her symptoms of depression and the frequency of her crying spells. At termination, she described her reconnection with her spiritual life as the most important element of the treatment and her greatest strength in making changes. Her self-rated spiritual distress was 1 out of 7, her husband had begun to walk with her each morning, and their marital conflict dropped to once a week. At a 6-month follow-up, Jeanine had maintained her spiritual practices at 30 minutes each day (with some alteration of the specific spiritual activities), she was sleeping 7 to 8 hours each night, and she had not had a recurrence of crying spells. She reported that at times she still struggled with self-doubt and with her decision to stay at home with the kids. However, she stated that she considered those difficulties as motivators to continue her spiritual pursuits rather than topics requiring a return to therapy.

COMPLEX CASES

This case provides one example of how spirituality may be intertwined with mental health treatment. Admittedly, this case was fairly simple; Jeanine was highly functional and motivated, and her spiritual life and cultural background were easily incorporated into a common Western version of mental health assessment and treatment. However, as Woody et al. (2003) noted, there are times when the process is more complicated. A fully collaborative approach may not be possible when clients are malingering, court-ordered to treatment, or not invested in certain mental health objectives. There may also be cases in which client pathology or stage of change (Prochaska, Norcross, & DiClemente, 1994) requires the therapist to add entries to the problem list without explicitly informing the client. Examples of this might include substance-abusing clients who vigorously deny substance-abuse problems, clients who externalize their problems and are not yet able to consider any personal ownership of their difficulties, and clients with personality disorders who might terminate therapy if a therapist's full assessment were revealed prematurely.

In these cases, a therapist may mentally maintain a separate problem list, final outcome, and treatment plan in parallel to the explicitly defined treatment (Woody et al., 2003). Because collaboration and negotiated goals are not completely explicit, however, the warnings from the multiculturalists are particularly relevant here. As discussed before, therapists are advised to critically evaluate their approach to ensure ethical and appropriate clinical care. Seeking peer consultation and maintaining clear documentation of decision making may also be valuable. Here is second case example to illustrate some of these issues.

CASE STUDY: MORE COMPLEX

William Schmidt, a 77-year-old Caucasian widower, was self-referred to an urban psychotherapy practice the day after he called a local crisis hotline. He explained during the crisis call, and later in his initial mental health interview, that he had experienced "nerve problems" his entire life and was at one time a "heavy drinker." He had cut his arms with a knife on several occasions, had dramatic fluctuations in mood when under stress, and had been hospitalized by his wife 30 years ago for threatening suicide. He stated firmly that he did not want medications or for anyone else to know that he was in treatment. At the completion of the initial assessment, Dr. Chris Bollware, a 40-year-old, male, African American therapist, decided that William was not currently a danger to himself or others, and together they agreed to meet regularly for therapy. The initial cultural assessment was discussed with William and documented.

Cultural Assessment

Age and generational influences: 77 years old; World War II generation; served stateside after being drafted in the Army Air Corps.

Developmental or acquired disabilities: Eyesight and hearing mildly impaired though able to maintain independent living.

Religion or spiritual orientation: Raised Catholic and married in the Catholic church; reported a strong current aversion to organized religion and other sources of "authority." He defined himself as "spiritual but not religious"; previously associated with Alcoholics Anonymous (AA) and has appreciation of the AA conception of spirituality and "Higher Power."

Ethnicity: Ancestry is German; reported that he took pride in his heritage prior to World War II but since then has downplayed this connection.

Socioeconomic status: Previously middle class before retirement; currently on fixed income; medication costs place him near poverty line.

Sexual orientation: Heterosexual; was married for 48 years before wife died of cancer.

Indigenous heritage: None

National origin: Third-generation German American; all ancestors were German except for one grandmother who was Finnish.

Gender: Male; middle child of three boys; no children.

A thorough exploration of the client's past and present functioning led Chris to diagnose William with recurrent major depressive disorder and alcohol dependence in full remission. Careful additional questioning revealed the possible underlying presence of a personality disorder. The initial problem list was discussed and agreed on. Issues such as client–therapist differences (age, race, socioeconomic status), the salience of William's German heritage to treatment, and Chris's status as a practicing Catholic were discussed. William stated that these issues were not barriers to working together, though Chris suggested that the conversation be left "open" in case an issue was to arise in the course of treatment.

William's presenting issue was then addressed. His general label of "nerve problems" was explored and then translated into more concrete descriptors after a thorough discussion.

Problem List

The problem list included the following:

- daily depressed mood
- daily low energy
- daily feelings of worthlessness
- suicidal thoughts once per week
- conflict with others (neighbor clerks landlord) 2 to 3 times per week
- daily "overreaction to stress"
- lack of social interactions
- lack of exercise

Chris formed his additional problem list mentally:

- low affect tolerance
- poor communication skills
- interpersonally hostile stance
- intellectualized coping style

Strengths List

William's list of strengths was a collaborative venture that required several discussions. They settled on three strengths: wisdom from many experiences, analytical thinking style, and interest in learning.

Setting and Measuring Goals

William initially described his overall hope for treatment as "feeling better." With some further discussion, this was refined to "reduce depression and get along better with people."

Selecting and Implementing Interventions

The first treatment plan for William was negotiated and written as shown in Exhibit 7.3.

Review of Progress

After five sessions, William's depression scale scores were unchanged. He had attended one AA meeting but complained that he did not know any of the people there, and he reported that he had lost his old sponsor's phone number. William also appeared to be uncomfortable discussing emotionally laden topics in session; he fell silent and appeared irritated when Chris identified the pattern in session.

William and Chris then explicitly discussed their therapeutic impasse and agreed that they both felt "stuck." To change gears, Chris began asking about those aspects of life that William found meaningful. William provided an enthusiastic description of his love of reading. Specifically, he described reading dozens of books on spirituality and spiritual ways of understanding psychology. As Chris displayed interest and asked more questions, William wondered aloud whether his own problems were really spiritual problems. With more

---

EXHIBIT 7.3
Treatment Plan 1 for William

Client's Goal 1: Reduce depressive symptoms by 50%

Measurement: Center for Epidemiologic Studies Depression Scale administered weekly to assess depression (baseline 50/60)

Strategies:
1. Read general handout on depression and discuss in session
2. Read handouts on cognitive distortions and discuss in session
3. Take one walk each day
4. Attend one AA meeting
5. Call old AA sponsor

Review: 3 to 5 weeks

Therapist's Goal 2: Increase affect tolerance and self-reflection in session; increase social support and connection outside of session; monitor therapeutic relationship and reassess periodically

Measurement:
1. Informal assessment in session based on therapist observation
2. Client attendance at group activities per week

Strategies:
1. Periodically direct course of therapy to emotionally laden topics
2. Encourage development of emotional language
3. Introduce initial formulation of client's chronic interpersonal problems
4. Encourage group participation through AA or other opportunities
5. Explicit check in with client about quality of alliance periodically

Review: Weekly

---

discussion, they decided to change the treatment plan to reflect this new direction. Chris's mentally held treatment goal entry that addressed group participation was moved to the explicitly negotiated treatment plan (see Exhibit 7.4).

Over next few months, William was able to connect with a spiritually focused AA meeting and to look forward to that social contact. His nephew also showed him how to access spiritual resources on the Internet. After some typing practice, William joined a Course in Miracles study group online. In session, discussion often focused on constructing a framework to understand William's mood, learning history, and interpersonal problems. A combination of the AA perspective on "stinking thinking," an evolving conviction that his fundamental identity was spiritual and eternal, and a need to "walk the walk" rather than just intellectually understand spiritual concepts, became the overt framework for treatment. Eventually, William adopted a "practicing virtues" goal for therapy to replace his emotional reactivity, interpersonal conflict, and dysfunctional thinking. His depression scale scores trended downward, although occasional setbacks periodically produced elevated symptoms.

Health problems forced William to forgo his regular sessions during the 2nd year of therapy. During one of the final therapy sessions, he described the early refocus on spirituality as the only thing that kept him coming back to treatment. He also stated that looking for "the light rather than the darkness" was important for him, as well as his new mantra that he is a "spiritual being having a human experience rather than a human being having a spiritual

EXHIBIT 7.4
Treatment Plan 2 for William

Client's Goal 1: Reduce depressive symptoms by 50%
Measurement:
1. Center for Epidemiologic Studies Depression Scale administered weekly (most recent rating 51/60)
2. Frequency of group-oriented spiritual activities and AA meetings
Strategies:
1. Read one book each week on spirituality and mental health and discuss in session
2. Attend three AA discussion meetings each week until a meeting is found that focuses on spiritual issues
3. Inquire about spirituality groups or classes in community and bring results to session Pick one spiritual activity to practice daily
Review: 3 to 5 weeks

Therapist's Goal 2: Increase affect tolerance and self-reflection through spiritual pursuits; monitor therapeutic relationship and reassess periodically
Measurement: Informal assessment in session based on therapist observation
Strategies:
1. Incorporate interventions into client's spiritual worldview
2. Encourage self-reflective spiritual pursuits
3. Explicit periodic check-in with client about quality of alliance
Review: Weekly

---

experience." In other words, focusing on his spiritual strengths was more powerful than trying to reduce his depressive symptoms, and finding a core spiritual identity was a stabilizing and positive influence on his development.

As a final word, Makover (1992) offered advice to therapists when the process of therapy has broken down. He suggested that the prerequisites for a successful treatment plan are the clarity of the client's request for help, the ability of the therapist to provide appropriate treatment, and the realistic agreement between them about how their work will achieve that goal. Often, failure to make progress in treatment means that the therapist does not know what the client is actually seeking, the two have not agreed on how to work together, or they are unable to carry out the plan they generated. When stuck, Makover suggested, revisit these three treatment planning issues.

TWO FUTURE DIRECTIONS

There remain a number of issues yet to explore in the realm of spirituality and treatment planning. As mentioned before, empirically supported treatments that incorporate spiritual issues and strengths are currently rare, and further advances in this direction would be quite welcome. Also valuable would be research that might distill the differential effects of treatment plan elements (e.g., degree of structure, frequency of review, display of measurement data) and offer guidelines about which aspects are critical and which are unrelated to clinical outcomes.

Advances in client–treatment matching may also be applicable to treatment planning with spiritual clients. There are already efforts to match treatment to client personality variables (Harkness & Lilienfeld, 1997; Maruish, 2002) and to use computerized methods to match client characteristics to types of psychotherapy (Fisher, Beutler, & Williams, 1999). Such efforts might be extended to religious orientations (Batson, Schoenrade, & Ventis, 1993), religious coping styles (Pargament, 1997), or dispositional variables related to spirituality, such as devoutness or honesty (Paunonen & Jackson, 2000).

CONCLUSION

The quest to provide spiritually sensitive mental health treatment is a noble and vital one for therapists. In addition to various ethical obligations, this quest is pragmatically useful. Spiritual issues are often intertwined with mental health problems, strengths, and solutions. Many scholars are working to define ways in which to accomplish this goal, and our chapter is one such effort in the cause. We believe that therapists can adopt a respectful and useful method of working with diverse spiritual populations through the use of formal treatment planning embedded within a multicultural framework.

To refer back to the first case example, had the therapist, Jill, used a basic but formal treatment planning method, she may have opened up a helpful discussion into Edward's spiritual and religious life. Instead, Edward left treatment prematurely and did not return until years later, when he arrived at the office of the first author (Brian J. Zinnbauer) and related his past "therapy horror story."

We began the chapter with a quote by Woody et al. (2003, p. 1), "successful treatments rarely occur by chance," and would add that unsuccessful treatments also rarely occur by chance. It is true that there are limits to what mental health professionals can control and predict in any given therapeutic encounter. They can and should, however, strive to know themselves, know their clients, and provide help from a sensitive and informed perspective.

REFERENCES

American Counseling Association. (2005). *Bylaws*. Retrieved November 15, 2006, from http://www.counseling.org/AboutUs/ByLaws/TP/Home/CT2.aspx

American Psychiatric Association. (2000). *Diagnostic and statistical manual of mental disorders* (4th ed., text rev.). Washington, DC: Author.

American Psychological Association. (2003). Guidelines on multicultural education, training, research, practice, and organizational change for psychologists. *American Psychologist, 58*, 377–402.

Arthur, N., & Stewart, J. (2001). Multicultural counselling in the new millennium: Introduction to the special theme issue. *Canadian Journal of Counselling, 35*, 3–14.

Batson, C. D., Schoenrade, P., & Ventis, W. L. (1993). *Religion and the individual: A social–psychological perspective*. New York: Oxford University Press.

Beiser, M. (2003). Why should researchers care about culture? *Canadian Journal of Psychiatry, 48*, 154–160.

Blanter, A. (1997). The implications of postmodernism for psychotherapy. *Individual Psychology: Journal of Adlerian Theory, Research and Practice, 53*, 476–482.

Blanton, H., & Jaccard, J. (2006). Arbitrary metrics in psychology. *American Psychologist, 61*, 27–41.

Butter, E. M., & Pargament, K. I. (2003). Development of a model for clinical assessment of religious coping: Initial validation of the process evaluation model. *Mental Health, Religion & Culture, 6*, 175–194.

Canadian Counselling Association. (2002). *Code of ethics*. Retrieved November 15, 2006, from http://www.ccacc.ca/coe.htm

Canadian Psychological Association. (1996). *Guidelines for psychological practice with ethnic and culturally diverse populations*. Ottawa, Ontario, Canada: Author.

Cardemil, E. V., & Battle, C. L. (2003). Guess who's coming to therapy? Getting comfortable with conversations about race and ethnicity in psychotherapy. *Professional Psychology: Research and Practice, 34*, 278–286.

Chinman, M. J., Allende, M., Weingarten, R., Steiner, J., Tworkowski, S., & Davidson, L. (1999). On the road to collaborative treatment planning: Consumer and provider perspectives. *Journal of Behavioral Health Services & Research, 26,* 211–218.

Daya, R. (2001). Changing the face of multicultural counselling with principles of change. *Canadian Journal of Counselling, 35,* 49–62.

Dunning, D. (2005). *Self-insight: Roadblocks and detours on the path to knowing thyself.* New York: Psychology Press.

Dunning, D., Heath, C., & Sols, J. M. (2004). Flawed self assessment: Implications for health, education, and the workplace. *Psychological Science in the Public Interest, 5,* 69–106.

Falvey, J. E. (2001). Clinical judgment in case conceptualization and treatment planning across mental health disciplines. *Journal of Counseling and Development, 79,* 292–303.

Falvey, J. E., Bray, T. E., & Hebert, D. J. (2005). Case conceptualization and treatment planning: Investigation of problem-solving and clinical judgment. *Journal of Mental Health Counseling, 27,* 348–372.

Fisher, D., Beutler, L. E., & Williams, O. B. (1999). Making assessment relevant to treatment planning: The STS clinician rating form. *Journal of Clinical Psychology, 55,* 825–842.

Fowler, J. W. (1981). *Stages of faith: The psychology of human development and the quest for meaning.* San Francisco: HarperCollins.

Fukuyama, M. A., & Sevig, T. D. (1999). *Integrating spirituality in multicultural counseling.* Thousand Oaks, CA: Sage.

Griffith, J. L., & Griffith, M. E. (2003). *Encountering the sacred in psychotherapy: How to talk to people about their spiritual lives.* New York: Guilford Press.

Harkness, A. R., & Lilienfeld, S. O. (1997). Individual differences science for treatment planning: Personality traits. *Psychological Assessment, 9,* 349–360.

Hathaway, W. L. (2003). Clinically significant religious impairment. *Mental Health, Religion, and Culture, 6,* 113–129.

Hathaway, W. L., Scott, S. Y., & Garver, S. A. (2004). Assessing religious/spiritual functioning: A neglected domain in clinical practice? *Professional Psychology: Research and Practice, 35,* 97–104.

Hays, P. A. (2007). *Addressing cultural complexities in practice: A framework for clinicians and counselors* (2nd ed.). Washington, DC: American Psychological Association.

Hill, P. C., & Hood, R. W. (1999). *Measures of religious behavior.* Birmingham, AL: Religious Education Press.

Hwang, W.-C. (2006). The psychotherapy adaptation and modification framework: Application to Asian Americans. *American Psychologist, 61,* 702–715.

Jongsma, A. E., & Peterson, L. M. (1995). *The complete adult psychotherapy treatment planner.* New York: Wiley.

Kazdin, A. E. (2006). Arbitrary metrics: Implications for identifying evidence-based treatments. *American Psychologist, 61,* 42–49.

Kirmayer, L. J., Groleau, D., Guzder, J., Blake, C., & Jarvis, E. (2003). Cultural consultation: A model of mental health service for multicultural societies. *Canadian Journal of Psychiatry, 48*, 161–170.

Koenig, H. G. (2005). *Faith and mental health: Religious resources for healing.* Philadelphia: Templeton Foundation Press.

Lo, H.-T., & Fung, K. P. (2003). Culturally competent psychotherapy. *Canadian Journal of Psychiatry, 48*, 161–170.

Makover, R. B. (1992). Training psychotherapists in hierarchical treatment planning. *Journal of Psychotherapy Practice and Research, 1*, 337–350.

Maruish, M. E. (2002). *Essentials of treatment planning.* New York: Wiley.

Miller, W. R. (Ed.). (1999). *Integrating spirituality into treatment.* Washington DC: American Psychological Association.

Mumma, G. H. (1998). Improving cognitive case formulations and treatment planning in clinical practice and research. *Journal of Cognitive Psychotherapy: An International Quarterly, 12*, 251–274.

Negy, C. (1999). A critical examination of selected perspectives in multicultural therapy and psychology. *Psychology: A Journal of Human Behavior, 36*, 2–11.

Neilson, S. L., Johnson, W. B., & Ellis, A. (2001). *Counseling and psychotherapy with religious persons: A rational emotive behavioral approach.* Mahwah, NJ: Erlbaum.

O'Donohue, W. T., Byrd, M. R., Cummings, N. A., & Henderson, D. A. (Eds.). (2005). *Behavioral integrative care: Treatments that work in the primary care setting.* New York: Brunner-Routledge.

Oman, D., & Thoresen, C. E. (2005). Do religion and spirituality influence health? In R. F. Paloutzian & C. L. Park (Eds.), *Handbook of the psychology of religion* (pp. 435–459). New York: Guilford Press.

Pargament, K. I. (1997). *The psychology of religion and coping.* New York: Guilford Press.

Pargament, K. I., Murray-Swank, N. A., & Tarakeshwar, N. (2005). An empirically-based rationale for a spiritually-integrated psychotherapy. *Mental Health, Religion, & Culture, 8*, 155–165.

Patterson, C. H. (2001). Multicultural counseling: From diversity to universality. *Journal of Counseling and Development, 74*, 227–231.

Paunonen, S. V., & Jackson, D. N. (2000). What is beyond the Big Five? Plenty! *Journal of Personality, 68*, 821–835.

Pedersen, P. B. (1997). Recent trends in cultural theories. *Applied and Preventative Psychology, 6*, 221–231.

Pedersen, P. B. (2001). Multiculturalism and the paradigm shift in counselling: Controversies and alternative futures. *Canadian Journal of Counselling, 35*, 15–25.

Peterson, C., & Seligman, M. E. (2004). *Character strengths and virtues: A handbook and classification.* Washington, DC: American Psychological Association.

Prochaska, J. O., Norcross, J. C., & DiClemente, C. O. (1994). *Changing for good.* New York: Avon Books.

Richards, P. S., & Bergin, A. E. (1997). *A spiritual strategy for counseling and psychotherapy*. Washington, DC: American Psychological Association.

Richards, P. S., & Bergin, A. E. (Eds.). (2000). *Handbook of psychotherapy and religious diversity*. Washington, DC: American Psychological Association.

Richards, P. S., & Bergin, A. E. (Eds.). (2004). *Casebook for a spiritual strategy for counseling and psychotherapy*. Washington, DC: American Psychological Association

Russell, S. R., & Yarhouse, M. A. (2006). Training in religion/spirituality within APA-accredited psychology predoctoral internships. *Professional Psychology: Research and Practice, 37*, 430–436.

Scott, S., Garver, S., Richards, J., & Hathaway, W. L. (2004). Religious issues in diagnosis: The V-code and beyond. *Mental Health, Religion, & Culture, 6*, 161–173.

Shafranske, E. P. (Ed.). (1996). *Religion and the clinical practice of psychology*. Washington, DC: American Psychological Association.

Speight, S. L., & Vera, E. M. (1997). Similarity and difference in multicultural counseling: Considering the attraction and repulsion hypotheses. *Counseling Psychologist, 25*, 280–298.

Sperry, L. (2001). *Spirituality in clinical practice: Incorporating the spiritual dimension in psychotherapy and counseling*. Philadelphia: Brunner-Routledge.

Stuart, R. B. (2004). Twelve practical suggestions for achieving multicultural competence. *Professional Psychology: Research and Practice, 35*, 3–9.

Sue, D. W., & Sue, D. (2003). *Counseling the culturally diverse: Theory and practice* (4th ed.). New York: Wiley.

Tarakeshwar, N., Stanton, J., & Pargament, K. I. (2003). Religion: An overlooked dimension of cross-cultural psychology. *Journal of Cross-Cultural Psychology, 34*, 377–394.

Weinrach, S. G., & Thomas, K. R. (2001). The counseling profession's commitment to diversity-sensitive counseling: A critical reassessment. *Journal of Counseling and Development, 74*, 472–477.

Westin, D., & Weinberger, J. (2004). When clinical description becomes statistical prediction. *American Psychologist, 59*, 595–613

Wilber, K. (2006). *Integral spirituality: A startling new role for religion in the modern and postmodern world*. Boston: Shambhala.

Woody, S. R., Detweiler-Bedell, J., Teachman, B. A., & O'Hearn, T. (2003). *Treatment planning in psychotherapy: Taking the guesswork out of clinical care*. New York: Guilford Press.

Yeh, M., McCabe, K., Hough, R. L., Lau, A., Fakhry, F., & Garland, A. (2005). Why bother with beliefs? Examining relationships between race/ethnicity, parental beliefs about causes of child problems, and mental health service use. *Journal of Consulting and Clinical Psychology, 73*, 800–807.

Zinnbauer, B. J., & Pargament, K. I. (2005). Spirituality and religiousness. In R. F. Paloutzian & C. L. Park (Eds.), *Handbook of the psychology of religion* (pp. 21–42). New York: Guilford Press.

8

HOW SPIRITUALITY CAN AFFECT
THE THERAPEUTIC ALLIANCE

J. SCOTT YOUNG, SONDRA DOWDLE, AND LUCY FLOWERS

A relationship is not a static thing; it is built and grows healthy or
unhealthy moment by moment.

—Richard Moss

The purpose of this chapter is threefold: to provide readers with a clear
understanding of the components that make up the therapeutic alliance, to
review research that explores how to build and maintain a therapeutically beneficial alliance, and to prepare readers to maximize the effectiveness of this fundamental factor of healing when working with clients' spiritually. Specifically,
readers should learn what research has revealed regarding the necessity of the
therapeutic alliance as a pan-theoretical component of all psychotherapeutic
efforts, as well as gain insight into the construction, maintenance, and repair of
the therapeutic alliance as it applies to clients' spiritually. Finally, practical steps
that therapists can take to facilitate the formation and maintenance of the therapeutic alliance are provided, as are "in their own words" reflections of therapists who work with spiritual issues in counseling and case examples.

Therapists should be concerned with the overall health of the clients with
whom they work; therefore, spirituality and religion can generally be viewed as
positive factors in the lives of clients. Nevertheless, it is clear that many therapists struggle to understand their role when the problems clients present involve
spiritual and religious issues or what, in the therapists' view, is an "unhealthy"
spiritual perspective or its opposite, the noticeable lack of a spiritual or values center. Therapists have reported both through research and personal

communications that highly conservative religious clients may be challenging (Young, Cashwell, Frame, & Belaire, 2002). This is not surprising given that therapists are trained to embrace a set of mental health values promoting tolerance of diverse opinions, diverse lifestyles, and the importance of self-determination, values that may at times be at odds with religious teachings. Yet, we believe that therapists can play a valuable function in facilitating positive change in the lives of their clients regardless of the clients' spiritual or religious orientation. Even with a great disparity of belief between clients and therapists, a deep connection can be fostered if the therapists are willing to adopt a multicultural stance and participate in focused self-reflection.

Throughout this chapter readers are asked to critically examine their assumptions and prejudices about spirituality and religion. The challenge is to dig deeply enough into oneself to reveal the often subtle biases one holds. There is clear evidence that value neutrality is not possible in therapeutic work (e.g., Tjeltveit, 1999); therefore, it is incumbent on all therapists to understand and fully own their projections so that these do not interfere with the therapeutic relationship. Regardless of their orientation toward spirituality and religion, therapists hold beliefs and opinions that will shape their work. No one is so clinically self-aware as to remove all residue of their personal values from the process—nor should one want to. Rather, the goal is to view clients' beliefs as a source of strength in counseling and to have enough spiritual self-awareness to foster a functional therapeutic alliance (Hagedorn, 2005).

GUIDING PRINCIPLES FOR SPIRITUALLY SENSITIVE THERAPEUTIC ALLIANCES

To provide organization and structure to this chapter, we developed a series of six guiding principles. The principles were created through conversations we had among ourselves and with other practicing therapists, whose comments may be found following a description of each principle. Readers will notice that many of these principles appear related to the American Psychological Association (APA) Division 36 (Psychology of Religion) "Preliminary Practice Guidelines for Working With Religious/Spiritual Issues" (see chap. 2, Appendix 2.1, this volume). As such, cross-references are provided after each principle has been described and before the therapist reflections are highlighted. These principles are similar to the APA Division 36 guidelines in that both provide general recommendations for working competently with spiritual and religious clients. However, these principles are unique in that they are targeted toward the therapeutic alliance, on which we believe most of the therapeutic process rests. Furthermore, the intent of the principles is to articulate what can be considered as foundational knowledge about the therapeutic alliance as well as the unique challenges and potential strengths present when building and maintaining such relationships with spiritually or religiously oriented clients. It is our hope that by carefully considering the implications of these principles, therapists can provide therapy with a renewed confidence with clients whom they previously found challenging.

Principle 1: Build a Strong Therapeutic Alliance

The fundamental importance of a strong therapeutic alliance holds true for all clients, including those with a spiritual or religious orientation. The therapeutic alliance has been referred to by various names within differing traditions of psychotherapy. These include the therapeutic relationship, the working alliance, therapeutic collaboration, the therapeutic contract, joining, the I—thou relationship, and the existential encounter. Despite the differences in terminology, there has been no dispute over the fact that the therapeutic alliance is a key variable in the healing process. As early as 1912, Freud recognized the importance of the *alliance*, a term he used in an attempt to portray the unique role the relationship played between healer and client. As the field progressed and the corpus of literature accumulated, practitioners, theorists and, later, *process-variable* researchers (e.g., Walborn, 1995) have all paid tribute to the centrality of a collaborative therapeutic relationship in human change processes. The therapeutic alliance is now universally accepted as a common relationship variable among all approaches to therapy (Bordin, 1994). This remains true regardless of any demographic uniqueness of clients, such as race, gender, age, diagnosis, spiritual, or religious orientation.

Research over the last 30 years has consistently indicated that the quality of the working alliance in the early stages of psychotherapy is predictive of a significant portion of the final outcome variance (Horvath & Greenberg, 1994). This holds true across diverse treatment orientations and modalities (Horvath & Bedi, 2002; Horvath & Symonds, 1991; Martin, Garske, & Davis, 2000). In fact, the early alliance has been found to be a better predictor of psychotherapy outcome than the alliance averaged across sessions or measured in the middle or late phase of treatment (Martin et al., 2000). Practically speaking, this means that, all things being equal, the therapists who attend fervently to the therapist–client relationship in the first through third counseling sessions are building a foundation that supports the work throughout the therapeutic process. This finding is no less true when the clients hold strong spiritual or religious values. In fact, it can be argued that the importance of a solid therapeutic alliance deserves equal if not more attention with this population because of the reality that by participating in secular psychotherapy spiritual clients are engaging in a process that creates a point of potential conflict. On the one hand, there exists the need for relief from suffering; on the other hand, there is the heightened sense of loyalty to one's spiritual or religious convictions that may emerge as the personality goes under the scrutiny and often-occurring feelings of upheaval brought on by the psychotherapeutic encounter.

The time and energy required to build and maintain the therapeutic alliance with the spiritually or religiously committed individual are nonetheless worth the effort. Only after the unique therapeutic collaborative relationship is formed does the possibility that relational dynamics and struggles come forward to be transformed by the therapeutic process. Given the uniquely personal and psychologically threatening nature of such atypical intimacy as is found in the therapist–client relationship, the importance of developing and maintaining a functional therapeutic alliance is unequivocal. Fortunately, many spiritual and religious traditions stress the importance of relationships (person's relationship to the divine, to the broader world, to the neighbor, and to the self). Therefore, many spiritually oriented clients have experienced the transformative power of a relationship with the divine, thus facilitating their engagement in the relational aspects of therapeutic processes so long as their views are treated respectfully (see chap. 2, Appendix 2.1: A-1, A-2, A-8, I-1, I-4, I-5, I-8, I-11, M-1, M-4, and M-7).

Therapist Reflections

To provide clinical relevance and application for this material, we interviewed four practicing therapists as to their thoughts about, and clinical experiences with, the guiding principles outlined herein. We asked these clinicians to reflect on the principles and openly offer opinions about them and how these tenets applied to clinical practice.

Therapist A

Therapist A is a 39-year-old woman who is a licensed professional counselor in full-time private practice. She has been a clinician for 10 years and is herself a Christian but not a conservative one. She readily admitted a bias that conservative religious clients (typically this meant conservative Christians) are more challenging clinically, yet she also reported that she often works successfully with these individuals in counseling. Regarding Principle 1, she indicated, "The fact that a client is highly religious does not affect my ability to form a therapeutic bond; however, I do have to work hard not to form a judgment that this person will not change. In other words, I have to work hard not to let my judgment that this rigidly religious person won't be successful." When pressed further to explain how she understood the importance of the therapeutic alliance with these clients, she stated, "I have to hold in my mind the sensitive tender place where I can see this person's humanity, where his (or her) hurts are to be honored and not judged. You just gotta love 'em."

Therapist B

Therapist B is a 52-year-old man who has been in full-time private practice for 4 years, following 10 years in community mental health. He is homosexual and very liberal. He grew up in a conservative religious tradition and reports that he is generally comfortable with highly religious or spiritually oriented clients because he understands their struggles to deal with the pressure of meeting high standards and others' expectations. When questioned about establishing the therapeutic alliance, he indicated, "Respect is the very beginning of everything. You have to be honored that someone is willing to come sit with you. Therefore, you have to be the hospitable one. I know I am changing for the client" (e.g., he adjusts his stance in therapy to support who and where the client is).

Therapist C

Therapist C is a 50-year-old woman who describes herself as "a Christian and a therapist but not a Christian therapist." She is a licensed psychologist in private practice. In her opinion, spirituality is part of therapy "only as far as the client needs it to be." "They need to know that they are valued, that I am open, and that I am not going to judge them. The client is saying, 'Allow me to believe what I believe and do not try to change me.' " When asked about forming a therapeutic alliance with diverse clientele, she indicated, "For example, gay and lesbian clients also want to know, 'Is she going to judge me? People beat them over the head with the Bible, so they want reassurance that I am not judgmental. I had a lesbian client whom I saw earlier when she was married. When she came out to me and I was not fearful, that was very powerful for her.' "

Therapist D

Therapist D is a 60-year-old male minister as well as a licensed mental health practitioner who has provided counseling services in a church-based counseling center for 5 years. He stated, "I rely on the ideas in Fowler's stages of faith.[1] I trust that the client is where they need to be. Also, I am aware of helping a person to not just work on their belief system, but to become . . . and I take seriously the idea of a soul or a true self and help the person to operate from within that soul or true self."

---

[1]The stage of faith model is a seven-stage developmental sequence that draws on the work of Piaget, Erickson, and Kohlberg to explain the meaning-making process over the life span (see Fowler, 1991).

Principle 2: Trust the Client's View of the Therapeutic Alliance

The client's view of the therapeutic alliance is more important than the therapist's view. Research has revealed that ultimately, it is the client's contribution to and perception of the therapeutic alliance that is indispensable to treatment outcomes (Connors, Carroll, DiClemente, Longabaugh, & Donovan, 1997; Horvath & Symonds, 1991; Luborsky, 1994). This is a point that deserves both full acknowledgment and careful reflection by all therapists. In a very real sense, this may mean that although in the therapist's opinion the therapeutic alliance is progressing nicely or has become well established, the client's experiences of the relationship are ultimately all that matters. It is not surprising that among trainers of therapists, this translates into the teaching that one must attend closely to clients' perceptions of the therapeutic encounter as it is forming and beyond (Teyber, 2006). There is much evidence, both anecdotal and research based, that clients quickly make determinations as to a therapist's ability to be helpful to them, which functionally looks like the client saying either aloud or to themselves, "You 'get' me and I want to keep paying you money to help me." This is no small matter to the suffering individual. To further complicate the matter, given the contentious history between religion and psychology, the potential exists for fear and misunderstanding on both sides of the relationship.

Clients who are deeply spiritually oriented bring with them into counseling their most closely held values and centers of meaning. These are the very perspectives that have historically been discounted or pathologized by many in the helping professions (Kelly, 1995). Although there has been a recent resurgence of serious scholarly attention to the role spirituality plays in the overall psychological adjustment of the individual, clients are generally sensitive to the fact that secularly trained therapists have historically viewed serious spiritual commitment minimally as a point of potential problem and maximally as blatantly dysfunctional. This tenuous history, regardless of whether it is viewed in such a manner by therapists as they sit with spiritual clients, is an important reality that cannot be ignored, because it may affect the clients' ability to form an effective therapeutic alliance. Needless to say, the more highly spiritual the clients, the more their skepticism may be activated by working with secular therapists.

As discussed earlier, research indicates a strong link between the therapeutic alliance early in the process and therapy outcomes, which speaks to the importance of attending to the client's perceptions of the relationship. This fact is in line with the experience of anyone who has ever been a client in therapy. Who cannot understand the feelings of a client who stops coming to counseling when that client (a) fails to connect to the therapist, (b) disagrees with the therapist as to what needs to be done to help him or her, and (c) is unable to form a sense of trust in the therapist? Therefore, the necessity of attending to the quality of the relationship that is forming as therapy begins is a truism that should be universally accepted among therapists because it is indeed accepted among clients. Furthermore, would not this be of even more acute importance to clients who hold deeply personal spiritual beliefs and are entering a process in which they may fear challenge or misunderstanding by the person who is designated as the helper? Therefore, to facilitate a positive therapeutic encounter with the highly spiritually oriented individual, we suggest that therapists do the following:

1. Adopt a stance of open curiosity when discussing clients' spiritual beliefs.
2. Attend closely to how spiritually oriented clients perceive the therapist's view of their beliefs.
3. Work to deeply understand clients' unique interpretations of spiritual or religious teachings.
4. Provide multiple opportunities for the clients to discuss their perceptions of the therapeutic encounter.
5. Take seriously any indications from clients that the therapist does not accurately understand the clients' spiritual perspectives.

Given that the clients' experience of the relationship with the therapist is so fundamental, the first order of business in therapy is to demonstrate a deep sense of respect for clients, including their beliefs, faith, and spiritual practices. As is often discussed in psychotherapeutic training, many variables may activate transference for clients; however, we argue that the therapists' prejudices about spirituality need not be one. It is paramount to respect clients' spiritual lives without a hidden agenda, even if something within clients' belief systems are contributing to their problems. Needless to say, clients will recognize any insincerity in therapists, and untruthfulness will damage the bonding that must take place for a working therapeutic alliance to develop. Said simply, therapists cannot lie, directly or indirectly, and expect clients to feel safe.

Therapists who work with this population must, at some point, do their own soul searching in regard to their ability to find a place of neutrality between their own and their clients' spiritual stances. Therapists trained in secular settings are likely to have had experiences in training or in clinical practice whereby clients' interpretations of spiritual teachings were viewed as problematic either by an instructor or a supervisor or by the therapists themselves. Nevertheless, each client must be treated as an individual. Therefore, a self-aware objectivity on the therapists' behalf will increase the likelihood that a therapeutic alliance can form, and subsequently, that the clients' authentic beliefs may be brought forward in the session and dealt with if need be. Furthermore, objectivity resulting from therapists having worked through their own issues related to spirituality allows a greater capacity for tolerance, thereby decreasing the likelihood the therapists will interpret clients' beliefs through their own filter. Hagedorn (2005) suggested that the process of therapists developing such a spiritual self-awareness involves answering a series of questions. First, "How have my values developed across my life span?" Second, "What are my personally held biases, fears, and doubts?" Third, "How do I understand the assimilation of spirituality and religion with the counseling process?" Finally, "How comfortable am I in exploring religious and spiritual matters with clients?"

By way of example, I (J. Scott Young) was raised in a highly religious family, and much of my psychological work has been to find a balance between an internal sense of freedom while remaining true to my faith, which I value deeply. Part of the growth process for me involved seriously challenging my family-of-origin rules and expectations as well as my religious training, so that I could come back to each with a personally owned sense of participation in both. One bias that I hold on the basis of my personal experience is the value of challenging what one was taught. Obviously, as a therapist, I must be extremely cautious not to expect this as a necessary step for every spiritual client who is struggling. Some may need to go through such a process of challenging their beliefs, but many will not. If, however, a client with whom I work sensed that I am encouraging the client to challenge his or her beliefs and this is not the client's desire, then the therapeutic relationship faces an unnecessary hurdle. In sum, a therapist must either find a way to accept as valid the client's spiritual life as the client lives it or openly acknowledge his or her personal biases so the client may then make a choice about continuing therapy with full knowledge of the therapist's perspective. Without such transparency it is unlikely the client would be able to develop a therapeutic alliance that is functional (see chap. 2, Appendix 2.1, this volume: A-1, A-2, A-8, I-4, I-8, I-11, and M-2).

Therapist Reflections

Therapist A

When asked about how she attends to the client's perceptions of the therapeutic alliance when working with a highly religious or spiritually oriented client, Therapist A stated, "I discuss the idea that they should be genuine with me and express their feelings without concern for my reactions. I tell them, 'You pay me to take care of my feelings and I guarantee you I will.' I watch closely their reaction and use immediacy often."

Therapist B

Therapist B responded, "I model for them a relationship in which they can be who they are. I use their language and reference points as much as possible, and I attend closely to what they say and what they do not say. I check in often. If at any point I sense they are uncomfortable I move to the basic listening skills and reflect and paraphrase very carefully."

Therapist C

When asked about the client's perceptions of the relationship, Therapist C indicated, "Probably 75% of my clients are interested in whether I am a Christian. They want reassurance that I am, but are usually not interested in my denominational affiliation. Personally, I don't think what I believe is that important; it is about where the client is."

Therapist D

Therapist D responded, "The mental health professional's job is not to fix the client's religious beliefs but expand the range of possibilities within the client's frame of reference."

Principle 3: Use Relational Experiences of the Spiritual Perspective

The clinical behaviors that facilitate the formation of a solid therapeutic alliance entail the activation of relational experiences consistent with a spiritual perspective. This principle is good news to therapists in that it highlights a point of convergence in perspective between secularly trained therapists and most spiritually sensitive individuals. Many spiritual traditions have much to say about the importance and power of relationships to actualize human potential (Kluckhohn & Strodtbeck, 1961; Smith, 1965). According to many spiritual traditions, it is a person's relationship to the divine that is the agent of transformation, whereas in the counseling office, the concern is with the therapist–client relationship as the catalyst for change. Yet both perspectives emphasize that the quality and type of relationships one engages in are in and of themselves potentially activating for change. Furthermore, many spiritual teachings and traditions embrace the idea that people are made for intimate relationship and communal living and are made more whole by connections characterized by trust, integrity, and respect. An important strength often present when working with these individuals is that the language and concepts of relationships as a transformative reality are often deeply woven into their spiritual lives. This offers an opportunity to draw on this sensitivity when forming counseling relationships.

Many commonly used therapeutic approaches share the philosophy of the central power of relationship. More than most styles of therapy, the existential and humanistic approaches emphasize the power of the relationship as a healing mechanism (Corey, 2004). Adherents to these approaches argue that the relationship between therapists and clients is the most impactful element of the counseling process, more than technique or clinical acumen. Although this may not be a perspective shared by many therapists today, the underlying idea that relationship plays a key role in healing is a value shared by most approaches to therapy.

Consider the similarities of emphasis about relationship as discussed in the healing professions and as discussed in spiritual writings, texts, and scriptures. Although each emphasizes the issues of relationship from a particular perspective, they share many commonalities that are familiar to individuals who hold spiritual beliefs. The following list outlines the shared perspective of psychology and spirituality as it relates to the role of relationships:

1. Being in a state of health (or balance) involves the capacity for good relationships.
2. Certain quality of relationships holds the power for healing and redemption.
3. Broken relationships lie at the heart of much human suffering.
4. Humans are created for interdependence and relationship.
5. Humans have free will in relationships.
6. Human potential is maximized in community rather than in isolation.

To explore more specifically the formation and maintenance of the therapeutic alliance, it is helpful to consider what the extant literature says about the behavioral factors that, when displayed by therapists, facilitate healthy therapeutic relationships. These include the following:

1. The therapist maintains a here-and-now focus (Bordin, 1994).
2. The therapist engages in affiliative but nondominant behaviors (Bordin, 1994).
3. The activities of counseling are thematically focused (Bordin, 1994).
4. The therapist makes interpretations that deal with the client's current wishes (Bordin, 1994).
5. The therapist responds to the client's religious beliefs and practices with deep respect and genuine compassion (Basham & O'Connor, 2005).

As discussed in Principle 2, it is also beneficial to consider clients' perspectives in therapeutic relationship formation. The following list taken from the Helping Alliance Counting Signs (Luborsky, 1994) measure offers a set of factors that, when present, support the client's experience of joining with the therapist:

1. The client feels the therapist is warm and supportive.
2. The client believes the therapist is helping him or her.

3. The client feels changed by the treatment.
4. The client feels a rapport with the therapist.
5. The client feels respected and valued by the therapist.
6. The client conveys a belief in the value of the treatment process.

There have been some surprising findings among researchers in this area related to the therapists' contribution to the therapeutic alliance. For example, the experience level of the therapist has not been found to correlate with his or her ability to form an effective alliance. Specifically, a study of therapists' levels of experience by Dunkle and Friedlander (1996) found experience not to be predictive of clients' alliance ratings. This finding should be comforting to both graduate students and newly practicing therapists. By contrast, this finding does speak to the likelihood that relationship formation is more an innate personal trait shared by effective therapists and is somewhat difficult to learn.

In terms of qualities of clients that affect their ability to form therapeutic bonds, researchers have linked insecure attachment styles with poor-quality initial therapeutic alliances in psychotherapy (Eames & Roth, 2000; Mallinckrodt, Coble, & Gantt, 1995; Ogrodniczuk, Piper, Joyce, & McCallum, 2000; Satterfield & Lyddon, 1995). Evidence from the attachment literature suggests that the quality of clients' early relational or family experiences may influence their ability to form an alliance early in individual psychotherapy. These findings speak to the need for therapists to assess the early experiences of all clients, including those who are highly spiritually oriented, to determine if there are experiences that will make the formation of a therapeutic alliance difficult. If there are, these clients will require a longer time to form a sense of safety and closeness with the therapists. Therapists will need to pay careful attention to any indication that the clients are not feeling connected. Teyber (2006) emphasized the need for clients to have a corrective emotional experience in counseling, which involves therapists treating clients in a manner that is unlike that which they would normally experience from others. It is interesting to note that clients' psychiatric symptoms do not appear to predict alliance formation (Mamodhoussen, Wright, Tremblay, & Poitras-Wright, 2005). (See chap. 2, Appendix 2.1, this volume: A-1, A-2, I-8, I-9, I-11, M-2, M-3, and M-4.)

Therapist Reflections

Therapist A

When asked about how she attempts to activate a quality relationship with religious client, Therapist A reported, "Modeling about the therapeutic relationship is very helpful. I use immediacy and transparency myself so the clients can have permission to do this themselves. A colleague and I are doing cotherapy with a couple right now who are highly religious. We ask them often, 'Do you feel understood, so I hear you correctly? The husband has been able to say, No.' "

Therapist B

Therapist B responded, "I expect them (highly religious clients) to want more rational approaches to counseling. I become hyperaware of using the basic listening sequence. I become very technical, moving back into the basics. I rely on the clients to show me if they are comfortable (with the counseling process). I also ask them, 'Did you get what you wanted?' (from the counseling session). I check in more."

Therapist C

Therapist C made an interesting observation as to which clients struggle more to form a therapeutic alliance: "People most comfortable with their spirituality, with their spirituality intact, tend to be the ones who seem to form a relationship more quickly and are not really concerned about my spiritual beliefs. The ones who ask questions about my personal beliefs tend to be shaky and more rigid. They want to know they are right."

Therapist D

Therapist D stated succinctly, "All problems are relationship problems."

Principle 4: Respect Clients' Spiritual Ideals

Because clients' spiritual ideals symbolize their closely held personal truth, they deserve the greatest compassion and respect by therapists. It is not uncommon for individuals to be hesitant to express their doubts, concerns, and uncertainties related to their spiritual beliefs. Generally, such matters are not topics people speak about in the public settings of everyday life. I (J. Scott Young) have found that, when asked directly about their spiritual perspective, even graduate students quite interested in the area of spirituality in counseling report difficulty expressing themselves because these are such highly personal communications. I typically ask students to write a spiritual autobiography as a part of a course on Spirituality in Counseling, and consistently students report this exercise to be emotionally exposing and personally powerful. At its core, one's spiritual beliefs, practices, doubts, and victories are often woven together with the most impactful events of one's life. Whether we think about it, if one has ever been spiritual, one's current relationship to spirituality is an artifact of the experiences of one's life. If one has left religion, there is often a story of hypocrisy or betrayal. If one has moved more deeply into spirituality, there are often stories of faith affirmation, of turning points, and of a deep sense of meaning. In sum, for people who are spiritually oriented, though they may be hurt or angry about religion, their spiritual story encompasses the totality of who they are.

Imagine then a spiritual client who comes into counseling in a distressed state in which it is not easy for the therapist to recognize how complicated and anxiety provoking it might be for the client to discuss spiritual issues. Yet, for many people, spiritual uncertainties are the very issues they need and want to express. For spiritually committed individuals, personal problems are typically filtered through their understanding of the religious teachings they have received. Questions such as "Where is God?" "Why is this happening to me?" "Is God angry with me?" and "Is this a punishment for sin?" are existential ruminations these individuals might pose to themselves. Still they enter the office of a therapist, which is not an overtly spiritual environment, and are uncertain about what to say or how it will be received. Richards and Bergin (1997) described the struggle of such clients as follows:

> Because religious people often experience ridicule, if they do share their spiritual beliefs they do so apprehensively. Therapists should remember this, and if their clients disclose some of their beliefs and special experiences, from whatever cultural and family history they may come, therapists should treat this information with as much empathy and respect as they can. It may be useful to acknowledge to clients explicitly, when they have disclosed such information, that it is not always easy to discuss such sensitive, private matters and they respect the client for having the trust and courage to do so. (p. 126)

In my clinical practice, I (J. Scott Young) have encountered spiritually committed clients who come into counseling in a state of great confusion regarding their relationship with God and what role God plays in the psychological turmoil they are facing. Individuals in this state have frequently been hurt by their religious experiences or have come to feel God is punishing them. Clients who are wounded or hurt around religion may (a) feel oppressed and weighed down by religion; (b) hold guilt and fear of not being good enough; (c) feel a fundamental sense of betrayal by church members or religious leaders; (d) focus on God's judgment of them; (e) distrust their own power and freedom to direct their life; and (f) need to work through anger at God, at the church, at their parents, and so on. Such clients need to be treated with the utmost respect by therapists. They are not unlike individuals who have been hurt in a relationship, yet in this case the relationship is between the client and his or her God. Not only will respect facilitate the formation of the therapeutic alliance, but respect will also preserve the therapeutic alliance. Researchers consistently find that the therapeutic alliance, if well established early in the process, will sustain the work throughout, even if there are later difficulties in the relationship (Bordin, 1994). Furthermore, such compassion and respect, if given to clients early, will sustain the relationship even if mistakes are made later. Kelly (1995) spoke eloquently to the understated yet powerful role the therapists' holding of the clients' struggles can be when he stated, "In the spiritual domain, the contribution of the client's spirituality is fundamentally indirect, achieving its effect through the relational elements of the counselor–client bond, without conveying any personally specific beliefs about his or her spirituality" (p. 96). (See chap. 2, Appendix 2.1, this volume: A-1, A-2, A-7, A-8, I-1, I-4, I-8, I-11, M-2, and M-4.)

Therapist Reflections

Therapist A

When asked about respecting clients' spiritual ideals, Therapist A responded, "I match the clients' language, and I communicate that I will not discount or judge where they are. I want them to know that I accept them in their struggle. I will draw on Bible stories and images to frame their situation. It is about creating a safe space from them to not have it all together."

Therapist B

Therapist B answered, "My advice to mental health professionals (to support client's disclosures about religious or spiritual issues) is question, reflect, reflect . . . use the basic counseling skills. Trust the power of the skills and the concept of powerful questions. Be more present and show respect."

Therapist C

When asked about the therapists' compassion for clients spiritual disclosures, Therapist C stated, "I pray for my clients but not with them. Some of my clients might not like to think that I pray for them so I would not like for this to be advertised. In my opinion the therapist's spiritual discipline is probably as important as dealing with spirituality in the session."

Therapist D

Therapist D had an interesting take on the role of the therapist's compassion for clients' disclosures of spiritual struggles. "Even though we know that people use their faith understanding to give meaning to their lives, how can clinicians really make sense of how a patient understands his or her illness and gives meaning to it?"

Principle 5: Use a Less Judgmental Approach

The more rigid clients are in terms of their spiritual or religious perspective, the less judgmental therapists need to be. It should be well-known to therapists that individuals who hold strong beliefs will also have a significant emotional investment in maintaining the belief that compels them to protect and defend their belief structures. If, while in counseling, clients who are highly charged around spirituality feel threatened about these beliefs, they will almost certainly defend their position, develop heightened resistance, or experience increased emotional distress. Subsequently, direct confrontation of clients' beliefs or even their perception of a subtle attempt to undermine or change beliefs is generally a therapeutic blunder and will strain the therapeutic relationship. Needless to say, dealing with therapeutic issues that are related to clients' religious orientation can present challenging clinical situations for therapists. During the development of a working alliance with religious clients, Kelly (1995) suggested therapists should strive to (a) foster a relational space that respects the clients' spiritual or religious dimension and that allows them to explore spiritual themes, both positive and negative, as they relate to therapeutic issues; (b) help clients to integrate personally beneficial spiritual or religious material so they can expand and transform their perspective on the issues and problems as well as clarify or eliminate negative spiritual or religious elements; and (c) use positive religious resources as appropriate.

Each therapist we interviewed in some way addressed the fact that clients who are highly spiritual or religious may also be more rigid in their thinking about religious precepts and ideals, though obviously this is not always the case. As Fowler (1991) and others have shown, people who are actually more developed spiritually become more at peace with their beliefs as the beliefs become internalized. In other words, as people's beliefs are lived from within as well as without, they provide a deep sense of purpose that does not depend on the approval of others. Nevertheless, in clinical environments one challenge therapists sometimes face is highly religious clients who are also rigid about their beliefs. Such individuals may either be hyper-religious, filtering nearly all of their experiences through a religious frame of reference, or have compartmentalized thinking, referencing religious rules to make decisions. These are the types of individuals that we, as well as all the therapists interviewed, found most challenging to work with, not because of the spiritual aspects per se but rather because of the black-and-white thinking patterns that sometimes occur. The following list outlines characteristics of rigidly religious individuals that make them challenging to work with clinically:

1. They tend to be convinced they are right.
2. They feel the need to convince others that they hold the truth.
3. They are closed to contrasting viewpoints.
4. They become easily threatened when their views are questioned.

5. They tend to surround themselves with like-minded people.
6. They use religious doctrine as a means to avoid considering new information or perspectives.
7. They are judgmental toward views differing from their own.

The question then becomes how to work with such individuals, particularly if there are clinical issues that need to be addressed that may challenge religious perspectives. As with any other problematic pattern of thinking, therapists must provide both challenge and support. This means the therapists must offer appropriate alternative reframing of the clients' thinking while at the same time provide deep support for the clients and their personhood. What this entails is the ability to feel and communicate heartfelt compassion for rigidly religious clients while at the same time asking them to consider alternative interpretations of their beliefs or perspectives that do not require them to reject their faith.

In clinical practice, I (J. Scott Young) have found this to entail working from within the clients' current frame of reference to bring forth a transformed perspective of their beliefs. This can only happen, however, if the clients first truly believe that I respect and care for them. For example, I once worked with a young man who was highly religious and depressed. As I moved further into the counseling, it was clear that the young man's movement into more religious behaviors and involvement was an attempt to deal with his depression. I sensed he very much needed his religion and that it was helpful to him, but he had such perfectionistic standards of himself and others that he was frequently disappointed. He was also very angry and judgmental. Through a careful process of validation of his perspectives and allowing him to project and blame others for not being what they should be, we were able to form a secure therapeutic alliance. He would criticize and vilify his former girlfriend, friends, people at church, and even himself. Slowly, however, I was able to introduce the idea that his thinking was distorted and that he was actually using religious idealism as a weapon to separate himself from others. We talked about grace, love, acceptance, and God's sovereignty as ways to help him relax his righteous anger about people he perceived as hypocritical or who had hurt him. I remember vividly one day when he came into counseling and said, "You know I have realized that when I work to change my thinking, I feel better. There are still things happening that could upset me but I am working to not let them." He indicated that it was like the whole world looked different. We talked in detail about the idea that his showing more forgiveness and compassion with himself was making his relationship with others different. He was learning that his sense of "rightness" actually made him angry and pushed others away. Essentially in this case I was using religiously based cognitive–behavioral therapy. Similar to any other problematic thinking pattern, religiously based cognitive distortions can be addressed clinically, but because of the sensitive nature of such patterns this can only occur if the client is first wrapped in a blanket of nonjudgmental acceptance from the therapist that cannot be faked.

Therapists must decide for themselves if and how they can find a therapeutic stance whereby they can work with rigidly religious clients and still maintain deep compassion for the individual. As authors, it is our position that clients require high levels of patient acceptance because they are so highly rigid. Yet, similar to any other form of rigidity, clients can only move to a more cognitively complex stance gradually and in an environment that is not threatening. It may be helpful for therapists to frame clients' religion as not only a strength but also to gently offer possible reinterpretations. However one frames this, it benefits the therapeutic relationship for therapists to find a place of nonjudgmental acceptance toward clients' beliefs, including the cognitive distortions and inconsistencies, or to refer clients elsewhere.

We realize that readers of this book might personally ascribe to a strong spiritual faith themselves or might just as well be personally nonspiritual. Similarly, readers might view themselves as highly spiritual or have no real need to think in terms of spirituality. Nevertheless, it is imperative that therapists observe their own motives and intentions closely when working with clients who are highly committed to a spiritual perspective. We offer the following statement that therapists might make to clients or to themselves that would reassure the clients and would require the therapists to adopt an open stance in terms of clients' belief systems:

> You do not have to argue or defend your religious positions with me. You are free to believe whatever you wish, as I have no interest in undermining your spiritual life. I view faith commitment that is based in love as a positive factor for a person's overall mental health. So, let us agree to openly explore together how you think about spiritual ideas, adopting a joint attitude of relaxed curiosity, so we might learn how your beliefs affect your psychological life. If I offer any interpretations about your thinking in this area, it is only to expand your options in understanding your faith.

Perhaps one of the most difficult situations therapists might encounter is one in which clients' specific religious rigidity strikes the therapist as dysfunctional to the point that it warrants intervention, even though the client may not view it as such (see chap. 10, this volume). As in any clinical situation, we cannot take clients places they do not wish to go, yet we can make gentle attempts to assist clients in enlarging their scope of thinking if the narrowness of their thinking is hurtful to themselves or to others. If therapists wish to do such work, the following is offered as a possible place to begin:

1. Spend a great deal of time exploring how clients conceptualize their beliefs.
2. Think in terms of expanding clients' options (e.g., more freedom, more flexibility, more love) versus fixing the dysfunctional beliefs.

3. Use gentle confrontation followed by support.
4. Offer new conceptualizations from within the clients' religious frames of reference (e.g., religious stories, language, concepts).
5. Work at clients' cognitive levels of complexity or slightly beyond.
6. Work with religiously based cognitive distortions such as other rigid psychological structures (e.g., beliefs, thoughts, and schemas).

(See chap. 2, Appendix 2.1, this volume: A-6, A-7, A-8, I-8, I-11, M-2, M-6, and M-7.)

Therapist Reflections

Therapist A

When asked about using a less judgmental approach with clients, Therapist A responded, "I use their language. I tune into their words. That helps the client. I have to work to get them out of their heads, but I have to honor their need to have something concrete. They often want an A-B-C, 1-2-3 change." She has noticed these individuals lack an "openness of language about sin," which creates a challenge in helping them not judge themselves too harshly.

Therapist B

Therapist B stated, "I ask them, what about the words *forgiveness* and *grace*, how do you see those concepts in your life? I use this when they (the highly religious clients) have trouble accepting sin in their lives. Yet I have also had people with PhDs who are very concrete. I have had atheists who were rigid."

Therapist C

Therapist C replied, "I try to honor and not make judgments about my clients' religion and spirituality."

Therapist D

Therapist D responded, "The counselor does not have to buy into the client's belief system to work effectively, but instead can operate from within the counselor's own perspective on spirituality without letting on to the client that the counselor is at a different place. For Christians who believe the Bible is divinely inspired and literally true, if they keep studying they will see different viewpoints in the Bible and work to reconcile them in any way possible or move to a view of the Bible with inspiration that transcends dichotomies. They may resist because they believe they will go to hell. So the work is to help to see that the Bible can be inspired and inspiring without necessarily being consistent throughout."

Principle 6: Explore Client Resistance

Resistance as a broader clinical issue is widely researched and discussed in the literature and is defined as all attitudes or behaviors of a client that are counter to the process of change (Raue & Goldfried, 1994). There are numerous expressions of resistance, including the following:

1. The belief that therapy will not be effective.
2. Considering change impossible.
3. Opposition to sharing feelings, thoughts, or behaviors that are integral to one's problems.
4. An unwillingness to engage in the activities of therapy within or outside of sessions.
5. Rejecting therapist feedback.
6. A failure to engage in self-observation and self-monitoring of thoughts, feelings, and behaviors (Goldfried, 1982). (Raue & Goldfried, 1994, pp. 134–135)

In the context of this chapter, however, resistance to discussing spirituality is not necessarily an indication of an overall pattern of resistance, although it certainly can be. At times, it may be clear to a therapist that a spiritual issue may be underpinning a client's presenting concerns although the client may be reluctant to address his or her spirituality. This presents a therapeutic and relational challenge. There are certainly many times in therapy when a therapist must provide direct feedback to a client even though it is difficult for the client to hear. As Carl Whitaker, a pioneer in the field of family therapy, once suggested, good therapy is often bloody, but similar to surgery, it is the only way to get the disease out of the person. Although this is a somewhat dramatic way of stating it, there are indeed times when clients may need to be confronted on their spiritual perspective, for example, a client who uses spirituality as a reason to avoid connection to others, a client who spends so much time with spiritual pursuits that other areas of his or her life suffer, or a client who is in a spiritual bypass (i.e., attempts to avoid addressing psychological problems by using spiritual solutions). In any of these cases, it is clinically necessary to directly address the role of the client's spiritual perspective or practices in the maintenance of his or her psychological difficulties. As with any feedback or confrontation, the clinical task is to be clear and specific about the behaviors or cognitions that are problematic while being supportive of the personhood of the client.

Individuals seeking therapy possess a range of openness to addressing spiritual issues that must be taken into consideration. For example, some clients simply do not think of themselves as religious and therefore assume that any talk of spirituality indicates a move toward religion. By contrast, some clients who are highly religious do not wish to have their religious views challenged; therefore, they are unwilling to discuss their beliefs in session. In fact, Kelly (1995) indicated that there are indeed clients who will respond with hostility to any discussion of spirituality or religion or topics that are perceived as such. Furthermore, there are those clients who consider spirituality and religion as unreal and therefore are not relevant to their understanding of their lives. For these clients, discussing spirituality may be damaging to the therapeutic alliance and ethically problematic because it is never appropriate for the therapist to impose his or her values on the client. In general, however, most client resistance to this domain of human experience is born out of a lack of understanding as to what spirituality involves, as well as a lack of awareness as to how it may benefit them to explore this dimension therapeutically. Therefore, clinicians should be prepared to explain to a client how issues of meaning, purpose, connection, and transcendence are relevant to people's lives regardless of their religious orientation.

Clinicians can take the following steps when facing a client who is reluctant to address spiritual issues in therapy:

1. Explore the client's feelings about openly discussing his or her spiritual beliefs.
2. Explain the relevance of including spirituality as a component of psychological treatment.
3. Slowly explore the client's spiritual perspective.
4. Address directly with the client your perceptions of how the client's psychological issues are related to his or her spiritual perspectives.
5. Spend adequate time using therapeutically supportive interventions (i.e., reflective listening, processing of feelings) to assist the client in exploring the relationship between his or her spiritual perspective and psychological difficulties.

(See chap. 2, Appendix 2.1, this volume: A-1, A-3, A-5, I-1, I-6, I-11, M-3, and M-4.)

Therapist Reflections

Therapist A

When asked about client resistance, Therapist A noted, "Generally, clients who resist spiritual issues have wounds around religious experiences or their life experience has left them afraid to have hope in anything, thus hope in something greater than themselves is too risky. Hope is my ultimate objective. If they are able to hope and believe in themselves and the world around them again, that is the most important foundation for spirituality one can have."

Therapist B

Therapist B responded, "Resistance is to be celebrated, meaning you have hit on something that is deep and needs to be explored. One way I explore directly a client's spiritual perspective is to say something such as, 'To help you, it is important that we bring more of your worldview, spirituality, or religious views into this process.' I might ask the client questions about the purpose of life, even how life started, the nature of the universe, or a favorite image of God. If they quote dogma or scripture to me, I may gently question them to ascertain if they have ever questioned those beliefs or if they believe it because they were taught to. If a person is particularly rooted in the scriptures of his or her religion, I might ask them to pick a story or passage that seems to apply to this situation. I ask very specifically what it means, how does it apply, and what does it require of them and their Creator."

Therapist C

Therapist C reflected, "There are clients who do not consider themselves spiritual and don't care to explore it in session. If the presenting problem is directly influenced by spiritual issues, I usually wait a while (often several sessions) and let the client get comfortable with therapy and establish a trust relationship with the therapist. I find that the relationship between the client and therapist is often the thing that most influences comfort in discussing any subject and especially things that are the most painful. Clients often will mask pain and use religion or spirituality as a way to avoid the real issues. With these clients, 'I will pray about this' is often used instead of 'let's discuss this' or 'I will work on this.' However, the pain, even with a spiritual mask, can become unbearable, whether it is a relationship issue or depression or something else. My approach is always to focus on the client–therapist relationship and build on that. I find that if a client really wants to get better and feels that the therapist can be trusted, most topics are open for discussion eventually."

Therapist D

In response to the question about client resistance, Therapist A replied, "I assume that whenever clients are dealing with the meaning of life and values that give life meaning, they are in touch with spiritual issues. Most resistance seems to revolve around emotionality attached to particular doctrinal or religious concepts or language. I try to use clients' language and religious concepts to work with these issues, and this usually reduces resistance. I do find among some evangelical Christians a preoccupation with literal interpretations, salvation status, and heaven-when-you-die focus that lends itself to judgmental attributions and emotional rigidity. However, I can usually find within their own tradition ample biblical concepts to relate to their issues in a healthy way."

CASE STUDY

Carolyn and Marshal had been married for over 25 years at the time they came for counseling to deal with ongoing marital issues that led Carolyn to threaten divorce, a possibility Marshal desperately hoped to avoid.[2] There were several factors that presented potential challenges to the formation of a therapeutic alliance, which are presented in relation to each guiding principle outlined in the chapter.

Carolyn and Marshal were lifelong members of a fundamentalist Christian denomination in which Carolyn's father had been a minister. The church leaders taught the inerrant truth of the Bible and that women should not be in positions of authority within the church. At the time therapy began, Carolyn felt betrayed by her husband for his unwillingness to end his service as a board member for a church-based mission that she had formed 10 years earlier. In fact, Carolyn had worked for 10 years as the primary energy of the mission but had grown increasingly dissatisfied with her role within the organization and eventually felt pushed out by the leaders of the church. Solely on the basis of her being a woman, it was decided by the male leadership of the church that it was inappropriate for Carolyn to act as the overseer of the ministry, even though she had competently established the ministry and its system for developing orphanages in Eastern Europe and adopting underprivileged children to American families. Carolyn had tolerated this frustration for many years but grew to find this arrangement unbearable. Therefore, she broke all ties with the mission she had founded. Marshal's feeling was that Carolyn had brought him into the ministry with her, and he did not feel he should walk away from it after he had become involved. As a result of the rejection by the church leadership and her perception of a lack of support by her husband, Carolyn began moving away from the church but was searching for a spiritual identity to which she could connect. Marshal wanted to continue his involvement with the congregation and very much wanted Carolyn to return to church with him.

---

[2]For the case presented in this chapter, pseudonyms are used, and identifying details have been altered for confidentiality.

Principle 1: Build a Strong Therapeutic Alliance

Challenge: The therapist was a man and in a role of authority, which could trigger defensiveness in Carolyn as she was sensitive to the perception that men manipulated and controlled her. Marshal was older than the therapist and was forced into counseling by his wife's threats.

Response: By adopting a patient and nonjudgmental attitude toward both the couple's conservative church affiliation and traditional marital style, the therapist made Carolyn and Marshal feel accepted and helped them to explore their marital issues from within their conservative frame of reference.

Principle 2: Trust Clients' View of the Therapeutic Alliance

Challenge: When the therapist would validate Marshal's view of the marriage, Carolyn would sometimes shut down, feeling as though her husband and the therapist were not validating her experience. However, she had been taught that men in positions of authority should be deferred to, so the therapist was aware it would be difficult for Carolyn to disagree with him (a male therapist).

Response: By patiently exploring Carolyn's feelings as they related to both her familial and church history, the therapist was able to maintain his alliance with her.

Principle 3: Use Relational Experiences of the Spiritual Perspective

Challenge: The therapist, although a Christian, was a member of a liberal Protestant church that had a female minister, was socially very liberal, and downplayed the authority of religious leaders and the inerrant truth of the Bible.

Response: The therapist worked diligently to provide nonjudgmental acceptance of the couple through patience, reflective listening, and compassionate feedback, so they could experience the therapeutic relationship as safe, warm, and purposeful. Furthermore, the therapist intentionally did not disclose his theological views in the counseling sessions both because they were not asked for by the clients and because they were not relevant to the couple's marital and spiritual struggles.

Principle 4: Respect Clients' Spiritual Ideals

Challenge: Carolyn was angry and often felt misunderstood, yet avoided conflict. Furthermore, there existed a complicated dynamic within her spiritual perspective such that her religious history both provided her support and caused her psychological difficulty.

Response: Carolyn's conflicted feelings around the role of male authority in the church and in her marriage were explored gently but in depth, without being challenged as harmful to women or antiquated. If she wished to change her beliefs, the impetus must come from her rather than from the influence of the therapist's more liberal perspective.

Principle 5: Use a Less Judgmental Approach

Challenge: Marshal was less psychologically minded than his wife and came to counseling because he felt as though he had no choice. The possibility existed that if he did not feel an ongoing bond with the counselor, his resistance could be activated.

Response: The therapist emphasized Marshal's skills as a good provider, as a problem solver, and as highly supportive of his wife, so that he would feel adequate in the therapeutic relationship and feel supported in his need to be the leader in the home.

Principle 6: Explore Client Resistance

Challenge: The couple was initially open to discussing religion but did not differentiate spirituality as a separate phenomenon. It became clear, however, that Carolyn was in need of a spiritual connection that did not reinforce her feelings of inferiority.

Response: In the early stages of therapy, the language used by the therapist to discuss any spiritual or religious topic was from the couple's religious perspective. After the establishment of a solid therapeutic alliance, the therapist was able to explore with Carolyn her desire for a spiritual connection through means other than her church. Over time, with careful exploration of her experience of the church, Carolyn was able to differentiate her religious experiences from her spiritual connection to God. Eventually, she came to feel she could more readily develop her spiritual life outside of the church. Subsequently, Carolyn stopped attending church. Marshal, although initially concerned about her choice, slowly came to accept or at least tolerate her decision, but he maintained his connection to and involvement with the church. The couple is still married and doing well at the time of this writing.

CONCLUSION

Our purpose in this chapter was to assist therapists in developing and maintaining therapeutic alliance with spiritually oriented clients or with clinical issues of a spiritual nature. Clinicians are encouraged to view the therapeutic alliance as the precious center of therapy that takes precedence over other therapeutic concerns and include spirituality as a domain worthy of clinical attention. In the clinical encounter, therapists should meet clients' spirituality and spiritual orientations with an attitude of patience and openness, assisting clients in maximizing the benefits of their beliefs and practices as an adaptive component of their total personality.

REFERENCES

Basham, A., & O'Connor, J. (2005). Use of spiritual and religious beliefs in pursuit of clients' goals. In C. S. Cashwell & J. S. Young (Eds.), *Integrating spirituality and religion into counseling* (pp. 144–145). Alexandria, VA: American Counseling Association.

Bordin, E. S. (1994). Theory and research on the therapeutic working alliance: New directions. In A. O. Horvath & L. S. Greenberg (Eds.), *The working alliance: Theory, research and practice* (pp. 13–37). New York: Wiley.

Connors, G. J., Carroll, K. M., DiClemente, C. C., Longabaugh, R., & Donovan, D. M. (1997). The therapeutic alliance and its relationship to alcoholism treatment participation and outcome. *Journal of Consulting and Clinical Psychology, 65*, 588–598.

Corey, G. (2004). *The theory and practice of counseling and psychotherapy*. Belmont, CA: Thomson Brooks/Cole.

Dunkle, J. H., & Friedlander, M. L. (1996). Contribution of therapist experience and individual characteristics to the working alliance. *Journal of Counseling Psychology, 43*, 456–460.

Eames, V., & Roth, A. (2000). Patient attachment orientation and the early working alliance: A study of patient and therapist reports of alliance quality and ruptures. *Journal of Psychotherapy Research, 10*, 421–434.

Fowler, J. W. (1991). Stages in faith consciousness. *New Directions for Child Development, 52*, 27–45.

Goldfried, M. R. (1982). Resistance and clinical behavior therapy. In P. L. Wachtel (Ed.), *Resistance: Psychodynamic and behavioral approaches* (pp. 95–114). New York: Plenum Press.

Hagedorn, W. B. (2005). Self-awareness and self-exploration of religious and spiritual beliefs: Know thyself. In C. S. Cashwell & J. S. Young (Eds.), *Integrating spirituality and religion into counseling* (pp. 63–84). Alexandria, VA: American Counseling Association.

Horvath, A. O., & Bedi, R. P. (2002). The alliance. In J. C. Norcross (Ed.), *Psychotherapy relationships that work: Therapist contributions and responsiveness to patients* (pp. 37–69). New York: Oxford University Press.

Horvath, A. O., & Greenberg, L. S. (Eds.). (1994). *The working alliance: Theory, research and practice*. New York: Wiley.

Horvath, A. O., & Symonds, B. D. (1991). Relation between working alliance and outcome in psychotherapy: A meta analysis. *Journal of Counseling Psychology, 38*, 139–149.

Kelly, E. (1995). *Spirituality and religion in counseling and psychotherapy: Diversity in theory and practice*. Alexandria, VA: American Counseling Association.

Kluckhohn, F. R., & Strodtbeck, F. L. (1961). *Variations in values orientations*. Evanston, IL: Row, Peterson.

Luborsky, L. (1994). Therapeutic alliances as predictors of psychotherapy outcomes: Factors explaining the predictive success. In A. O. Horvath & L. S. Greenberg (Eds.), *The working alliance: Theory, research and practice* (pp. 38–50). New York: Wiley.

Mallinckrodt, B., Coble, H. M., & Gantt, D. L. (1995). Working alliance, attachment memories, and social competencies of women in brief therapy. *Journal of Counseling Psychology, 42*, 79–84.

Mamodhoussen, S., Wright, J., Tremblay, N., & Poitras-Wright, H. (2005). The Couple Therapy Alliance Scale Revised: Empirical issues. *Journal of Marital and Family Therapy, 31*, 159–169.

Martin, D. J., Garske, J. P., & Davis, K. M. (2000). Relation of the therapeutic alliance with outcome and other variables: A meta-analytic review. *Journal of Consulting and Clinical Psychology, 68*, 438–450.

Ogrodniczuk, J. S., Piper, W. E., Joyce, A. S., & McCallum, M. (2000). Different perspectives of the therapeutic alliance and therapist techniques in 2 forms of dynamically oriented psychotherapy. *Canadian Journal of Psychiatry, 45*, 452–458.

Raue, P. J., & Goldfried, M. R. (1994). The therapeutic alliance in cognitive–behavior therapy. In A. O. Horvath & L. S. Greenberg (Eds.), *The working alliance: Theory, research and practice* (pp. 131–152). New York: Wiley.

Richards, P. S., & Bergin, A. E. (1997). *A spiritual strategy for counseling and psychotherapy*. Washington, DC: American Psychological Association.

Satterfield, W. A., & Lyddon, W. J. (1995). Client attachment and perceptions of the working alliance with counselor trainees. *Journal of Counseling Psychology, 42*, 187–189.

Smith, H. (1965). *The religions of man*. San Francisco: Harper & Row.

Teyber, E. (2006). *Interpersonal process on therapy: An integrative model*. Belmont, CA: Thomson Brooks/Cole.

Tjeltveit, A. C. (1999). *Ethics and values in psychotherapy*. New York: Routledge.

Walborn, F. S. (1995). *Process variables: Four common elements of counseling and psychotherapy*. Pacific Grove, CA: Brooks/Cole.

Young, J. S., Cashwell, C. S., Frame, M. W., & Belaire, C. (2002). Spiritual and religious competencies: A national survey of CACREP accredited programs. *Counseling and Values, 47*, 22–33.

9

IMPLEMENTING TREATMENTS THAT INCORPORATE CLIENTS' SPIRITUALITY

LEWIS Z. SCHLOSSER AND DAVID A. SAFRAN

An idea that is developed and put into action is more important than an idea that exists only as an idea.

—Gautama Buddha

Given the increased awareness and public expression of spirituality and religion embraced by many Americans, it follows that spirituality should be included in mental health treatment. Moreover, many techniques used by therapists have a spiritual component already embedded within their theoretical approach, and therapists would be wise to use these facts in connecting with clients who may be in search of the sacred. Hence, in this chapter we focus on the implementation of spirituality into treatment. Specifically, we discuss (a) the commonalities between spirituality and therapy, (b) a pantheoretical approach to integrating spirituality into treatment, (c) how spirituality can be implemented into traditional theories of therapy, (d) spiritually accommodative and spiritually oriented approaches, and (e) case examples of implementing spirituality into four different treatment approaches (i.e., cognitive–behavioral, interpersonal, humanistic, and psychodynamic).

CONCEPTUALIZATION OF SPIRITUALITY AND MENTAL HEALTH TREATMENT

It is our contention that one's beliefs directly influence the way one interprets one's experience and that this notion is central to the idea of spirituality

193

as well as many forms of counseling and psychotherapy. Greenson (1967) noted that a therapeutic process refers to an interrelated series of psychic events within the client, a continuity of psychic forces and acts that have a remedial aim or effect. Hence, we assert here that mental health treatment shares a great many things with spirituality, and therapists can use this knowledge in working with the clients in their care. Consider that spirituality and the most well-known models of mental health treatment (e.g., humanistic, psychodynamic, and cognitive–behavioral) share the goals of increased self-knowledge, reduction in suffering, and an understanding of one's place in the world (Sperry & Shafranske, 2005). Therefore, when people have difficulties in these domains, they may seek out a spiritual advisor or a therapist. Perhaps the stigma associated with mental health treatment could be reduced if it were seen in this light. Given the blurring of distinctions between spirituality and psychotherapy in the amelioration of an individual's personal angst, we believe that therapists have to recognize that spirituality is not that far removed from the goals of therapy. If the goal of therapy is to help clients attain a sense of personal well-being, then therapy is the resolution of conflicts related to the soul and the mind. Finally, it could even be argued that the purpose of therapy is to help clients along their spiritual journey, if one adheres to the definition of spirituality put forth by Frame (2003; see also chap. 1, this volume). In this way, the therapist serves as a guide to the client who is on a spiritual path of sorts. This definition, of course, is similar to the Jungian notion of the wounded healer (Sedgwick, 1994).

Therapists have to be cognizant of these constructs to better assist clients in reducing psychosocial stressors that may contribute to egodystonic behaviors; this process can also facilitate a greater sense of client self-awareness. The incorporation of spirituality into the therapeutic process allows therapists to help clients explore their own attitudes and beliefs in a safe environment. Does it matter whether this process is attained through personal spirituality or in a therapist's office where psychotherapy interventions will assist the client? The ends used to achieve the means may be less relevant; what matters is that many therapy clients bring a sense of spirituality that needs to be addressed.

INTEGRATING SPIRITUALITY INTO TREATMENT IMPLEMENTATION

It is our belief that a person's spirituality (or lack thereof) influences his or her life philosophy (Halbur & Halbur, 2006), which in turn influences the person's choice of preferred theoretical orientation as a mental health professional. Regardless of one's approach to therapy, the concept of spirituality can be present during treatment. As such, it is incumbent on therapists to accept the differences between themselves and their clients with regard to the importance of spirituality within the therapeutic context and to do so without bias or prejudice. For example, spirituality and behaviorism may be seen as antithetical to one another; however, behaviorist therapists must be cognizant that clients may attribute behavioral change to spiritual factors. In this way, awareness is a key component of integrating spirituality into therapy, and we discuss this concept in greater detail later. Awareness alone is not enough, as therapists must also have the requisite knowledge and skills to incorporate spirituality into the therapeutic process. Although spirituality and religion have been mentioned as important cultural variables in the multicultural literature, heretofore there has not been an explication of how spirituality in particular can affect therapy (Schlosser, Foley, Poltrock, & Holmwood, in press). We begin with an overview of the therapist influences of spirituality in treatment by incorporating spirituality into the multicultural awareness/knowledge/skills paradigm outlined by Sue (1982).

Awareness

To effectively integrate spirituality into treatment, therapists must first be aware of spirituality within themselves and their clients (see chap. 3, this volume). That is, they must take the time to examine their own beliefs and feelings regarding the role that spirituality plays in their own lives, in the lives of their clients, and in the therapeutic process. To accomplish this, therapists need to increase their comfort with the role of spirituality in everyday life and examine their willingness to bring this issue into the therapeutic process. There are three potential therapist responses to this examination.

The first is when therapists accept spirituality as a relevant construct vis-à-vis psychotherapy. In this case, the therapist must be attuned to the spiritual nature of the client's content. At the same time, however, caution should be exercised so that nonspiritual content is not erroneously interpreted as spiritual in nature. That is, therapists who welcome spirituality into the therapeutic process must concern themselves with not making assumptions regarding spirituality until these issues have been explored with the client.

The second type of response is when therapists reject spirituality as a relevant construct for the therapeutic process. For these clinicians, the task is to consider, and hopefully accept, that there may be a spiritual component to clients' presenting problems. In this case, it is imperative that therapists be cognizant of their own feelings regarding spirituality (i.e., be aware of any possible countertransference) and consider the role that spirituality may play for the client. These therapists must be careful not to underinterpret the importance or presence of spirituality in the client's content.

The third response is when therapists espouse neutral feelings regarding the role spirituality plays in therapy. It is our contention that absolute neutrality is not possible because we believe that people have leanings, and they might simply be out of awareness or not previously considered. Hence, these clinicians should explore their own feelings about spirituality in greater detail. In this way, they can determine in which of the two response groups discussed earlier they best fit.

Therapists must also be sure that they have a good awareness of the differences between spirituality and religion. Failure to possess adequate knowledge about these issues could lead to erroneous labeling of behaviors as psychopathology when in fact they may be quite appropriate for a particular faith community.

It is also important for therapists to understand their own thoughts and feelings regarding spirituality and religion. One way to accomplish this would be to engage in the construction of a "spiritual autobiography" (Curtis & Glass, 2002, p. 5). Basically, therapists engage in a self-reflective process regarding events in their own life that may be facilitative or inhibitory in relation to their work with clients. Therapists must seek to understand themselves fully (e.g., Zinnbauer & Pargament, 2000), including their views of psychopathology and religious and spiritual function or dysfunction. Without this self-examination, the potential for bias to enter the therapeutic endeavor goes unchecked and unexamined, which may eventually lead to unethical and potentially harmful treatment to certain clients (Knox, Catlin, Casper, & Schlosser, 2005).

In fact, Zinnbauer and Pargament (2000) suggested that therapists must share their own personal values with clients as appropriate so that clients can make truly informed decisions regarding their own treatment. Worthington and Sandage (2001) further noted that religious clients might inquire about the therapist's religious beliefs and values. This open and honest modeling by the therapist may be inconsistent with certain approaches to mental health treatment; however, we are in agreement with Zinnbauer and Pargament in that clients should have the opportunity to make informed consent decisions with all of the facts needed to make sound choices about their mental health treatment. Indeed, the findings by Knox et al. (2005) supported this idea: Therapists who were perceived as open, accepting, and safe were able to facilitate discussions of spiritual content. This was above any match of religious or spiritual beliefs between clients and therapists. Hence, it appears clear that an open and accepting stance from the therapist is critical for the implementation of spirituality into treatment. It is important to note, however, that therapists do not have to be spiritual themselves to implement spirituality effectively into treatment. However, therapists do need to know how their own attitudes about spirituality, as well as any personal beliefs, influence their clinical practice.

It is critical to remember the larger context in which the implementation of spirituality into treatment affects the lives of therapists and clients. In the United States, for example, there is a backdrop of Christian domination that has significant effects on Christians and non-Christians alike. These effects, termed *Christian privilege* by Schlosser (2003), provide unequal access and unearned benefits to Christians and can lead to oppression and discrimination against non-Christians (e.g., Jews, Muslims, atheists, agnostics). The effects of Christian privilege on those who do not benefit from it are numerous and must be considered during the implementation of spirituality into mental health treatment. In addition, there may be fundamental differences in beliefs between therapists and clients that could negatively affect the treatment if not addressed (Worthington & Sandage, 2001). Finally, cultural norms are likely to vary on the basis of geography; this could dictate the degree to which spirituality is implemented into therapy. (See chap. 3, this volume, for more information on self-awareness.)

Knowledge

As part of the self-assessment process, therapists also should take stock of their knowledge regarding spirituality and its potential place in therapy. If therapists believe that their own knowledge is insufficient, then it is incumbent on them to ensure continuing education in this area; failure to do so could be considered unethical (American Psychological Association, 2002). Such knowledge can be gained from a variety of sources. Some examples include workshops or classes on spirituality, spirituality or spiritual texts, exposure to or interaction with leaders or members of spiritual communities, and periodic reexamination of their own spiritual beliefs garnered from their own religious beliefs. Personal psychotherapy that includes an examination of one's own views of spirituality can also be helpful. The last example may also facilitate skill development to a degree through modeling.

Certain clinical issues may naturally lend themselves to the inclusion of spirituality into treatment. Some examples include loss and major life changes. Attending to spirituality when these issues come up may be easier for the therapist because they naturally pull for clients to consider their place in the world and, this is a task commonly associated with spirituality. In addition, clients may turn to a faith community during these difficult times as a means of coping. Results from an empirical investigation revealed that clients covered a broad range of topics related to spirituality in secular therapy, including exploring existential issues (Knox et al., 2005). This tells us that therapists need to be aware of spiritual issues from clients who present with a variety of concerns. Furthermore, Knox et al. (2005) found that clients in their study did not finely distinguish their psychological problems from their religious and spiritual concerns. Finally, Knox et al. (2005) found that these discussions tended to be positive in the context of clients raising these topics. Hence, it is important for therapists to consider these findings when spiritual issues appear related to presenting problems. However, it is important to remember that some clients may be deferential to the therapist because of the inherent power differential within psychotherapy; these clients may welcome the therapist's introduction of spiritual concerns into treatment. At the same time, it is important to note that some clients may be against the inclusion of spirituality and religion in the sessions (Worthington & Sandage, 2001).

Skills

Therapists need to be able to apply their awareness and knowledge of issues pertaining to spirituality in a skilled way with clients. Regardless of their own personal beliefs, therapists must gain experience with incorporating spirituality into sessions, of course with the caveat that its inclusion is appropriate given the client, content, and context. Skills can refer to integrating spirituality into established theoretical approaches, as well as expertise with spiritually accommodative or spiritually oriented approaches (Sperry & Shafranske, 2005). Implicit (e.g., therapist asking existential questions) and explicit (e.g., meditation, homework) spiritual interventions (see Tan, 1996) also would be subsumed within the category of skills. The self-awareness process is the foundation for being skilled in the implementation of spirituality into treatment. That is, to effectively use the aforementioned skills, therapists need to have an understanding of how spirituality can affect the lives of clients, as well as the most appropriate way of incorporating this construct into the sessions. Doing so should facilitate clients to attend to their presenting problems in a constructive fashion and increase clients' awareness of the role that spirituality may play in their everyday lives. Finally, competent therapists are aware of their own limitations and refer clients to another treatment provider when appropriate. Once therapists gain spiritual awareness and knowledge, these can then be translated into interventions. As we discuss in the next section, therapists do not necessarily need to learn completely new theories, because spirituality can be incorporated into the commonly use theories of counseling and psychotherapy.

When implementing spirituality into treatment, therapists need to be thoughtful in choosing appropriate spiritual techniques or interventions. There are a variety of specifically spiritual interventions and techniques that therapists can consider incorporating into their treatment (see Table 9.1). Of course, this incorporation can take place within or outside of the session, depending on the professional's own feelings about spirituality, as well as her or his theoretical orientation. Some of these techniques include prayer, meditation, worship, rituals, fasting, and quoting sacred texts (e.g., see Curtis & Glass, 2002). Therapists need to be thoughtful about whether to use these techniques in session because of the potential for misinterpretation and misunderstanding (i.e., because of the great variability within religious and spiritual communities). Outside of treatment, however, other techniques related to creativity can be used, such as journaling, art, and watching films. For example, clients who display some hesitancy about discussing spirituality in session may be more likely to discuss it as part of a larger homework assignment related to their treatment. Discussion of the written assignments may pose an interesting inroad to the

TABLE 9.1

Examples of Spiritual Interventions and Techniques

Intervention	Sample readings
Prayer (therapist or client guided)	Frame (2003), McCullough and Larson (1999), Tan (1996)
Teach spiritual concepts	Eck (2002), Fukuyama and Sevig (1999)
Forgiveness	Enright (2001), Worthington (2005)
Reference sacred writings	Frame (2003), Richards and Bergin (2005)
Meditation	Marlatt and Kristeller (1999), McMinn and McRay (1997)
Spiritual self-disclosure	Richards and Bergin (2005), Richards and Potts (1995)
Encourage altruism and service	McMinn and McRay (1997); Schwartz, Meisenhelder, and Ma (2003)
Spiritual confrontation	Richards and Bergin (2005), Richards and Potts (1995)
Spiritual assessment	Gorsuch and Miller (1999), Hodge (2005)
Spiritual history	Chirban (2001), D'Souza (2003)
Spiritual relaxation and imagery	Frame (2003), Richards and Bergin (2005)
Clarify spiritual values	Fukuyama and Sevig (1999)
Use spiritual community and spiritual programs	Oman and Thoresen (2003), Tan (1996)
Spiritual journaling	Frame (2003)
Experiential focusing method	Frame (2003), Hinterkopf (1994, 1998)
Encourage solitude and silence	Long, Seburn, and Averill (2003); McMinn and McRay (1997)
Use spiritual language and metaphors	Fukuyama and Sevig (1999), Prest and Keller (1993)
Explore spiritual elements of dreams	Bullis (1996), Fukuyama and Sevig (1999)
Spiritual genogram	Frame (2003), Hodge (2001)

inclusion of spirituality into their lives. Similarly, others may prefer to engage in artistic expression, such as drawing, writing poetry, or sculpting; films related to meaning could also be useful.

Next we briefly review how spirituality can be incorporated into a number of traditional theories of therapy followed by spiritually oriented and spiritually accommodative treatments. We then present a clinical case study, followed by a discussion of how to implement spirituality into the treatment of these cases from several different theoretical approaches.

IMPLEMENTATION OF SPIRITUALITY INTO TRADITIONAL THEORIES OF THERAPY

Several traditional therapy theories naturally lend themselves to the implementation of spirituality; for example, existential psychotherapy and spirituality have much in common. However, professionals have failed to explain specifically how to conduct existential psychotherapy in the literature, and this prevents a demonstration of how to implement spirituality into said treatment. In fact, therapists who espouse an existential approach are likely to be implementing spirituality into treatment already, whether consciously or unconsciously.

Other theories can also include spirituality, such as feminist thought, constructivism, and multiculturalism. Feminist therapies promote empowerment, and people who are spiritual can look to spiritual sources for empowerment. Constructivists adhere to focusing on understanding clients' constructions of the world and the subjectivity of these constructions. Hence, they are quick to listen for narratives that include spiritual themes and the meaning making behind the narratives. Multiculturalists, though not possessing a specific theory of change that has been empirically validated, also include spirituality as one of the cultural variables to consider in treatment. As mentioned earlier, the inclusion of spirituality grew from a multicultural framework. Of course, many other theories are not mentioned, but the purpose of this section is to introduce readers to the incorporation of spirituality into just a few of the commonly practiced therapies.

It is important to note that we are not suggesting that spirituality must always be incorporated into mental health treatment. There are obviously situations in which spirituality does not play a part in the treatment modality of choice. Rather, the critical notion we are espousing is awareness by therapists of the inclusion of spirituality in treatment, and that spirituality can be effectively implemented into most theoretical approaches to treatment. Some scholars go further; there have been some explications and evaluations of spiritually accommodative and spiritually oriented approaches to psychotherapy (McCullough, 1999; Sperry & Shafranske, 2005; Worthington & Sandage, 2001). We next review and summarize the literature on spiritually accommodative and spiritually oriented accommodative approaches.

SPIRITUALLY ACCOMMODATIVE
AND SPIRITUALLY ORIENTED APPROACHES

Although many therapists will choose to integrate spirituality into a traditional theoretical orientation, other therapists, depending on clients' beliefs, presenting problem, treatment setting, therapists' training, and therapists' comfort with spirituality, may choose to use a spiritually accommodative or spiritually oriented approach. Spiritually accommodative approaches typically combine a manualized treatment with practices and beliefs from a particular world religion, whereas spiritually oriented approaches are typically less standardized and more inclusive, making them applicable to a broader range of spiritual beliefs and traditions. Before implementing a spiritually accommodative or spiritually oriented approach to treatment implementation, therapists may find it helpful to ask themselves questions similar to the following: "What is the client's presenting problem and diagnosis?" "What is the client's level of spirituality and how might the client's spirituality be either a positive resource or a contributing factor to the presenting problem?" and "Does the setting I am working in have specific guidelines, expectations, or regulations about explicitly integrating spirituality into treatment?" Being mindful of these types of questions will help therapists determine the appropriateness of using a spiritually accommodative or spiritually oriented approach.

Within the spiritually accommodative and spiritually oriented subcategories, one of the most widely examined therapeutic approaches is Christian-accommodative cognitive–behavioral therapy (CBT; McCullough, 1999; Worthington & Sandage, 2001). In essence, this approach uses standard CBT methods in conjunction with aspects of Christianity (e.g., belief in Jesus Christ). Sometimes standard CBT methods are modified for the client; for example, the process of disputing negative cognitions is placed into a religious context (Johnson, DeVries, Ridley, Pettorini, & Peterson, 1994; Johnson & Ridley, 1992; Pecheur & Edwards, 1984; Propst, 1980; Propst, Ostrom, Watkins, Dean, & Mashburn, 1992). These authors described the use of Christian beliefs and imagery, biblical examples, and prayers in the sessions and as part of homework assignments. The literature on spiritually accommodative approaches remains in its infancy and is dominated by Christian approaches. There have been a few studies of Muslim-accommodative CBT (Azhar & Varma, 1995a, 1995b; Azhar, Varma, & Dharap, 1994); however, these studies have been conducted in Malaysia and need to be replicated with other Muslim populations. Building on the work of spiritually accommodative approaches, a number of spiritually oriented approaches have also begun to receive more attention in the literature. For example, Richards and Bergin (e.g., 1997, 2005) have written extensively on theistic-integrative psychotherapy (see chap. 11, this volume), which provides a theistic framework for understanding and addressing clients' spirituality. Similarly, Sperry (2005) also proposed an integrative spiritually oriented psychotherapy approach that is grounded in a biopsychosocialspiritual model, spiritual direction, attachment theory, and G-d-image research.

Overall, scholars (e.g., McCullough, 1999; Worthington & Sandage, 2001) have found no significant differences in the efficacy of treatment when comparing standard and spiritually accommodative and spiritually oriented approaches. Hence, what little we know suggests that standard approaches and spiritually accommodative approaches are equally effective, and as noted by McCullough, the issue becomes one of client preference. That is, highly spiritual or religious clients may seek out a mental health provider who they assume or know shares their values. In addition, these clients are likely to benefit from the use of spiritual or religious interventions (Worthington & Sandage, 2001).

Finally, it is crucial to remember that a host of other factors could affect the course of treatment in relation to spirituality in positive or negative ways. In the following case study, we introduce the client and his presenting concerns, and then we examine the issue of spirituality in treatment in the context of four psychotherapeutic frameworks.

CASE STUDY

Edward Peters is a 44-year-old married man. He is the youngest of three children born to an intact Orthodox Jewish couple living in Brooklyn, New York.[1] He reported no problems during his childhood years with regard to academic, social, and emotional functioning; he indicated having satisfactory relationships with all of his family members. There is no reported family history of mental illness or substance abuse. During his formative years, Mr. Peters attended a Jewish school for his elementary and secondary education. He and his family were also quite active in their religious community; this went beyond weekly attendance at services to include involvement with community service projects.

Mr. Peters decided to attend a secular college and earned his bachelor's degree in business administration. It was during his college years that he drifted away from his Orthodox upbringing, forgoing his religious upbringing for more conventional activities. During college he met his wife, a secular ethnic Jew, to whom he has been married for the past 19 years. They have two children, a 15-year-old boy and an 11-year-old girl. Religion has not been a major force for the family; only Mr. Peters attends religious services on major Jewish holidays.

Mr. Peters has been employed as an assistant vice president in a privately owned company for the past 10 years, having received two promotions during his tenure with this company. He was recently up for a promotion to vice president, a promotion that he did not receive. As a result, he began to feel emotionally lost, symptoms that he described as being dissatisfied with his life, losing interest in his marriage, and having difficulties at work; the last problem he attributed to not receiving a promotion that he felt was deserved. He also admitted to having an extramarital affair, a relationship that has caused him a great deal of consternation. Mr. Peters is torn between wanting to tell his wife about the affair (which has now ended) and keeping this from her forever. He is feeling a tremendous amount of guilt for his actions, yet sometimes thinks that disclosing the affair might cause more harm than good (i.e., it will hurt his wife and damage their relationship in an irreparable way). Mr. Peters decided

---

[1]For the case presented in this chapter, pseudonyms are used, and identifying details have been altered for confidentiality.

to seek psychotherapy for the first time so that he could try to understand why he is feeling as he does and what if anything he could do to resolve these issues.

IMPLEMENTING SPIRITUALITY IN FOUR APPROACHES

In this section, we present and discuss material related to the case study in terms of how to implement spirituality within some of the more well-known psychotherapeutic frameworks or schools of thought (i.e., cognitive–behavioral, interpersonal, psychodynamic, humanistic). However, before providing these examples, we encourage therapists to consider the following set of questions to facilitate the integration of spirituality into traditional psychotherapeutic frameworks:

1. Is the client interested in, or at least open to, discussing issues of spirituality as part of therapy?
2. How has spirituality been historically conceptualized from my theoretical framework of choice?
3. What values or underpinning beliefs does my theoretical framework of choice share with spirituality? What values or beliefs are at odds with spirituality?
4. How might spirituality be implicitly integrated into my theoretical framework of choice?
5. How might spirituality be explicitly integrated into my theoretical framework of choice?
6. Are there common practices or interventions inherent to my theoretical framework of choice that may appear similar to common spiritual practices or interventions? How might these practices or interventions be used to attend to the spiritual?

We also want to stress that variability exists within how these frameworks are applied by individual therapists. As a result, our subsequent discussions provide some possible ways of implementing spirituality into treatment, but this is not an exhaustive presentation. We discuss the first two theories (cognitive–behavioral and interpersonal) in greater depth and introduce the final two theories (psychodynamic and humanistic). This decision was made because of our own theoretical orientations and preferences for treatment approaches. Interested readers can obtain more information on psychodynamic and humanistic theories from several sources (e.g., Corey, 2004; Corsini & Wedding, 2007).

Cognitive–Behavioral

We present the use of CBT in terms of implementing spirituality into treatment. What follows is an excerpt from a fictionalized therapy session with

Mr. Peters followed by a discussion of the relevant issues vis-à-vis implementing spirituality into CBT. It is important to note that several questions and answers have been condensed here to give readers a general idea of how the approach can incorporate spiritual issues. In addition, we assume that readers can adapt the ideas they find here to a more give-and-take style of interaction.

> Therapist: From our initial discussion I understand the issues you are facing, and I feel the best way to address these issues is through an approach known as cognitive–behavioral therapy, or CBT. In using this method, we will break down the problems that you are experiencing and discuss each of them separately; this is done deliberately to make them more manageable. For each issue that we discuss, we will look at your thoughts and feelings to see how these interact to influence your behavior. I will then help you to understand how some of your thoughts may be based on cognitive distortions, and how these distortions of thinking can lead people to make poor behavioral decisions. We will then discuss how some of your thoughts can be changed to more helpful ones that will ultimately allow your actions to be more successful in the way in which you navigate your life. We are not going to delve into your past; rather, we will be focused on issues of the here and now. I believe that we can break down your issues into three different categories. The first issue you raised deals with your job dissatisfaction, the second issue deals with your marital problems inclusive of the fact that you have entered into an extramarital relationship, and finally you discuss feelings of a lack of pleasure in your daily life. The first issue we will discuss is your job situation; tell me how you feel about your current job and how things are going there for you.

> Client: I feel as though I am not recognized for the work I do. It seems as though everyone is getting ahead at work, and I am stuck in the same old rut. I feel that my family views me as a failure, and that my colleagues at work are all laughing behind my back because I did not get a promotion recently. I seem to lack motivation lately, which leads me to fall behind in my work. This course of events has led me to now dread going to the office each day, as I have almost no passion for the work that I am doing.

> Therapist: If I am hearing you correctly, then, it seems as if your present thoughts and feelings have not been helpful to you and have resulted in your actions at work being less than successful. The situation you present is as follows: You have had past success on your job, but because you did not get the promotion you are feeling embarrassed in front of your colleagues

and family and have lost focus at work, resulting in you not meeting your goals. Your present thought process is not helpful to you achieving positive feelings on your job. Let's discuss how your thoughts and feelings are not beneficial and how we can turn them into more helpful ones. At present, you are angry and feel bad that you did not get the promotion. Was there anything that you could have done differently so as to convince your supervisors that you were the one deserving of the promotion? Was the individual who received the promotion more deserving of the same than you? How can you refocus your energies at work and change the way you think about things?

Client: Well, I guess that I have lost my focus at work because of my marital problems. I have not been as productive as I had in the past, and in fact the person who received the promotion not only had more experience than me in the area into which she was promoted but over the last number of months she had been more productive than me, with her section outproducing mine by a significant number. I also think that I have been more aloof with my coworkers, isolating myself in my office and not participating in any office-related activities. I used to joke around with them and join them for lunch, things that I am no longer doing. I guess that my feeling of them laughing at me is more my perception of things because of how I am feeling and not really what they are feeling. I have to separate out my personal life from my professional life, with me devoting more energy to accomplishing tasks at work, and meeting if not exceeding expectations. I will make a conscious effort to interact more with my colleagues and to show them that I am part of the team. I will show my boss how good I am and work toward receiving a promotion in the future.

Therapist: Let's discuss your marriage—what kinds of thoughts and feelings are you having about this relationship?

Client: After 19 years I guess the passion has gone out of our relationship. I feel lost when I come home—as if no one is there for me. I feel that I have no one to turn to for support. She has taken me away from my parents and siblings because she is not religious and feels uncomfortable with all of the rituals and traditions adhered to by my parents. For example, my parents rarely come to our house because we don't keep kosher, and they never eat here. As you might guess, this has caused some friction between my wife and my parents. My wife, for one, resents their behavior and feels that my parents don't love our children or us; to make matters worse, they spend much more time with my siblings and their respective families. Now I've tried to explain to her that this is because my siblings (a) live near my parents, (b) still adhere to the Orthodox Jewish traditions, and (c) attend the same synagogue as my parents. My wife does not want to hear my explanation, and she thinks I am excusing their behavior. Perhaps as a reaction, she makes a big deal about her family and generally ignores mine. I also feel that my wife is no longer interested in me sexually or emotionally and spends more time with her friends and our children than she does with me. She hasn't noticed how badly I feel at work, and she never asks me how my day went. I just come home, eat dinner, watch TV, and go to bed. There seems to be nothing else for me. Even my kids seem to have drifted away from me and don't seem to want to spend time with me. I guess that's why I went outside of the relationship to find satisfaction that I wasn't getting at home.

Therapist: It seems as if your thoughts of being lost spiritually have translated into your feeling rejected by your parents and siblings as well as your wife and children. Rather than discussing your feelings with each family member, you have chosen to keep them inside of you, which has led you to feel sad and rejected and as if your home life is without passion. As you have distanced yourself from your family, you have sought out an extramarital relationship to make you feel better. However, this relationship caused a paradoxical effect in that it only contributed to you feeling more emotionally in turmoil.

Client: Are you Jewish? Do you understand what it means to be raised in an orthodox home and then break away from the faith?

Therapist: It sounds like you are concerned that I might not be able to relate to your experience? For now, I think it is important that we continue to focus on what you have shared. I understand that you feel as if your life has recently seemed to be a series of obstacles that have distracted you and prevented you from exploring your inner feelings. When you were younger you were able to use your religion as a way of getting in touch with your feelings and thoughts and help you cope with the stress of various life situations. In so doing you were able to find ways to resolve your inner conflicts and feel emotionally peaceful. Since you left the fold of Orthodox Judaism, I've got the sense that you've felt somewhat disconnected from your own spirituality. Would you agree?

Client: I think that is a fair assessment.

Therapist: It seems that you have closed yourself off from all things that have given you support in the past—God, your parents and siblings, and your wife and children. Hence, you may have lost your sense of spirituality that has caused you to lose a sense of awareness about yourself and your place in the world. When you were able to get in touch with these sources of support, they helped you with your thoughts and feelings. Now you seem to be riddled with feelings of guilt; thoughts you have problems dealing with that have left you feeling lost, alone, and unaware of the feelings inside of you. To become more self-aware, consider examining your emotional state of mind and your spirituality—this may help you gain insight. Consider asking yourself what can make you happy and satisfied in relationships with parents, siblings, wife, and children. Also consider asking yourself if you were happier when you had a relationship with your God, and does this relationship have to be done in the context of formal religion or can you achieve a sense of spirituality in the temple of yourself. What actions have you engaged in that have been less than productive? How can you change your thoughts and actions so that they can help you achieve healthier relationships?

Client: I guess you are saying that I have walled myself off from everything that had given me support in the past. I guess I have. My wife used to want to talk to me about work, but recently I have put her off, so I guess she stopped asking. I need to try and open the lines of communication between us. I haven't really spent much time with my kids lately, not asking them about school or what they are doing. It seems as though my lack of communication with them has created a wall between us. I have to do things to change that and bring them back into my life. I guess part of the sexual problem is that I think that my wife doesn't want me—but the truth is I have not recently expressed an interest in having sex with her. Maybe I have to think about how she feels about me differently and try to bring romance back into our relationship. I guess I have to stop looking outside of the relationship for satisfaction. I also never told my wife how I feel about my parents and them not being an important part of my life is bothering me. Is it possible that my parents don't feel comfortable in my home because we do not keep kosher? I never thought of this. Maybe I have to make more of an effort to get close to my parents. I could extend myself more to them, and perhaps tell them that I will order out kosher food when they come over and have a special set of dishes to be used for them when they come over so that they feel more comfortable. I was raised in a home where achievement was paramount and I feel that my family does not understand me since I left the religious practices that I was raised with. My family has always associated religion with a sense of belonging, and I guess the fact that I don't practice my faith anymore means that I don't belong. I feel that I let everyone down and that no one understands me, not even God. I feel like a hypocrite when I enter a synagogue, as if they know that I drifted from my Orthodox roots.

Therapist: Have you considered incorporating your religious/spiritual beliefs into your everyday life? It seems that you have inculcated a good deal of personal stress and you have a less-than-positive image of yourself. When you had the formalized belief system of Orthodox Judaism, there was a covenant of faith that you could follow. However, since you have separated your spiritual life from your secular life, this fragmentation has caused you to feel less than in touch with your feelings, feeling adrift as if you do not belong anywhere. Identify your thoughts that have led to these feelings so we can examine them. You can still find your sense of spirituality and incorporate this into your everyday life.

Client: Are you saying that I have to attend synagogue?

Therapist: No, I am suggesting that you have a sense of guilt over events in your life, from your lack of religious identification to your marriage and your job. Search for what is important to you in your life and how you relate to these issues. If you feel that such a search can be facilitated by attendance at a religious service, that is fine, but please recognize that this search can also be facilitated by a personal search of your own thoughts and feelings—getting in touch with all of them and incorporating all of them into your life.

Client: I guess I have to change a lot of thoughts I have. I have to start to feel connected to people and events in my life so as to feel whole, and this includes accepting my religion, my parents, my wife, my children, and my job as all important elements of my life.

At the midpoint in this session, Mr. Peters noted several thoughts, feelings, and actions, which the therapist was able to help him differentiate between in terms of what was helpful and what was not. The therapist did a good job in refocusing Mr. Peters's thoughts as they relate to his job. However, the therapist did not address the issue of the client's loss of passion. The initial failure to do so prevented a discussion of the client's spiritual well-being. As the session progressed, the therapist recognized the importance that Mr. Peters's faith had in his life and the fact that the separation of his spirituality from his secular life contributed to a sense of anomie and lack of meaning that contributed to problems at home and at work. If the therapist had ignored this aspect of the client's life, an important element of the client's past that helped him feel integrated and whole would have been ignored, possibly resulting in an inability on the client's part to formulate positive thoughts that would ultimately lead to positive actions. When the therapist helped the client change his thought pattern, the client was able to view his life and the actions he took in a more egosyntonic fashion.

Interpersonal

Integrating spirituality into interpersonal psychotherapy is presented next. Before we begin, it is important to acknowledge that many different approaches to psychotherapy identify themselves as "interpersonal." Our own thinking lies closest to that of those therapists who believe that clients present to and behave with them in treatment as they do with other people in their world. As a result, the therapist experiences the client as others do in her or his life and can provide the client with valuable feedback about how she or he is perceived by others. To effectively implement spirituality into this kind of interpersonal psychotherapy, therapists need to be tuned into issues from clients with a spiritual nature, as well as their own thoughts and feelings about spirituality; the former helps the therapist recognize when spirituality is a necessary part of the discussion, and the latter helps ensure that the therapist's own biases do not interfere with the process (e.g., for those who hold a less-than-positive view of spirituality and religion). There are many techniques associated with our understanding of interpersonal psychotherapy; one example is detailed inquiry. Next we present the use of this technique vis-à-vis the implementation of spirituality into Mr. Peters's treatment.

In helping Mr. Peters better understand himself and the origins of his difficulties, the therapist can use detailed inquiry as a means to bring spirituality into the discussion. Detailed inquiry is a process by which the therapist explores aspects of the client's experiences to get a full picture of the situation, with a specific focus on the interpersonal aspects of the issues at hand. To effectively implement spirituality into counseling and psychotherapy, however, the therapist needs to listen for key words and phrases (e.g., peace, sacred) or ideological expressions (e.g., fatalism) that signal the potential presence of an underlying spiritual concern. The detailed inquiry can then be used effectively and empathically to facilitate the client's exploration of this material in session. Following is an interpersonal therapy case vignette that shows how a skill such as detailed inquiry can lead to the incorporation of spirituality in Mr. Peters's treatment.

Client:	Things are just not going well at work, and things at home are not any better. There is no peace in my life, and I just feel lost.
Therapist:	Tell me more about your problems at work. How are things with your supervisor? Your coworkers? How do you feel you've been performing on the job lately?
Client:	Well, I get along with everyone fine, and I think I am doing my job OK. However, I was just passed over for a promotion, so I guess my supervisor does not think too highly of me, but I've never talked with her about it.
Therapist:	So perhaps there is an outlet for you to get some feedback from your supervisor on how you are doing on the job, and how you can increase the likelihood of getting a promotion the next time one is available. And how about your problems at home? How are things with your wife? What are you typical interactions like lately? How are your relationships with your children?
Client:	Most of the family ignores me at home. I come home from work, eat dinner, watch TV, and go to bed. My kids typically ask my wife for whatever they need, and my wife seems more interested in her friends than me. So, I sit in front of the "boob tube" and fall asleep.
Therapist:	Sounds like you can always try to reconnect with your family by getting involved in their lives when you get home from work.

Here, after reflecting on the client's earlier use of words like "peace" and "feeling lost," the therapist realizes that spirituality could be playing a role in the client's problems and brings that into the detailed inquiry.

Client:	Things are just not going well at work, and things at home are not any better. There is no peace in my life, and I just feel lost.
Therapist:	I'd like to hear more from you about the problems you are having at work and at home. I am curious, however; what do you mean when you say there is no peace in your life? In what way or ways do you feel lost? I am getting the sense from listening to you that your overall perception is that you've somewhat lost your place in the world and are feeling disconnected from important people and activities in your life.
Client:	Well, I do think that I am alone, and perhaps that is partly because I am disconnected from my family; this disconnect is mainly caused by my leaving Orthodox Judaism and the

repercussions of that decision. These include my parents rarely visiting us, never eating at our home, and not being very involved in our life or the life of our kids. My spirituality was a strong component of my life when I was younger— it was very helpful to me during difficult times. Since I feel that nothing is going right in my life right now, I think my feeling lost is that I am without that stabilizing force and sense of security from which I can draw strength.

Therapist: Sounds like this loss is a pivotal issue for you that touches on all of your presenting concerns and something we need to discuss more.

Although these interactions are fairly brief, we hope the difference is clear in terms of the therapist's choice of focus. Whereas the initial focus sought to obtain more information regarding the difficulties Mr. Peters was having in vocational and interpersonal spheres of functioning, the latter focus recognized a potential spiritual component to his complaints, and as a result, led to a more holistic conceptualization of his difficulties. The course of the treatment in each vignette will take a different trajectory because of the attention to spirituality. In sum, interpersonal psychotherapy is a good fit for the implementation of spirituality. The provision of interpersonal feedback and facilitative exploration can assist clients with improving their psychological functioning; this is also likely to enhance their spiritual well-being.

Psychodynamic

Despite Freud's views regarding religion, it is quite possible for therapists who espouse a psychodynamic theoretical orientation to implement spirituality into their clinical work. Next we use two examples to illustrate this. First, we present an example of when a therapist misses an opportunity to incorporate spirituality into the treatment.

Client: Things are just not going well at work, and things at home are not any better. There is no peace in my life, and I just feel lost.

Therapist: Say more about these issues so we can explore your emotions further.

Client: I just feel like nothing in my life is going right. It seems like I am not recognized for anything I do, either at home or work. It's as if everybody is against me and ignoring my potential. At work I got passed over for a promotion, and at home my wife ignores me. In fact, she seems to pay more attention to everybody else other than me.

Therapist: It seems as if you are feeling adrift, lost in the world and mis-understood by everyone in your life, and this has led to some depression. You seem to have tried to cope by having an affair so as to reconnect with someone in the world, but this has not worked. In fact, it might have had a paradoxical effect and made you feel even more isolated.

Client: Part of this may be right, and I realized the part about why I had an affair, but this does not seem to deal with how I am feeling right now.

In the next segment, the therapist realizes that spirituality could be playing a role in the client's problems and addresses this in the session.

Client: Things are just not going well at work, and things at home are not any better. There is no peace in my life, and I just feel lost.

Therapist: It seems as if you are feeling adrift and lost in the world. It seems that you think these feelings are due to issues at work and home, and to some degree you are correct. However, it is interesting that you omitted the absence of spirituality and religion in your life over the past 25 years. Perhaps your feelings and behaviors are related to a disconnection from your spiritual self.

Client: I guess I didn't think of that. I used to get a great deal of personal satisfaction from going to services, as it allowed me to engage in self-reflection regarding the issues and events from my life. This is something that I have not done for a long time and is probably why I sought out mental health treatment at this point in my life. My drift from my religion of origin has contributed significantly to the psychological distance between my parents and me. They don't visit very often, and everyone is uncomfortable during their few short visits. I feel bad about this; I love my parents and would like to have a better relationship with them. I also think that my marital problems are linked to this as well.

In the first segment, the client let the therapist know that there was some content missed in the interpretation delivered. Specifically, the connection was not made between the client's feeling lost and his disconnection from his family and religion of origin. In the second segment, the interpretation provided by the therapist incorporated the spirituality component, which tapped into the client's core issues. By attending to issues related to spirituality and religion, psychodynamically oriented therapists have the potential to facilitate increased insight in their clients. In fact, we would posit that the search for spiritual well-being is akin to psychodynamic treatment—to understand oneself better.

Humanistic

Therapists who espouse a humanistic approach to treatment typically conceptualize their clients in terms of Maslow's (1958) hierarchy of needs. However, these humanistic professionals can use their therapeutic skills (e.g., reflection) to tap into religious and spiritual content. In thinking about Mr. Peters, it would be fair to say that his problems would place him in the Love/Belonging stage of Maslow's hierarchy. This is because he evidences inter-personal difficulties at work and at home and generally is having problems with feeling loved and feeling like he belongs. Although this conceptualization is accurate, it fails to recognize the spiritual component to Mr. Peters's difficulties. By attending to the underlying feeling of spiritual disconnection, the human-istic therapist can work with the client on all of the areas of dysfunction. That is, Mr. Peters's problems at home and work, along with his inability to cope effectively with them, seem to be a result of his disconnection from his religion and family of origin. Of course, the skills of empathy, genuineness, and uncon-ditional positive regard would still be of use here. In fact, for the therapist to be genuine, she or he must understand her or his own feelings about spirituality and religion. In sum, conceptualizing Mr. Peters's problems more holistically and reflecting them as such would be an effective way to incorporate spiritual-ity into the humanistic approach to mental health treatment.

CONCLUSION

We see the implementation of spirituality into treatment the way Yalom (1980) saw existential issues: Spirituality and spiritual issues are present in a lot of clients if both client and therapist are open to seeing or hearing about those issues. This task may not be easy at times; however, we feel that this approach can bear great fruit for those therapists willing to try. In addition, for those seeking a spiritually accommodative or spiritually oriented approach to treatment, it is clear that we need a greater diversity of models that represent the broad spectrum of spiritual beliefs and worldviews beyond Christianity (e.g., Buddhism, Hinduism, and Judaism). Understanding the spiritual and religious needs of clients allows therapists to use a more complete battery of treatment approaches and options.

REFERENCES

American Psychological Association. (2002). *Guidelines on multicultural education, training, research, practice, and organizational change for psychologists*. Washington, DC: Author.

Azhar, M. Z., & Varma, S. L. (1995a). Religious psychotherapy as management of bereavement. *Acta Psychiatrica Scandinavia*, *91*, 223–235.

Azhar, M. Z., & Varma, S. L. (1995b). Religious psychotherapy in depressive patients. *Psychotherapy and Psychosomatics*, *63*, 165–173.

Azhar, M. Z., Varma, S. L., & Dharap, A. S. (1994). Religious psychotherapy in anxiety disorder patients. *Acta Psychiatrica Scandinavia*, *90*, 1–3.

Bullis, R. K. (1996). *Spirituality in social work practice*. Philadelphia: Taylor & Francis.

Chirban, J. T. (2001). Assessing religious and spiritual concerns in psychotherapy. In T. G. Plante & A. C. Sherman (Eds.), *Faith and health: Psychological perspectivas* (pp. 265–290). New York: Guilford Press.

Corey, G. (2004). *Theory and practice of counseling and psychotherapy* (7th ed.). Belmont, CA: Wadsworth.

Corsini, R. J., & Wedding, D. (Eds.). (2007). *Current psychotherapies* (8th ed.). Belmont, CA: Wadsworth.

Curtis, R. C., & Glass, J. S. (2002). Spirituality and counseling class: A teaching model. *Counseling and Values*, *47*, 3–12.

D'Souza, R. (2003). Incorporating a spiritual history into a psychiatric assessment. *Australasian Psychiatry*, *11*, 12–15.

Eck, B. E. (2002). An exploration of the therapeutic use of spiritual disciplines in clinical practice. *Journal of Psychology and Christianity*, *21*, 266–280.

Enright, R. D. (2001). *Forgiveness is a choice: A step-by-step process for resolving anger and restoring hope*. Washington, DC: American Psychological Association.

Frame, M. W. (2003). *Integrating religion and spirituality into counseling: A comprehensive approach*. Belmont, CA: Brooks/Cole.

Fukuyama, M. A., & Sevig, T. D. (1999). *Integrating spirituality into multicultural counseling*. Thousand Oaks, CA: Sage.

Gorsuch, R. L., & Miller, W. R. (1999). Assessing spirituality. In W. R. Miller (Ed.), *Integrating spirituality into treatment: Resources for practitioners* (pp. 47–67). Washington, DC: American Psychological Association.

Greenson, R. R. (1967). *The technique and practice of psychoanalysis*. New York: International Universities Press.

Halbur, D., & Halbur, K. V. (2006). *Developing your theoretical orientation in counseling and psychotherapy*. Boston: Allyn & Bacon.

Hinterkopf, E. (1994). Integrating spiritual experiences in counseling. *Counseling and Values*, *38*, 165–175.

Hinterkopf, E. (1998). *Integrating spirituality in counseling: A manual for using the experiential focusing method*. Alexandria, VA: American Counseling Association.

Hodge, D. R. (2001). Spiritual genograms: A generational approach to assessing spirituality. *Families in Society*, *82*, 35–48.

Hodge, D. R. (2005). *Spiritual assessment: Handbook for helping professionals*. Botsford, CT: North American Association of Christians in Social Work.

Johnson, W. B., DeVries, R., Ridley, C. R., Pettorini, D., & Peterson, D. R. (1994). The comparative efficacy of Christian and secular rational–emotive therapy with Christian clients. *Journal of Psychology and Theology, 22,* 130–140.

Johnson, W. B., & Ridley, C. R. (1992). Brief Christian and non-Christian rational–emotive therapy with depressed Christian clients: An exploratory study. *Counseling and Values, 36,* 220–229.

Knox, S., Catlin, L., Casper, M., & Schlosser, L. Z. (2005). Addressing religion and spirituality in psychotherapy: Clients' perspectives. *Psychotherapy Research, 15,* 287–303.

Long, C. R., Seburn, M., & Averill, J. R. (2003). Solitude experiences: Varieties, settings, and individual differences. *Personality and Social Psychology Bulletin, 29,* 578–583.

Marlatt, G. A., & Kristeller, J. L. (1999). Mindfulness and meditation. In W. R. Miller (Ed.), *Integrating spirituality into treatment: Resources for practitioners* (pp. 47–67). Washington, DC: American Psychological Association.

Maslow, A. H. (1958). Higher and lower needs. In C. L. Stacey & M. DeMartino (Eds.), *Understanding human motivation* (pp. 48–51). Cleveland, OH: Allen.

McCullough, M. E. (1999). Research on religion-accommodative counseling: A meta-analysis. *Journal of Counseling Psychology, 46,* 92–98.

McCullough, M. E., & Larson, D. B. (1999). Prayer. In W. R. Miller (Ed.), *Integrating spirituality into treatment: Resources for practitioners* (pp. 85–110). Washington, DC: American Psychological Association.

McMinn, M. R., & McRay, B. W. (1997). Spiritual disciplines and the practice of integration: Possibilities and challenges for Christian psychologists. *Journal of Psychology and Theology, 25,* 102–110.

Oman, D., & Thoresen, C. (2003). Spiritual modeling: A key to spiritual and religious growth? *International Journal for the Psychology of Religion, 13,* 149–165.

Pecheur, D. R., & Edwards, K. J. (1984). A comparison of secular and religious versions of cognitive therapy with depressed Christian college students. *Journal of Psychology and Theology, 12,* 45–54.

Prest, L. A., & Keller, J. F. (1993). Spirituality and family therapy: Spiritual beliefs, myths, and metaphors. *Journal of Marital and Family Therapy, 19,* 137–148.

Propst, R. L. (1980). The comparative efficacy of religious and non-religious imagery for the treatment of mild depression in religious individuals. *Cognitive Therapy and Research, 4,* 167–178.

Propst, R. L., Ostrom, R., Watkins, P., Dean, T., & Mashburn, D. (1992). Comparative efficacy of religious and non-religious cognitive–behavioral therapy for the treatment of clinical depression in religious individuals. *Journal of Consulting and Clinical Psychology, 60,* 94–103.

Richards, P. S., & Bergin, A. E. (1997). *A spiritual strategy for counseling and psychotherapy.* Washington, DC: American Psychological Association.

Richards, P. S., & Bergin, A. E. (2005). *A spiritual strategy for counseling and psychotherapy* (2nd ed.). Washington, DC: American Psychological Association.

Richards, S. P., & Potts, R. W. (1995). Using spiritual interventions in psychotherapy: Practices, successes, failures, and ethical concerns of Mormon psychotherapists. *Professional Psychology: Research and Practice, 26*, 163–170.

Schlosser, L. Z. (2003). Christian privilege: Breaking a sacred taboo. *Journal of Multicultural Counseling and Development, 31*, 44–51.

Schlosser, L. Z., Foley, P. F, Poltrock, E. S., & Holmwood, J. R. (in press). Why does counseling psychology exclude religion? A content analysis and methodological critique. In J. G. Ponterotto, J. M. Casas, L. A. Suzuki, & C. M. Alexander (Eds.), *Handbook of multicultural counseling* (3rd ed.). Thousand Oaks, CA: Sage.

Schwartz, C., Meisenhelder, J. B., & Ma, Y. (2003). Altruistic social interest behaviors are associated with better mental health. *Psychosomatic Medicine, 65*, 778–785.

Sedgwick, D. (1994). *The wounded healer: Countertransference from a Jungian perspective*. New York: Routledge.

Sue, D. W. (1982). Position paper: Cross-cultural counseling competencies. *The Counseling Psychologist, 10*, 45–52.

Sperry, L. (2005). Integrative spiritually oriented psychotherapy. In L. Sperry & E. P. Shafranske (Eds.), *Spiritually oriented psychotherapy* (pp. 307–329). Washington, DC: American Psychological Association.

Sperry, L., & Shafranske, E. P. (Eds.). (2005). *Spiritually oriented psychotherapy*. Washington, DC: American Psychological Association.

Tan, S. Y. (1996). Religion in clinical practice: Implicit and explicit integration. In E. P. Shafranske (Eds.), *Religion and the clinical practice of psychology* (pp. 365–387). Washington, DC: American Psychological Association.

Worthington, E. L. (Ed.). (2005). *Handbook of forgiveness*. New York: Brunner-Routledge.

Worthington, E. L., & Sandage, S. J. (2001). Religion and spirituality. *Psychotherapy, 38*, 473–478.

Yalom, I. D. (1980). *Existential psychotherapy*. New York: Basic Books.

Zinnbauer, B. J., & Pargament, K. I. (2000). Working with the sacred: Four approaches to religious and spiritual issues in counseling. *Journal of Counseling and Development, 78*, 162–171.

10

SPIRITUALITY IN THERAPY TERMINATION

JAMIE D. ATEN, MICHAEL W. MANGIS, CLARK CAMPBELL, BRENT T. TUCKER, AHMED NEZAR KOBEISY, AND RANDALL HALBERDA

Termination of therapy is as important as the initial phase
—Gerald Corey

Some people believe that therapy never ceases, that clients continue their dialogues with us for the rest of their lives.
—Jeffrey Kottler

Termination is meant to solidify the transition from clients' reliance on therapists to bring change in their life to a reliance on internalized strengths and insights that maintain the progress realized in therapy. Although the termination stage is an important part of the therapeutic process and some researchers have focused attention on termination in more recent years (e.g., Joyce, Piper, Ogrodniczuk, & Klein, 2006), termination has received relatively little attention in the mental health literature. The topic of termination has traditionally been the "dirty little secret" of counseling and psychotherapy, and novice therapists are often left to figure out the process on their own accord (Schlesinger, 2005). For these very reasons, it is important that termination be addressed in this book, not only by highlighting this understudied stage of treatment but also by bringing attention to an even further understudied topic: the role of spirituality in termination. Thus, the purpose of this chapter is to provide a strategy for addressing spirituality during termination. Common spiritual issues that are often encountered by therapists during termination are also highlighted. Before discussing how spirituality can be integrated into this stage of the therapeutic process, we provide a conceptual framework for understanding termination.

CONCEPTUALIZATION OF TERMINATION

Whether a client pursues short- or long-term counseling, termination is the goal of every psychotherapy relationship. Termination should be viewed as a unique stage of therapy, not simply just the pronouncement of completion at the last therapy session. Psychotherapy is considered successful when sufficient changes have been made in the client's life that therapy is no longer needed, at least on a continual basis. In many respects, termination can be viewed as a launching of sorts for clients, because one of the primary objectives of therapy is to foster client independence (Bertolino & O'Hanlon, 2002). Another core objective of termination is to provide clients with a healthy ending to the therapeutic relationship, thereby modeling appropriate behaviors for saying goodbye. Termination can also provide a summarizing of clients' progress and growth and prepare clients for challenges they may face in the future (Corey, 2005).

Termination can occur at the instigation of either the mental health professional or the client. Many therapists have a mental picture of an ideal termination situation, creating a deceptive impression that all or even most therapies come to a textbook ending. In reality, terminations take many forms, ranging from no formal termination (i.e., client does not return to therapy) to a termination experience extending over multiple sessions (Murdin, 2000). In fact, most therapists will acknowledge that some clients simply disappear without termination even being acknowledged or brought to completion. Another common experience among therapists is the "surprise ending," in which the client comes to a session and announces that he or she does not need to come back to therapy. If the goals are short term in nature, this may be appropriate. Yet, in this scenario, a list of possibilities typically runs through the mental health professional's mind that may account for the unexpected announcement, including "Have I been ignoring the client's readiness for termination?" or "Is the client dissatisfied with therapy?" It is usually preferable at such times to request another session to discuss the ending of the therapy unless external pressures do not allow for it (e.g., sudden job transfer).

Although it is common for clients to terminate prematurely, therapists can increase the likelihood of having a more therapeutic and planned termination with clients by beginning to prepare for and discuss termination throughout the entire therapeutic process (Hill & O'Brien, 1999). In these more ideal instances, the intensity and length of the therapeutic relationship usually define the length of the termination phase. A 6-week series of sessions aimed at phobia desensitization hardly necessitates the same type of termination process as a 3-year course of intensive psychotherapy facilitating recovery from childhood parental abandonment. Overall, the termination stage of therapy often varies across a continuum, depending on the client's presenting problem(s). On one end of the continuum, termination may be quite brief and require little planning or preparation. On the other end, termination may cover several weeks and stimulate some of the most intensive work of the entire course of therapy (Walsh, 2007). For example, a client with particular vulnerabilities to loss resulting from bereavement and abandonment issues may benefit from a more gradual termination than, say, a client who sought brief solution-focused therapy for vocational issues. Likewise, therapists may consider transitioning from weekly to biweekly sessions, to monthly sessions, to a formal termination session (Cormier & Hackney, 2005).

Given the client's presenting problem(s), the termination stage of treatment can even look qualitatively different and have different goals from the sessions leading up to termination. The way the termination stage will look and the goals that are set largely depend on the level of closure needed by the client. For example, Freud and other theorists have often likened psychotherapy to surgery; closure of the surgical field marks the end of the surgery and the transition to the stage whereby the body can begin healing the wound and readjusting to the changes that have been made (Stepansky, 1999). This analogy is apt when applied to psychotherapeutic termination, as clients may have experienced dramatic changes in their internal and external worlds during therapy. To abruptly end the therapeutic relationship can be similar to the surgeon leaving the operating room without closing up the surgical opening. Like surgeries, some therapies have been brief and minimally invasive and therefore require minimal closure because the wound was small. The more in-depth the therapy, the more time is required to reduce the intensity of the therapeutic relationship for the client and to help the client adjust and end the relationship.

TEMPLATE FOR ADDRESSING SPIRITUALITY IN TERMINATION

The termination stage of treatment can provide opportunities for spiritually attuned therapists to address spiritual issues and matters. Most clients lack appropriate interpersonal models for ending healthy relationships (Schlesinger, 2005). Thus, clients may rely on their spiritual beliefs or past experiences with spirituality or spiritual communities to make sense of the therapeutic relationship that is coming to an end. Clients may also on some level, whether consciously or unconsciously, draw from these resources as models for gaining closure. For example, most spiritual traditions offer rituals or experiences to help people find closure, from a corporate prayer being said at the end of a spiritual meeting to a benediction at a funeral being offered by a spiritual leader. Even nonspiritual clients have likely encountered these types of spiritual rituals (e.g., a spiritual ceremony at a wedding) and may draw from these experiences because of their familiarity. Clients who are more spiritually committed may even expect the spiritual to be used or incorporated into termination. That is, spiritually committed clients who use their beliefs to interpret and facilitate endings in other situations will likely want to do the same in the termination stage, even if spirituality has not been explicitly addressed in the earlier stages of treatment. The following sections offer a template to assist therapists in their efforts at successfully addressing spirituality in termination.

Therapists Engage in Self-Reflection

Therapists should engage in self-reflection when approaching termination to reflect on their previous experiences with spirituality and endings, both professionally (e.g., termination sessions with clients) and personally (e.g., loss of a close friend; see chap. 3, this volume, on self-awareness for specific strategies). For a number of different reasons, many therapists report that they feel uncomfortable with the termination process. This may occur because termination is a form of loss for both clients and therapists, which tends to recapitulate unresolved or painful issues from previous losses from the clients' and therapists' lives (Capuzzi & Gross, 2007). For instance, the experience of termination for clients and therapists may lead to revisiting difficult situations and strong emotions connected to spiritual strain. According to Exline and Rose (2005), spiritual strain often occurs when people feel abandoned by God or blame God for negatively perceived events. Consider a therapist who lost a parent to illness as an adolescent, which caused her to reject her faith tradition out of anger toward God. If this therapist has not engaged in self-reflection and tried to work through this experience, then any experience of loss during termination could potentially trigger negative responses connected to her unresolved spiritual strain. In return, she may be unable to properly attend to her clients' needs.

Another reason that therapists avoid termination is because they have had a negative past experience with a client in the termination process, which can make them feel apprehensive and even doubt their mastery over this final stage of treatment. These feelings of apprehension and doubt can be heightened even more by particular topics such as spirituality. For instance, a colleague once shared a time when he was nearing the end of a termination session when suddenly the client began to pray a blessing on behalf of the therapist. Taken completely off guard, the therapist awkwardly ended the session just moments into the client's prayer and quickly walked the client in silence out to the waiting room. This therapist said he had always regretted how he dealt with this client's spirituality and always dreaded that a similar situation might reoccur with another client. A few years later, through deep self-reflection, this therapist realized not only that he was afraid spiritual matters might surface during termination but also that he had been unwittingly blocking his clients from expressing their spirituality during this phase of treatment. He acted to protect his needs likely at the cost of some of his clients' needs. Thus, self-reflection is useful in assessing therapists' motives to assure that the clients' interests are placed ahead of the interests of the therapists. As one could imagine from the aforementioned examples, the ending of the therapeutic relationship can also have an impact on therapists' affect and may increase the likelihood of counter-transference occurring.

Engaging in self-reflection before terminating with clients is also of particular importance for spiritually oriented therapists who seek to reaffirm their own spiritual understanding of healing through their therapeutic work. Just as therapists who have had negative or less than ideal experiences with spirituality during endings may have their objectivity clouded, therapists who have had positive experiences are also at risk. For example, a spiritually oriented therapist may assume that because a client has discussed spiritual matters over the course of therapy, the client will offer some form of spiritual expression as a symbol of the help received. If the client then makes no such gesture, such as disclosing that he feels God used the therapeutic relationship to bring healing, the therapist may feel hurt. Or, if the therapist is determined to focus on spiritual matters during the last session, the therapist may neglect other important aspects of termination, such as helping the client find closure. Because of their own spiritual beliefs, spiritually oriented therapists may also feel the need to introduce spirituality into the last session because this is how they make meaning of endings. If this has not been discussed prior to the actual termination session, then the client could be caught off guard by such a gesture and made uncomfortable or feel as though the therapist was proselytizing.

Therapists who engage in self-reflection during the termination process also serve as useful models for clients. Therapists can model a variety of ways to address spirituality during the termination process. One way therapists can model spiritual sensitivity for clients is through the use of self-disclosure. If spirituality has been a part of therapy or if therapists suspect a spiritual matter may surface during termination, therapists can share with their clients about how spiritual matters have surfaced in prior therapy relationships. Likewise, if therapists have had a similar spiritual experience as their clients, they may choose to share an experience through appropriate self-disclosure. This could consist of therapists sharing how their spirituality helps them to make meaning and find purpose in endings. Of course, anytime a therapist self-discloses, it must be done with careful consideration of clients' needs and the potential negative effect on clients.

Another way therapists can model self-reflection is by "thinking out loud" with their clients. For instance, take a therapist who is working with a client who had previously been resistant to discussing spirituality but suddenly reports thinking about deep spiritual issues. The therapist could model self-reflection by saying, "I have to admit, I am a little surprised. Before today, it seemed as though you were kind of against anything spiritual. I'm wondering if these spiritual questions you have began asking could somehow be connected to our relationship coming to an end?" Therefore, clients may tacitly observe therapists practicing self-reflection and realize the benefit of this practice for their own ongoing mental health.

Therapists Explore Clients' Existential and Spiritual Questions

Termination is an opportunity to bring closure to a significant emotional and interpersonal experience for clients. Termination also provides an opportunity for enhanced meaning making among many clients as they see the end of the therapeutic relationship approaching. It is not unusual to see a microcosm of the psychotherapy experience play out in the termination process. Thus, termination presents therapists with an opportunity to solidify and enhance therapeutic gains for clients related to spirituality. Intentionally bringing an end to a significant relationship is an unusual experience for anyone. People tend to try and maintain relationships that are fulfilling and only eliminate those that are unfulfilling. Knowing that a relationship is ending can raise several existential and spiritual questions for clients (Mann, 1973).

One question clients may ponder during termination is, "What does my therapy mean about my past, present, and future?" This is a significant question of identity as clients seek to make meaning of their new understanding of themselves. Clients will vary in their awareness of this existential processing, but most, if not all, clients seem to want to put therapeutic insights into a meaningful context in their life stories. As clients approach the end of therapy, there is a heightened effort to solidify meanings gleaned from therapy into a broader life context.

A second existential and spiritual question aroused through termination is, "What do my self-insights mean about my life purpose and relationship to God?" This may directly lead to questions about the nature of the sacred. "What kind of a God would allow bad things to happen?" and "How does God want me to use my distressing experiences in positive ways?" may be questions clients consider as termination approaches. Certainly, the degree to which clients ponder spiritual issues in general will affect the degree to which these questions are addressed directly by clients. However, many clients raise these questions over the course of therapy, and it is common for these questions to be reengaged in the termination process.

Another question clients raise in termination is, "How should I now live?" In other words, once clients have processed distressing emotions, experiences, or memories in therapy, they seek to learn how these experiences may affect their lives now. This question is related to the previous question but is more inwardly focused for clients, whereas the previous question was more focused on God. The previous question also addressed the nature of God, whereas this question addresses the nature of clients' relationship to God. This may lead spiritually open clients to ask themselves and their therapists how God wants them to live their lives with their new understanding of themselves.

A fourth existential or spiritual question involved in termination pertains to clients' relationship with therapists. Because the therapeutic relationship accounts for a significant amount of change obtained through psychotherapy, clients may ask about the nature of their ongoing relationship with their therapists and how this will affect their spirituality. This is especially true for clients who feel that the psychological insights gained from therapy have also led to a deepened sense of spirituality. In other words, clients may ask, "What will my experience with the sacred be like after I stop coming to therapy?" and "How will ending my relationship with my therapist affect other relationships that have provided me purpose and connectedness?" Because psychotherapy involves a unique kind of relationship, clients attempt to understand how this relationship may affect their current and subsequent relationships with others.

Although these existential and spiritual questions may be raised throughout therapy, these questions are intensified through the termination process. Thus, most forms of psychotherapy recommend anticipating the emotional significance of termination and framing it as both a task and a process (Charman & Graham, 2004).

Therapists Facilitate Clients' Spirituality

Therapists should facilitate clients' spirituality in the termination process. As with any other spiritual aspect of psychotherapy, the spiritual orientation and values of the client should be supported and integrated within the termination process. As discussed previously, clients will likely want to explore the transcendent meaning of their insights and behavioral changes. Therapists should enhance and encourage this meaning exploration as a way of solidifying broader therapeutic gains. Spirituality almost always involves particular rituals such as prayer and meditation. These rituals can be affirmed by the therapist as a way of enhancing the spiritual aspect of termination, for example, by allowing a client to say a prayer at the end of a termination session.

For those clients who have expressed a desire to integrate spiritual practices in their lives, termination provides a time for review and application of such practices. To the extent possible earlier in therapy, clients may have already begun to use spiritual practices to accentuate and solidify their gains in treatment. For clients who have struggled with worry and anxiety, meditation may be part of the treatment strategy for reducing baseline anxiety level (Rausch, Gramling, & Auerbach, 2006). The form of meditation used can be drawn from clients' spiritual tradition, and clients may be more likely to use such a relaxation strategy if it ties in with their spiritual lives. Yoga and tai chi can also be encouraged for appropriate clients; for example, research has found that Hindu participants were more open to religious pathways such as yoga (Tarakeshwar, Pargament, & Mahoney, 2003).

Having clients consult spiritual texts for passages of inspiration provides another possible way to integrate spiritual practices into termination. Clients can be encouraged to locate passages of a sacred text that deal with a topic relevant to their presenting issues, such as jealousy, finances, or worry. Clients can be instructed to create a brief list of inspirational teachings they can read over when feeling discouraged. Therapists may also want to consult a leader from the client's spiritual community to discover appropriate passages related to various topics, being careful to protect the client's confidentiality. Sacred texts dealing with transition or taking new responsibility may be particularly appropriate to help clients during the termination process. However, care should be used in referencing spiritual texts outside a therapist's own spiritual tradition because of possible misapplication of texts.

On the whole, sensitivity to the clients' needs and desires will determine the best practice for incorporating spiritual practices and rituals in this process. Therapists should also consult their state and professional ethical codes and guidelines for determining the appropriateness of using spiritual practices. Proper training and supervision are also necessary before using these practices. Lastly, therapists should be informed that although research has shown that spiritual practices can have a positive effect on client mental health, there still remains a great deal of debate over their use in therapy (Chappelle, 2000; Richards, 1995). For instance, Richards and Bergin (2005) noted that arguments have been raised regarding therapist-led spiritual practices that go beyond therapists' scope of professional competency. Additionally, others have stated that engaging in spiritual practices with clients can cloud clients' understanding of therapists' professional role. It has also been noted that making certain spiritual practices a routine in therapy can take away the significance of such practices. Therapists who use spiritual practices may also be at risk for causing clients to perceive therapists as being more spiritual, causing the client to be inhibited or to become dependent on the therapist for spiritual direction (McMinn, 1996). Although more research is needed in this area to bring clarity to this debate, it appears that if handled appropriately, there are major benefits to be had for clients (Tan & Dong, 2001).

Therapists Identify Purpose and Meaning of Clients' Behavior

Therapists should identify the purpose or meaning of their clients' behavior in anticipation of termination. For those clients who identify a spiritual worldview, their behaviors often have spiritual implications (Rose, Westefeld, & Ansely, 2001). As noted earlier, some clients draw from their spiritual experiences or traditions in an effort to make meaning from endings. It is common practice for clients from Christian, Jewish, and Islamic faiths, for example, to engage in spiritually oriented behaviors such as praying as means for managing the transition involved with terminating therapy. This largely stems from the fact that most major spiritual traditions instruct believers to engage in prayer as a means of parting and as a way to show gratitude, provide protection, and share blessings. Clients may wish to express thanks through prayer and continue to outline what and how they need to maintain gains in their communication with God.

Gift-giving behaviors are another way clients often make meaning out of the therapeutic experience (Shapiro & Ginzberg, 2002), which can also stem directly from clients' spiritual beliefs. Almost every major spiritual tradition teaches the importance of giving to others. For example, in Buddhist belief, *dana* (generosity) is considered a universal virtue, and people are expected to give a gift to the monk who has provided spiritual guidance. Not only is giving expected to repay, but Buddhists believe that giving will help a person move further on the path of freedom. In this example, a therapist could offend or even do harm by not accepting the gift (Kaviratna, 1980).

Clients may also give thanks to a Supreme Being for the progress made in therapy during termination, attributing success to the divine. Therapists should not confuse this practice with ungratefulness on the part of clients but rather should understand it as gratitude in an indirect way. In Islam, for instance, when Muslims thank God for the help they receive, they are thanking God for sending a good person (in this case, a therapist) their way (Kobeisy, 2004; Podikunju-Hussain, 2006).

Thus, clients may use and wish to integrate their spirituality into termination through behaviors, such as engaging in a spiritual ritual or practice, as a way to signify the end of the therapeutic relationship. Such behaviors often stem from good intentions and can help clients garner deeper meaning and purpose from the therapy experience. Some clients may wish to engage in a ritual for other reasons, however, such as trying to convert their therapists to a particular spiritual tradition. Therefore, it is important for therapists to identify the purpose and meaning of clients' behavior. Therapists should be cautious not to be reactive toward spiritually latent behaviors in termination. Rather than making assumptions and reacting in a hasty manner, therapists should talk with the client and explore the purpose of the behavior. The reason for this is that some behaviors may look similar on a surface level but have deeper underpinning messages that need to be discussed before intervening.

Therapists Practice Authenticity

Therapists should be genuine and authentic in response to expressions of spirituality during the termination process. Authenticity is a term some therapists use to describe integrity or personal integration. Consistency or integration of thoughts, feelings, and behaviors allows therapists to respond authentically and genuinely. Conversely, inconsistency in these areas of functioning portrays fragmentation and is likely seen by clients as inauthentic (J. B. Miller et al., 2004). Because many clients have experienced interpersonal distress, including deception and lies in their interactions with others, they are particularly sensitive to dishonesty and inconsistencies in therapists' responses. If therapists are not authentic in their responses to clients' spirituality or spiritual issues, clients will likely be able to sense this incongruence. Through genuine and honest therapeutic responses to spirituality in termination, therapists affirm a strong therapeutic alliance and promote interpersonal trust. This is by no means an easy task, especially if therapists feel uncomfortable with how clients are displaying or talking about spirituality. Taking a risk by being open in the here and now makes therapists vulnerable to a number of possible reactions from clients. Therapists may fear that if they share discomfort with spirituality during termination, this may somehow undo the progress clients have made or may upset clients. However, researchers have found that using self-disclosure and immediacy can be useful tools (Farber, Berano, & Capobianco, 2004). This is not to say that being real with clients around spiritual matters will always be perceived positively by clients. Yet, it would appear that if clients are already aware that therapists are not being congruent, not stating so would likely cause more harm to the therapeutic relationship. Likewise, if therapists have a strong negative inner response, this may be indicative that either a new issue has been brought up that should be addressed and resolved during the session or perhaps an additional session is necessary to work through what occurred. The reason for suggesting that an additional session may be warranted is that many clients present "door-knob" statements (e.g., when a client discloses crucial or significant information while leaving the session) during termination (Sommers-Flanagan & Sommers-Flanagan, 2002), which in the framework of this chapter may have a spiritual context.

Although the focus of therapists is always on clients and on how they might benefit most from the therapeutic relationship, therapists are also encouraged not to compromise their own values. Therapists are not required to agree with clients' spiritual beliefs or participate with clients in spiritual practices that they feel uncomfortable with or that conflict with their own worldviews; however, they may find it useful to take an accommodating approach (Worthington & Sandage, 2002). If differences are present, therapists need to decide whether it would be therapeutic to address these differences with clients. It would be counterproductive for therapists to point out every area of disagreement around spiritual issues, just as it would be to overfocus on political differences in therapy.

In most cases, therapists should acknowledge their clients' belief systems and affirm how important those beliefs are for their clients. This may be done as simply as using reflection or restatement skills, such as "I can tell how important your beliefs are to you. It sounds like your faith really helped you through all the struggles you were facing at that time." Therapists then can respect their clients' spiritual beliefs while maintaining their own belief systems by clearly delineating between client and therapist beliefs (Schultz-Ross & Gutheil, 1997). Another way therapists can address differences is to attempt to find commonalities in overarching beliefs, such as valuing hope, optimism, and forgiveness, which most psychotherapies and spiritual traditions teach. Discrepancies between therapists' and clients' beliefs can also be addressed through compromising actions. For example, if a therapist feels uncomfortable with spiritual practices, he or she could allow a client to read an encouraging passage from a sacred text rather than the therapist reading the text out loud, or could allow a client to say a prayer in session rather than the therapist saying the prayer. As noted earlier, many clients want to pray during the last session, yet many therapists feel uncomfortable with this practice. In this case, therapists might say, "I think that you saying a short prayer would be a very kind and meaningful gesture symbolizing our work together. If it is okay, I would like to spend that moment reflecting in silence on our relationship and on what was accomplished." If a client directly asks the therapists to say a prayer, some therapists may also be inclined to respond, "Would you mind saying a prayer for both of us?"

Still, there may be times when the differences between therapists' and clients' beliefs are so discrepant that the differences need to be addressed. Although perhaps a rather extreme example, I (Jamie D. Aten) once worked with a client in a correctional facility whose pagan spirituality was very important to him but was also connected to his racist White supremacy beliefs; it was clear that there were incompatible differences in our worldviews. I communicated that I disagreed with his racist beliefs stemming from his religion but that I thought other aspects of his faith (e.g., thought watching, a form of meditation) could serve as valuable resources for coping and change. I also conveyed that when he disclosed racist attitudes, it made me feel uncomfortable and that it was not appropriate to use words of hate in the session. I gave my client the opportunity to respond and processed our conversation. In cases when there are significant differences in beliefs, therapists should openly and adequately communicate their feelings to their clients without diminishing their clients' beliefs. Therapists should discuss with clients their reasons for feeling uncomfortable and make sure clients understand their reasons for not participating. To avoid turning the conversation into an argument over beliefs or practices, therapists should focus more on the process that has made them uncomfortable rather than on the specific content. Using self-disclosure appropriately in this way will help avoid scenarios that could potentially make clients feel offended and rejected (Genia, 1995). Furthermore, being authentic with clients demonstrates therapists' ability to effectively deal with spiritual issues and validates clients' spirituality.

Therapists Develop Relationships With Spiritual Leaders

Therapists should develop and maintain ongoing relationships with spiritual leaders from diverse faith backgrounds. Researchers have shown that in most cases therapists have overlooked and underused the resources spiritual leaders have to offer (Edwards, Lim, & McMinn, 1999; McMinn, Runner, & Fairchild, 2005; Weaver, 1998). Spiritual leaders, such as clergy, priests, and rabbis, are trained professionals who have unique training and specializations (e.g., spiritual guidance) in spirituality and religion that most therapists lack (Aten, 2004). Although therapists may collaborate with spiritual leaders at any point throughout the therapeutic process (e.g., a client asks that his or her rabbi be included in the treatment process), the importance of such relationships becomes particularly evident during termination. Having ongoing relationships with spiritual leaders can help therapists better anticipate spiritual issues that might arise during termination and identify spiritual opportunities for continued support for clients after termination.

Even though ongoing collaborative relationships between therapists and spiritual leaders are encouraged, therapists who lack an established relationship may find it helpful to collaborate with spiritual leaders during termination in the following instances:

1. Clients request a spiritual leader be used during the termination process (e.g., consultation).
2. Therapists and clients reach a stumbling block in the relationship over spiritual concepts or practices as they are preparing for termination.
3. Therapists do not possess knowledge about spiritual issues, concerns, traditions, teachings, practices, terminology, hopes, or fears presented by clients during the termination process.
4. Clients are interested in getting connected to a spiritual community following treatment.
5. Clients want to receive spiritual guidance from a spiritual leader once treatment is ended.
6. When a spiritual leader or religious services will be part of the posttreatment plan.

Yet, before collaborating with spiritual leaders, therapists must assess how essential collaboration will be to positive client outcomes, the appropriateness of collaboration based on clients' needs and wants, and if collaboration can be done without compromising clients' rights or professional ethical guidelines.

In addition, therapists should consider whether collaborating with spiritual leaders would be beneficial for clients. Numerous examples in the literature demonstrate how therapists collaborating with spiritual leaders can have a positive impact on clients (Flannelly, Stern, & Costa, 2006; McMinn & Dominquez, 2005). However, collaboration is not always appropriate or needed (e.g., clients report no spirituality). For instance, stigma around mental health issues may be stronger in some spiritual communities, particularly minority groups (e.g., Muslims). Some Muslim clients have reported that they would not want to directly involve a spiritual leader who knows them or knows other people who know them for the fear of breaching their confidentiality (Kobeisy, 2004).

When deciding to collaborate with spiritual leaders, therapists need to also determine whether their clients' consent is necessary. In most cases, therapists do not need to receive consent if they simply call a trusted spiritual leader in an effort to better understand an unfamiliar spiritual teaching when no client case information is exchanged. Still, therapists should take caution, as confidentiality can be compromised without giving explicit information (Welfel, 2002). One therapist, for instance, contacted a spiritual leader to ask advice on how to help a woman from the leader's own faith community whose husband was murdered in a brutal robbery. Because the incident was reported in the news and because the woman was a member of the congregation of the spiritual adviser, the spiritual leader was able to identify the client even though no identifying information or context was provided. However, if clients ask to have therapists consult with spiritual leaders about treatment received, then appropriate consent and release forms need to be obtained. Even in these cases when clients request spiritual leaders be included in some form of their treatment, therapists should help clients weigh the potential positives and negatives, as well as revisit the issue of confidentiality before taking action.

Therapists Provide Avenues for Continued Support

Therapists should consider ways to provide clients with continued support that use clients' spirituality after termination. Interpersonal support within the therapeutic alliance provides the foundation for therapeutic gains, and relapse or regression can occur when this support is removed at termination. To prevent this unfortunate circumstance, therapists should consider ways of facilitating support for clients after termination is complete (Cormier & Hackney, 2005). Continued support may involve some periodic contact with therapists, such as prearranged telephone check-ins or notes. A common practice simply involves discussing ways in which clients can develop and enhance their own support system after termination. Clients may be encouraged to communicate their needs more clearly or to identify people who will likely be supportive of their concerns. Moreover, clients can be encouraged to think about how they may garner continued support by using their spirituality (e.g., Senter & Caldwell, 2002; Watlington & Murphy, 2006). As mentioned earlier in this chapter, one way that clients may use their spirituality to find comfort and experience a sense of ongoing support is to continue to engage in the spiritual practices they have found helpful. Getting clients connected to a spiritual community or trusted spiritual leader is another example of how therapists can help clients to use their spirituality as a source of continued support once therapy is terminated (these strategies can also be used from the onset of therapy).

When facing termination, depending on the clients' presenting issue and expressed desire for involvement in spiritual communities, some clients (e.g., clients who are deeply spiritual) make the transition easier when they become more integrated into a spiritual community. Hence, therapists may consider encouraging clients to continue participation in healthy spiritual communities. When doing so, therapists should encourage clients who are interested in getting connected to a spiritual community to search for communities or organizations that match their stated values to increase consistency with ideal and real aspects of self. For example, a Native American client who has reported wanting to get more in touch with his cultural heritage may benefit from participating in powwows and other Native American tribal traditions (Nebelkopf & Phillips, 2004; Trujillo, 2000). Overall, participation in spiritual communities provides opportunities for greater social support, improved meaning-making strategies, enhanced well-being, and more opportunities for facilitating spirituality (e.g., Frazier, Mintz, & Mobley, 2005; McCullough, 2001). Depending on the client's presenting issue and expressed desire for involvement in spiritual communities, such involvement can ease the process of termination. For instance, therapists may encourage clients to begin or continue involvement with a religious organization, such as a local church, synagogue, or temple. Or, therapists may suggest that clients get involved with groups, for example, Alcoholics Anonymous, which have long encouraged connection with participants' Higher Power as part of the recovery process. Furthermore, groups such as Alcoholics Anonymous often facilitate participants' spirituality and use spirituality to help prevent relapses (Galanter, 2006).

Having clients meet with trusted spiritual leaders may also help clients find additional support (Chappelle, 2006). The following are some examples of benefits clients may experience from getting connected to a trusted spiritual leader: (a) receiving pastoral counseling and spiritual guidance; (b) finding out about support systems and resources available in spiritual communities; (c) gaining insight into spiritual practices, doctrines, beliefs, customs, behaviors, and concepts; and (d) developing a deeper understanding of diverse spiritual traditions. Such meetings may also provide clients with a way to gain information about particular spiritual communities prior to getting involved. It gives clients the opportunity to learn of the issues facing those organizations and decide if they still want to participate. Additionally, contacts with trusted spiritual leaders may facilitate easier integration into spiritual communities. Clients may be able to tell if they would be interested in a particular spiritual community or spiritual organization from the style of the leader. If a positive relationship develops, these contacts can facilitate consolidation of skills gained in the therapy process. Psychologically minded spiritual leaders may also be able to help monitor the behaviors of clients once they finish therapy and can recommend further psychotherapy if it appears warranted.

Although connecting or reconnecting with a spiritual community or spiritual leader may prove beneficial for some clients, therapists must exercise caution to avoid adding to clients' expectations. Therapists should encourage clients to consider the potential costs of involvement with a spiritual community or spiritual leader. For example, sometimes congregations or communities caught in division can create additional stress for people forced to choose sides on a controversial issue. Hence, clients should be encouraged to take the initiative and recognize potential positives as well as pitfalls.

Therapists Maintain Boundaries

Therapists should maintain appropriate boundaries throughout and after the termination process. Interpersonal boundaries represent the rules and expectations that regulate relationships. These expectations are often unstated and perhaps unconscious. Firm boundaries provide a therapeutic frame, which in turn supports a strong therapeutic alliance (Akhtar, 2006). Maintaining these boundaries through the termination phase allows clients to continue trusting therapists and provides clients with a firm relational foundation from which to launch out of therapy successfully. Yet, some boundaries, such as engaging in multiple relationships, may not be as clear for clients because of their spiritual backgrounds (Bernstein, 2001; Boyd-Franklin, 1989). For example, clergy often are sought out by parishioners for pastoral counseling and spiritual guidance. It is common for clergy to maintain multiple roles with their parishioners, such as pastor, pastoral counselor, and even friend. Likewise, many spiritual leaders who provide pastoral care or spiritual guidance will continue to engage in ongoing relationships even after individual meetings are finished with counselees. Therefore, clients who have received counsel from spiritual leaders may expect much the same tenuous termination from therapists. To avoid these types of potential problems, therapists should establish clear boundaries from the onset of the therapeutic relationship and reiterate expectations as termination is approaching.

Attending the same place of worship can also pose a unique boundary challenge for therapists who are a part of a spiritual community. Although this challenge is rarer for therapists in large urban and metropolitan areas, it is a much more common occurrence in rural areas or geographical locations where certain spiritual communities are scarce. As Campbell and Gordon (2003) noted, circumstantial contact is not only difficult to avoid but may be inevitable. For instance, there are only a few synagogues in the entire state of Mississippi. Therefore, Jewish therapists in this state may find it difficult to avoid at least minimal contact with former clients of the same tradition. This dilemma can be viewed as analogous to addiction counselors who are often in recovery and have a high probability of attending meetings with clients after termination (W. R. Miller, 1999). According to the Ethical Principles of Psychologists and Code of Conduct (American Psychological Association, 2003), "Multiple relationships that would not reasonably be expected to cause impairment or risk exploitation or harm are not unethical" (Ethical Standard 3.05). For example, if a therapist attends a Bat Mitzvah in a nearby town for his niece and sees a former client and learns that she attends that synagogue, no violation has occurred because this is solely circumstantial. However, if the therapist then plans to join the same synagogue, the opportunity for possible multiple roles may move beyond just chance encounters (G. A. Miller, 2005). In most instances no ethical codes will have been breached nor will any harm have been caused to former clients (Peterson, 1992). Still, therapists need to think carefully about what type of impact it might have on former clients if they are involved in the same spiritual community. A series of probing questions originally developed by W. R. Miller (1999) for addiction counselors who attend 12-step groups have been adapted and are offered to help therapists critically examine boundary issues that can occur when therapists and clients are a part of the same spiritual community:

1. What are the different roles I have with this former client in my spiritual community?
2. Are these roles conflictual with one another or potentially confusing or damaging for my former client?
3. What is the least number of roles I can feasibly have with this former client while attending the same spiritual community?
4. What is my role in this spiritual community with this former client?
5. Are there personal needs of my own that I am trying to have met with my client by being involved in the same spiritual community?
6. Should I consult with another professional about the roles I carry with my former client because we attend the same spiritual community? (p. 275)

If therapists suspect that there may be a chance that they could come into contact with former clients because of the reasons stated earlier, they need to take the initiative to have a conversation to prepare clients for such an occurrence. Therapists who are aware that a client is part of a shared spiritual community in the early stages of treatment may consider referring if other therapists are available. Overall, much of the awkwardness that could surface can be avoided if therapists talk with clients to discuss how possible interactions outside of therapy in public settings will be handled (Backlar, 1996). For example, therapists may tell clients that they generally wait until clients approach them before saying hello in public and that interactions typically do not go beyond a brief greeting. Therapists can also educate clients on what is appropriate and what is not appropriate. This may take the form of therapists informing clients that it is not appropriate to seek guidance or counseling in settings outside of the therapy room. Even if therapists have these discussions with clients, clients may forget or ignore the ground rules laid out. In these instances, therapists will need to revisit the conversation in the here and now with clients to remind them of what was agreed on. If a former client and therapist end up attending the same spiritual community, and the client has a difficult time respecting the established boundaries, the therapist should revisit their ethical codes and guidelines and obtain outside supervision and consultation for how to best approach the issue.

Case Study

The following case brings attention to the way spirituality can surface during termination by highlighting the experience of Tyson, a community mental health therapist who specializes in treating childhood attention-deficit/hyperactivity disorder (ADHD).[1] Specifically, this case recounts how Tyson was caught off guard by the parents of one of his child clients who drew on their spiritual beliefs to make meaning of the termination process, which Tyson felt differed starkly from his atheistic worldview. The case also gives insight into the internal reaction Tyson initially felt and his reported self-talk when the parents introduced the spiritual. How he was able to remain authentic to his beliefs while learning to respect the beliefs of his client's parents is also discussed.

Tyson had spent nearly 9 months working intensely with Billy, an elementary school-age boy who had a severe case of ADHD. At the onset of therapy, Billy's parents brought Billy to therapy feeling hopeless and powerless because their child's symptoms seemed to be worsening. Billy's teachers were always sending notes of frustration home and scheduling what felt like constant parent–teacher conferences. In fact, Billy's parents had begun looking into alternative school programs and the possibility of home schooling. Although change was slow at the beginning of therapy, Billy had begun to respond to the cognitive–behavioral treatment Tyson was using and to drug therapy under the care of a local family practice doctor. However, it was the extra time Tyson put into helping Billy outside of their normal therapy sessions that seemed to really pay off. Through numerous consultation sessions between Tyson and Billy's parents and teachers, Tyson was able to help those in Billy's life stick to a strict behavioral program to which Billy responded well. Tyson also spent numerous hours over that period talking with and consulting with Billy's family doctor about how he was reacting to the prescribed medications and drug therapy.

After months of hard work, to the amazement of Billy's parents, the ADHD symptoms that had caused them so much stress and worry seemed to be under control. For example, Billy had made fantastic progress at school; his grades had improved dramatically as well as his classroom behavior. Thus, Tyson

---

[1]For the case presented in this chapter, pseudonyms are used, and identifying details have been altered for confidentiality.

began preparing Billy and his parents for termination. He talked with them about the purpose of the last session and what the session would be like. Tyson told them he wanted to spend some time looking back at the progress Billy had made, to talk about strategies for continued support, and to say goodbye to one another. Overall, Tyson felt proud of the work he had accomplished with Billy and his parents, as well as the strong therapeutic bond that had evolved. Working with Billy and seeing the type of progress Billy had made helped to reaffirm Tyson's self-efficacy as a therapist. On difficult days, Tyson would often think about the work he had done with Billy as a form of encouragement.

It was finally time for Tyson to formally terminate with Billy and his parents. As they all sat down to start the session, Tyson noticed that Billy's parents had a small wrapped gift. About halfway into the session, Billy's parents began to reflect on the progress Billy had made and offered the wrapped gift to Tyson as a symbol of their appreciation. As Tyson opened the gift, Billy's parents stated that they felt like God had put them all together for a reason and were thankful God had finally helped their little boy. Tyson was completely taken off guard; this was the first time any talk of God or spirituality had surfaced over the past 9 months. Moreover, as an atheist who had negative experiences with spirituality, Tyson felt bothered by what Billy's parents were saying. "What did God have to do with it?" thought Tyson. Other thoughts quickly followed as he distractedly finished opening the gift: "I'm the one who had to start off doing therapy with this kid as he bounced around under the desk and chairs. I'm the one who spent all those hours playing phone-tag with his teachers and doctor." Tyson tried to push these thoughts and his feeling aside when he realized what Billy's parents had bought him, a Christian book called *The Purpose Driven Life* by Rick Warren, an Evangelical Christian pastor.

Billy's parents quickly urged Tyson to look at the words they had inscribed on the front page of the book, thanking him for the work he had done with their child. Still, Tyson had a hard time accepting the gift as he struggled to process their earlier comments. Tyson was familiar with the book, which he felt represented an entirely different set of beliefs and worldview from his atheistic perspective. Tyson did not know how to handle his feelings or confusion; he felt blindsided. He graciously accepted the book from Billy's parents and refocused the attention back onto the progress Billy had made and on their role as parents. The rest of the termination session was rather uneventful, yet after Billy and his parents left, Tyson remained sitting in his office pondering what just happened. He felt irritated with how the session had gone; it did not go as he had expected. "Where did this whole God-thing come from?" he questioned. "Were they trying to convert me or something?" he asked himself. Overall, he found his feelings of frustration juxtaposed with feelings of gratitude, as the words penned inside the book meant a great deal to him.

Feeling distraught, Tyson sought out consultation from a colleague. His colleague helped Tyson see that Billy's parents really did appreciate all he had done for them. Tyson's colleague helped him shift his perspective to see that Billy's parents were saying thank you in the best way they knew how, drawing from their spiritual background. They were not out to convert him but rather were sharing a deep and personal side of themselves, their spiritual side. In essence, Billy's parents had taken a risk by making themselves vulnerable through the gift they shared with Tyson. He left the consultation meeting with a renewed appreciation for how the session ended, and his feelings of frustration began slowly to be replaced with feelings of contentment. Although Tyson no longer has the book, he had carefully removed the page with the penned thank-you letter from Billy's parents. Years later, the page with the penned thank-you letter continues to serve as a source of encouragement for Tyson and has become a cherished reminder of clients he has helped.

The case highlights an example of how spirituality can surface during the termination process, even when it appeared absent during subsequent sessions. This case also highlights the internal struggle and questioning Tyson faced as he sought to understand the behavior of his client's parents and to make meaning for himself about their relationship and his role as the therapist. Tyson learned that his client's parents used their spirituality to make meaning of their relationship with him and that their gift was meant to symbolize the help he offered. By seeking to understand the underlying purpose of Billy's parents through consultation, Tyson grew to appreciate the way they ended the therapeutic alliance. Although occurring after therapy was over, Tyson also found a way to remain authentic and true to his beliefs.

CONCLUSION

The topic of termination has long been overlooked by most therapists, as has the topic of spirituality in termination. Yet, as demonstrated throughout this chapter, whether they have discussed spiritual matters or not, many clients may draw from spiritual beliefs and experiences to make meaning of endings. Unfortunately, few therapists have been trained to approach or address spirituality during this important phase of therapy. It is important, then, for therapists to anticipate how the spiritual may surface during the termination process and consider how they might address the various scenarios outlined in this chapter. Therapists should also remember to remain true to their own personal belief systems while respecting their clients' spirituality. Overall, spirituality and spiritual practices can provide a number of unique opportunities for therapists to help clients successfully end and find meaning in the termination process as well as provide a foundation for continued support. It is hoped that the template and strategies offered in this chapter will enhance therapists' ability to work with spirituality during the termination process.

REFERENCES

Akhtar, S. (Ed.). (2006). *Interpersonal boundaries: Variations and violations*. Lanham, MD: Jason Aronson.

American Psychological Association. (2002). Ethical principles of psychologists and code of conduct. *American Psychologist, 57*, 1060–1073.

Aten, J. D. (2004). Improving understanding and collaboration between campus ministers and college counseling center personnel. *Journal of College Counseling, 7*, 90–96.

Backlar, P. (1996). The three Rs: Roles, relationships, and rules. *Community Mental Health Journal, 32*, 505–509.

Bernstein, D. M. (2001). Therapist–patient relations and ethnic transference. In W. S. Tseng & J. Strelzer (Eds.), *Culture and psychotherapy: A guide to clinical practice* (pp. 103–121). Washington, DC: American Psychiatric Publishing.

Bertolino, B., & O'Hanlon, B. (2002). *Collaborative, competency-based counseling and therapy*. Boston: Allyn & Bacon.

Boyd-Franklin, N. (1989). *Black families in therapy: A multisystems approach*. New York: Guilford Press.

Campbell, C. D., & Gordon, M. C. (2003). Acknowledging the inevitable: Understanding multiple relationships in rural practice. *Professional Psychology: Research and Practice, 34*, 430–434.

Capuzzi, D., & Gross, D. (2007). *Counseling and psychotherapy: Theories and interventions* (4th ed.). Upper Saddle River, NJ: Pearson Prentice Hall.

Chappelle, W. (2000). A series of progressive legal and ethical decision-making steps for using Christian spiritual interventions in psychotherapy. *Journal of Psychology and Theology, 28*, 43–53.

Chappelle, W. (2006). An Air Force psychologist's collaboration with clergy: Lessons learned on the battlefield of Iraq. *Journal of Psychology and Christianity, 25*, 205–215.

Charman, D. P., & Graham, A. C. (2004). Ending therapy: Processes and outcomes. In D. P. Charman (Ed.), *Core processes in brief psychodynamic psychotherapy: Advancing effective practice* (pp. 275–288). Mahwah, NJ: Erlbaum.

Corey, G. (2005). *Theory and practice of counseling and psychotherapy* (7th ed.). Belmont, CA: Brooks/Cole.

Cormier, S., & Hackney, H. (2005). *Counseling strategies and interventions* (6th ed.). New York: Pearson Education.

Edwards, L. C., Lim, B. K., & McMinn, M. R. (1999). Examples of collaboration between psychologists and clergy. *Professional Psychology: Research and Practice, 30*, 547–551.

Exline, J. J., & Rose, E. E. (2005). Religious and spiritual struggles. In R. F. Paloutzian & C. L. Park (Eds.), *Handbook of the psychology of religion and spirituality* (pp. 315–330). New York: Guilford Press.

Farber, B. A., Berano, K. C., & Capobianco, J. A. (2004). Clients' perceptions of the process and consequences of self-disclosure in psychotherapy. *Journal of Counseling Psychology, 51*, 340–346.

Flannelly, K. J., Stern, R. S., & Costa, K. G. (2006). Rabbis and health: A half-century review of the mental and physical health care literature: 1950–1999. *Pastoral Psychology, 54*, 545–554.

Frazier, C., Mintz, L. B., & Mobley, M. (2005). Multidimensional look at religious involvement and psychological well-being among urban elderly African Americans. *Journal of Counseling Psychology, 52*, 583–590.

Galanter, M. (2006). Spirituality and addiction: A research and clinical perspective. *American Journal on Addictions, 15*, 286–292.

Genia, V. (1995). *Counseling and psychotherapy of religious clients: A developmental approach*. Westport, CT: Praeger/Greenwood.

Hill, C., & O'Brien, K. (1999). *Helping skills: Facilitating exploration, insight, and action*. Washington, DC: American Psychological Association.

Joyce, A. S., Piper, W. E., Ogrodniczuk, J. S., & Klein, R. H. (2006). *Termination in psychotherapy: A psychodynamic model of processes and outcomes*. Washington, DC: American Psychological Association.

Kaviratna, H. (Trans.). (1980). *Dhammapada: Wisdom of the Buddha*. Pasadena, CA: Theosophical University Press.

Kobeisy, A. (2004). *Counseling American Muslims: Understanding the faith and helping the people*. New York: Praeger.

Mann, J. (1973). *Time-limited psychotherapy*. Cambridge, MA: Harvard University Press.

McCullough, M. (2001). Religious involvement and mortality: Answers and more questions. In T. G. Plante & A. C. Sherman (Eds.), *Faith and health: Psychological perspectives* (pp. 53–74). New York: Guilford Press.

McMinn, M. R. (1996). *Psychology, theology and spirituality in Christian counseling*. Wheaton, IL: Tyndale House.

McMinn, M. R., & Dominquez, A. W. (Eds.). (2005). *Psychology and the church*. Hauppauge, NY: Nova Science.

McMinn, M. R., Runner, S. J., & Fairchild, J. A. (2005). Factors affecting clergy–psychologist referral patterns. *Journal of Psychology & Theology, 33*, 299–309.

Miller, G. A. (2005). *Learning the language of addiction counseling*. New York: Wiley.

Miller, J. B., Jordan, J. V., Stiver, I. P., Walker, M., Surrey, J. L., & Eldridge, N. S. (2004). Therapists' authenticity. In J. V. Jordan, M. Walker, & L. M. Hartling (Eds.), *The complexity of connection: Writings from the Stone Center's Jean Baker Miller Training Institute* (pp. 64–89). New York: Guilford Press.

Miller, W. R. (1999). *Integrating spirituality into treatment: Resources for practitioners*. Washington, DC: American psychological Association.

Murdin, L. (2000). *How much is enough: Endings in psychotherapy and counselling*. London: Routledge.

Nebelkopf, E., & Phillips, M. (2004). *Healing and mental health for Native Americans: Speaking in red*. Walnut Creek, CA: AltaMira Press.

Peterson, M. R. (1992). *At personal risk: Boundary violations in professional–client relationships*. New York: Norton.

Podikunju-Hussain, S. (2006). Working with Muslims: Perspectives and suggestions for counseling. In G. R. Walz, J. C. Bleuer, & R. K. Yep (Eds.), *Vistas: Compelling perspectives on counseling 2006* (pp. 103–106). Alexandria, VA: American Counseling Association.

Rausch, S. M., Gramling, S. E., & Auerbach, S. M. (2006). Effects of a single session on large-group meditation and progressive muscle relaxation training on stress reduction, reactivity, and recovery. *International Journal of Stress Management, 13*, 273–290.

Richards, P. S. (1995). Using spiritual interventions in psychotherapy: Practices, successes, failures, and ethical concerns of Mormon psychotherapists. *Professional Psychology: Research and Practice, 26*, 163–170.

Richards, P. S., & Bergin, A. E. (2005). *A spiritual strategy for counseling and psychotherapy* (2nd ed.). Washington, DC: American Psychological Association.

Rose, E. M., Westefeld, J. S., Ansely, T. N. (2001). Spiritual issues in counseling: Clients' beliefs and preferences. *Journal of Counseling Psychology, 48*, 61–71.

Schlesinger, H. J. (2005). *Endings and beginnings: On terminating psychotherapy and psychoanalysis*. Hillsdale, NJ: Analytic Press.

Schultz-Ross, R. A., & Gutheil, T. G. (1997). Difficulties in integrating spirituality into psychotherapy. *Journal of Psychotherapy Practice and Research, 6*, 130–138.

Senter, K., & Caldwell, K. (2002). Spirituality and the maintenance of change: A phenomenological study of women who leave abusive relationships. *Contemporary Family Therapy: An International Journal, 24*, 543–564.

Shapiro, E. L., & Ginzberg, R. (2002). Parting gifts: Termination rituals in group therapy. *International Journal of Group Psychotherapy, 52*, 319–336.

Sommers-Flanagan, R., & Sommers-Flanagan, J. (2002). *Clinical interviewing* (3rd ed.). New York: Wiley.

Stepansky, P. E. (1999). *Freud, surgery, and the surgeons*. Hillsdale, NJ: Analytic Press.

Tan, S. Y., & Dong, N. J. (2001). Spiritual interventions in healing and wholeness. In T. G. Plante & A. C. Sherman (Eds.), *Faith and health: Psychological perspectives* (pp. 291–310). New York: Guilford Press.

Tarakeshwar, N., Pargament, K. I., & Mahoney, A. (2003). Measures of Hindu pathways: Development and preliminary evidence of reliability and validity. *Cultural Diversity and Ethnic Minority Psychology, 9*, 316–332.

Trujillo, A. (2000). Psychotherapy with Native Americans: A view into the role of religion and spirituality. In P. S. Richards & A. E. Bergin (Eds.), *Handbook of psychotherapy and religious diversity* (pp. 445–466). Washington, DC: American Psychological Association.

Walsh, J. (2007). *Endings in clinical practice: Effective closure in diverse settings* (2nd ed.). Chicago: Lyceum Books.

Watlington, C. G., & Murphy, C. M. (2006). The roles of religion and spirituality among African American survivors of domestic violence. *Journal of Clinical Psychology, 62*, 837–857.

Weaver, A. J. (1998). Mental health professionals working with religious leaders. In H. G. Koenig (Ed.), *Handbook of religion and mental health* (pp. 349–360). San Diego, CA: Academic Press.

Welfel, E. (2002). *Ethics in counseling and psychotherapy*. Pacific Grove, CA: Brooks/Cole.

Worthington, E. L., & Sandage, S. (2002). Religion and spirituality. In J. C. Norcross (Ed.), *Psychotherapy relationships that work: Therapist contributions and responsiveness to patients* (pp. 383–399). New York: Oxford University Press.

11

CASE STUDY SHOWING INCLUSION OF SPIRITUALITY IN THE THERAPEUTIC PROCESS

KARI A. O'GRADY AND P. SCOTT RICHARDS

> For many, a concern with the sacred or transcendent goes to the heart of what it means to be human.
>
> —Thomas Plante and Allen Sherman

As Nick stood up to make his appointment for the next session, his therapist asked, "Nick, how tall are you?"[1] He replied that he was 6 feet and 3 inches. His therapist said, "That's pretty tall. How come you seem so small in my office sometimes?" Nick pondered the question for a moment before answering, "Maybe it's because my spirit is so small in ways."

Nick's response communicated a spiritual concern or struggle. Spiritual struggles represent significant inner conflict "when matters of the greatest value are at stake" (Pargament, Murray-Swank, Magyar, & Ano, 2005, p. 246). These struggles can be the source of tremendous angst for clients; however, spiritual concerns that are expressed and attended to during psychotherapy may serve as an important avenue for healing and growth. Such concerns can often help reveal the most fundamental and meaningful issues in clients' lives. Attending to the spiritual dimension of clients' lives can also significantly enhance therapists' ability to gain insight, develop a strong therapeutic alliance, and implement interventions for change (see chap. 1, this volume). Helping clients on a spiritual journey of growth and healing requires thoughtfulness and creativity at every stage of the therapy process.

---

[1]For the case presented in this chapter, a pseudonym is used, and identifying details have been altered for confidentiality.

THEORETICAL BACKGROUND

Our approach to integrating spirituality into psychological practice is grounded in a theistic framework for psychotherapy (O'Grady & Richards, 2007; Richards & Bergin, 2005). The conceptual framework for theistic psychotherapy includes theological premises that are grounded in a theistic worldview: philosophical assumptions, personality theory, and view of psychotherapy. The conceptual framework also provides a rationale concerning why spiritual interventions are needed in psychotherapy, what types of spiritual interventions may be useful, and how spiritual perspectives and interventions can be implemented throughout the course of psychotherapy.

The foundational conceptual assumptions of theistic psychotherapy "are that God exists, that human beings are the creations of God, and that there are unseen spiritual processes by which the link between God and humanity is maintained" (Bergin, 1980, p. 99). This approach also assumes that clients who have faith in God's power and draw on spiritual resources during treatment may find added strength and insight into how they can cope, heal, and grow. There are a number of other characteristics of theistic psychotherapy that are distinctive, including the view that (a) spiritual perspectives and interventions should be integrated into treatment in an integrative and treatment-tailoring manner, (b) therapists and clients may seek and on occasion obtain divine inspiration to assist them during treatment, and (c) psychotherapy is and ought to be a moral enterprise (Richards & Bergin, 2005). It is beyond the scope of this chapter to discuss these issues in detail, and so we refer interested readers to other sources (e.g., O'Grady & Richards, 2007; Richards & Bergin, 2005; Richards, Hardman, & Berrett, 2007).

Throughout the chapter we seek to describe and illustrate through the case example of Nick how we go about integrating spirituality throughout the course of treatment. We discuss how we typically go about (a) establishing a spiritually open and safe therapeutic relationship, (b) conceptualizing client issues and making a treatment plan, (c) conducting a religious and spiritual assessment, (d) implementing spiritual interventions ethically and effectively, and (e) including spirituality in the process of termination. We also discuss the role of self-awareness in therapy. We describe how the therapist worked with Nick at each stage of treatment, focusing particularly on how spirituality was integrated across each stage of the therapeutic process. We then provide a brief commentary about the therapist's rationale behind her actions, along with a description of how this case study is typical or atypical of our approach. We conclude with some general comments. Although we have chosen a spiritually devout client to highlight how we explicitly integrate spirituality across the therapeutic process, we wish to emphasize that the way in which we integrate spirituality into treatment varies considerably depending on the unique spiritual orientation of each client.

CASE BACKGROUND INFORMATION

At the time of services, Nick was a single, 24-year-old, Caucasian junior in college majoring in business economics. Nick was raised in the eastern United States, in an intact family. He described himself as an active member of the Church of Jesus Christ of Latter-day Saints. He presented for therapy with relationship difficulties as well as anxiety and feelings of inadequacy about making life decisions.

Nick was seen by Kari A. O'Grady (the first author) at the Counseling and Career Center at Brigham Young University (BYU) in Provo, Utah. The Counseling and Career Center is a full-service counseling center with an American Psychological Association (APA)–accredited internship site. It employs over 20 licensed PhD psychologists and approximately 10 to 15 other mental health professionals. At the time she worked with this client, Ms. O'Grady was a student in an APA-accredited doctoral program in counseling psychology at BYU. She identifies herself as a theistic integrative psychotherapist (Richards & Bergin, 2005) and is a devout member of the Church of Jesus Christ of Latter-day Saints.

ESTABLISHING AN OPEN AND SAFE ENVIRONMENT

In seeking to establish an open and safe environment for our clients, we have found it helpful to remember that therapy is typically a personal and vulnerable experience for our clients. It takes a great deal of courage for most clients to present for therapy and to share their struggles. We recognize that because spirituality and religion are often the most private and sacred aspect of our clients' lives, they can feel especially vulnerable exposing this side of themselves to others. Many clients feel uncertain about whether it is appropriate or safe to share spiritual issues in therapy (Richards & Bergin, 2000; Worthington, 1986). We try to help our clients feel safe to explore their spirituality because we believe spiritual and religious concerns can play a central role in our clients' emotional well-being, and because we feel that being an ethical therapist includes being sensitive to and respectful of this area of multicultural diversity (Crook-Lyon, O'Grady, Smith, Jensen, & Golightly, 2005; Fukuyama & Sevig, 1999; Richards & O'Grady, 2005; Smith & Richards, 2005).

We also feel it is important to be mindful of how our own views about spirituality and religion may be manifesting in therapy (see also chap 3, this volume). Discussing spiritual issues in therapy can generate feelings of vulnerability for therapists as well. When our clients wish to explore the spiritual aspects of their lives, we recognize that our experiences with and thoughts about spirituality may be brought to the surface. We have found that being sensitive to our own feelings about spirituality and religion and our comfort about including it as part of treatment help us to avoid countertransference that may constrain our clients' feelings of safety in exploring spirituality (see also chap. 8, this volume). Discomfort on the part of the therapist may manifest as overdirecting, minimizing, and avoiding spiritual content. Further discomfort by therapists may be communicated through tone of voice, choice of words, and interpretations (Chirban, 2001). We have discovered that being mindful about our views of spirituality and being thoughtful about what we are conveying to our clients allow us to be more open to what our clients are communicating.

In addition to keeping the issues mentioned earlier in mind, we often do a number of other specific things early in treatment in an effort to create a spiritually open and safe environment (see also chap. 4, this volume). For example, we mention to our clients during our informed consent procedures that we are willing to discuss and explore spiritual and religious issues if they wish. Sometimes we directly ask them whether their spirituality is important to them and whether they would like it to be included in therapy. We often reassure clients that we regard their spiritual beliefs as a potential resource for healing and growth, not as an indicator of psychopathology. We also often inform clients that with their consent we may use spiritual interventions during treatment if we think it could be helpful.

We typically avoid disclosing detailed information about our own spiritual and religious beliefs unless clients ask us directly about our beliefs or unless we think that such disclosures may be relevant to their issues and helpful to them (Richards & Bergin, 2005). To reduce the chance that clients will make assumptions about our spiritual or religious orientation, we also avoid wearing or displaying in our offices anything with religious symbols or content. When clients do disclose information about their spiritual background and beliefs with us, we communicate interest in and respect for what they share. If differences in spiritual or religious beliefs and values become apparent during therapy, we are careful to communicate to our clients that we respect their right to differ from us and that we accept them as a person regardless of what our differences in beliefs may be.

We have found that allowing spiritual issues to be a part of therapy usually enhances the therapeutic alliance, thus increasing the level of trust and safety clients feel in the relationship (see also chap. 8, this volume). The level of safety that is achieved when we create space for the spiritual helps our clients engage in a more open relationship with us (West, 2000). When our clients have experienced our openness to being transformed by the spiritual and have felt safe to explore the spiritual dimension of their lives within the relationship, they seem to progress more effectively in the healing process (Stone, 2005).

Case Illustration

In an effort to establish a spiritually safe environment for Nick, during the initial session the therapist let him know that, among other issues, she was open to discussing spiritual concerns in therapy. She also asked a few questions concerning his religious and spiritual life during intake. These questions included "Do you consider yourself to have a spiritual life? If so, how would you describe it?" Because Nick's description of his spiritual life included God, the therapist asked, "How would you describe your relationship with God?" She asked Nick whether he was affiliated with a religion and what that religion was. She also asked about his family's religious affiliation. This provided helpful information for case conceptualization, but it also let Nick know that the therapist considered spirituality and religion as potential areas for exploration in therapy.

Throughout the course of therapy, the therapist tried to be sensitive to Nick's spiritual concerns and help him know that it was okay to bring up spiritual issues. For instance, in one of the earlier sessions, Nick asked, "Is it okay to talk about my prayers in here or is that inappropriate for therapy?" The therapist recognized Nick's vulnerability in his desire to process something sacred in the therapy context. She asked Nick whether he felt safe doing so, and he noted that he felt comfortable doing so but was concerned about its place in therapy. She replied, "You have brought up the question of discussing prayer in therapy. Do you see prayer as possibly playing a role in either your problems or your healing?" He replied that he felt that his prayers were not very helpful recently and he wanted to explore why. He also expressed that he felt shame for not being able to have a more meaningful experience with prayer. The therapist said, "I am glad that you brought it up, Nick. Would you like to look at what is happening for you in your prayers in session?"

Authors' Commentary

This case illustrates some of the ways that we seek to create a spiritually open and safe environment with our clients. In the first therapy session, the therapist let Nick know that it was okay for him to discuss spiritual issues if he desired. She also asked Nick some open-ended questions that invited him to help her understand his global worldview (e.g., whether he believed in God, whether he was affiliated with a religious denomination, whether his spirituality or religion was important to him). As treatment progressed, the therapist continued to show interest in Nick's spiritual concerns whenever he discussed them, and she felt free to bring spiritual issues up when it seemed relevant to his presenting concerns and therapy goals.

Partway into treatment, the therapist also reassured Nick that it was okay to talk about specific aspects of his spiritual beliefs in therapy (i.e., his prayer life) when he expressed some uncertainty about doing so. It is not uncommon as treatment progresses for clients to seek reassurances about whether it is okay to discuss specific aspects of their spiritual beliefs, particularly beliefs that are especially sacred or sensitive to them. We find that if we respond with interest and reassurance to such inquiries, clients are often willing to go deeper and be more specific about sacred and sensitive aspects of their spirituality. As they do, we sometimes find that there are subtle and important connections between the sacred and sensitive aspects of their spirituality and their most challenging emotional and relationship issues. Once these connections are made manifest, opportunities arise for therapeutic exploration and the acquisition of emotional and spiritual insights and healing.

Consistent with chapter 3 of this volume, we have found that our own spiritual self-explorations, as well as our efforts to obtain continuing education about issues of spiritual diversity, have helped us feel more comfortable about discussing spiritual issues with clients from diverse spiritual backgrounds. In this case, the therapist's comfort about discussing spiritual issues helped Nick feel comfortable about discussing spiritual issues with her. The therapist's view that faith and spirituality may be a resource in treatment helped Nick recognize that it could be for him.

CONDUCTING A MULTIDIMENSIONAL ASSESSMENT

We conduct a spiritual and religious assessment as part of a multisystemic assessment strategy (Richards & Bergin, 2005; see also chap. 5, this volume). When we first begin working with clients, we globally assess all important systems or dimensions of human functioning: physical, social, behavioral, intellectual, educational–occupational, psychological–emotional, and spiritual–religious. During this phase of the assessment process, we rely primarily on client self-descriptions and our own clinical impressions about how clients are functioning in each dimension. We seek to understand whether clients' spiritual background and status may be relevant to their presenting problems and treatment planning. As recommended by Richards and Bergin (2005), we ask questions such as the following:

1. Are you willing to discuss religious and spiritual issues during treatment?
2. What is your current religious–spiritual affiliation? How important is this affiliation to you?
3. Do you believe your spiritual beliefs and lifestyle are contributing to your problems in any way?
4. Are you willing to participate in spiritual interventions if it appears that they may be helpful?
5. Do you believe that your religious and spiritual beliefs and/or community are a potential source of strength and assistance?

Depending on clients' presenting problems and goals, and the information obtained during the initial phase of assessment, we proceed with more in-depth religious–spiritual assessment only if it seems clinically warranted. The objective of our more in-depth spiritual assessment is to determine in what ways clients' spiritual and religious beliefs may be contributing to their problems and to determine whether their faith and spirituality may be a resource during treatment. We seek to gain insight into the following questions during our more in-depth religious–spiritual assessment.

1. How orthodox is the client in her or his religious beliefs and behavior?
2. What is the client's religious problem-solving style (i.e., deferring, collaborative, self-directing)?
3. How does the client perceive God (e.g., loving and forgiving vs. impersonal and wrathful)?
4. Does the client have a sound understanding of the important doctrines and teachings of his or her religious tradition?
5. Is the client's lifestyle and behavior congruent with her or his religious and spiritual beliefs and values?
6. Is the client's religious orientation predominantly intrinsic, healthy, and mature and/or extrinsic, unhealthy, and immature (and in what ways)?
7. In what ways are the client's religious and spiritual background, beliefs, and lifestyle affecting the client's presenting problems and disturbance?
8. In what ways might the client's faith, spirituality, and religious community be a resource to assist the client during treatment?

Most often, we seek insight into these questions during our clinical interviews. Occasionally, we find it helpful to use one or more standardized spiritual and religious measures, such as the Religious Commitment Inventory (Worthington et al., 2003) and the Spiritual Well-Being Scale (Paloutzian & Ellison, 1993). Many other spiritual and religious measures have been developed, mostly from within a Christian theological framework (Hill & Hood, 1999), but because most of these measures have not been validated in clinical situations, we recommend that therapists use them only with caution.

Case Illustration

Assessment and diagnosis of Nick were made through a thorough interview and case history during the intake session, as well as the Outcome Questionnaire (OQ–45.2). The OQ–45.2 is a 45-item outcome measure that assesses clients' functioning on three subscales: Symptom Distress (i.e., anxiety, depression, and substance abuse), Interpersonal Relations (i.e., relationship conflict), and Social Role (problems in work and school; Lambert & Burlingame, 1996). It is routinely administered to all clients at the BYU Counseling and Career Center.

In his initial session, Nick's speech was intense and pressured, and his overall presence was anxious, fast paced, and somewhat overwhelming. Nick explained in his initial interview that he was unable to maintain relationships with women for more than a couple of weeks. He wondered whether a flaw in his personality or an aspect of his presence scared people away. He described himself as friendly but unable to develop meaningful or lasting relationships with others. He also had difficulty making major life decisions. He felt a great deal of anxiety about making the right choice about where to live, what major and occupation to pursue, and how to conduct his life in relation to others. He expressed a wish to follow God's direction for his life and felt distress that he seemed unable to know what God wanted him to do. One of the reasons Nick presented for therapy was that he was experiencing distress about a decision he needed to make. Nick was trying to decide whether he should accept full-time employment as a manager of a restaurant or continue with part-time work and pursue his education full time. He needed to give the employer his answer by that evening. The therapist asked Nick what he would prefer to do, and he responded, "I do not know what God wants me to do." When asked again to share what he would prefer to do, Nick replied, "I want to do what God wants me to do. But I feel very stressed out because I cannot figure out what God wants me to do." He said that he had always had great difficulty making even simple decisions for his life.

Nick described a pattern of "down days" in which he felt symptoms of depression, including feelings of worthlessness and extreme loneliness. He also reported feeling unusually "high days" in which he experienced elevated levels of energy and a decreased need for sleep. Nick's initial OQ–45.2 score of 68 was slightly elevated beyond the normal range, indicating some symptoms of social and interpersonal distress. Testing and evaluation resulted in the following *Diagnostic and Statistical Manual of Mental Disorders, Fourth Edition, Text Revision* (American Psychiatric Association, 2000) diagnosis:

Axis I: 301.13 Cyclot hymic disorder, V62.89 Religious or spiritual problem

Axis II: No diagnosis

Axis III: None

Axis IV: None

Axis V: Global Assessment of Functioning scale = 65 (current)

Nick was the middle child of three children raised in an intact, middle-class family and described his family life in positive terms. His father worked in upper management and served in various positions in their church, and his mother stayed at home to care for the children and the home and was an active member of her church community. Nick felt loved and supported by both parents and reported a mostly positive relationship with his brother and sister, but he described feeling overshadowed by his older sister's accomplishments at times as well as feeling somewhat detached from his younger brother. Nick described himself as an active member of his church community and considered his relationship with God to be of great importance, but he often felt detached from God and feared His disapproval.

When he was in junior high, Nick's family relocated for employment purposes. Shortly after arriving at his new school, Nick was physically and verbally assaulted by his peers on numerous occasions. Although he was able to develop a few superficial relationships with peers, he mostly experienced rejection and bullying. These abusive experiences continued for 2½ years.

During assessment, the therapist learned that Nick considered himself a devout member of his church and that he had been raised in an orthodox home. When the therapist asked Nick to describe his relationship with God, he expressed a deep desire to please God in all of his choices and stated that he believed God loved him, but he was uncertain if God approved of him. Nick felt that because he believed God may not approve of him, he had difficulty having a meaningful relationship with God. It appeared that Nick's God image included a view of an omnipotent being who must be constantly pleased and whose favor was difficult to obtain. His description of God manifested an immature God-image development; God was not necessarily a resource in Nick's life but rather a means of distress. However, his strong faith in God and commitment to his religion suggested that, if repaired, Nick's relationship with God could become an important source of healing and growth for him.

Authors' Commentary

This case is typical for us in the sense that the therapist started with a global, multidimensional assessment of various dimensions of Nick's life, including his emotional, academic, interpersonal, biological, family, and spiritual and religious history and current functioning. She then proceeded with more in-depth assessments of some of these dimensions when it seemed clinically relevant. For example, when Nick brought up his prayer life, the therapist proceeded with a more in-depth assessment of that aspect of his spirituality. Because the BYU Counseling and Career Center does not include any questions about clients' religious or spiritual history on their intake questionnaire, the therapist was limited to gathering this information in her initial clinical interview, which is different from our preferred practice. In addition, because the center does not include any spiritual or religious measures in its assessment or outcome test battery, the therapist was unable to include such measures in her initial assessment procedures, which we normally include in other clinical settings. Owing to these limitations, the therapist relied exclusively on asking questions and listening carefully to information the client volunteered about his spirituality during the sessions.

CASE CONCEPTUALIZATION AND ESTABLISHING A TREATMENT PLAN

The multidimensional assessment we described earlier leads naturally to a multidimensional approach to case conceptualization and treatment planning, which includes a consideration of the spiritual and religious dimension of their lives (Richards & Bergin, 2005). We agree with Park and Slattery (chap. 6, this volume) that spirituality and religion provide a major source of meaning in many clients' lives. Understanding the meaning of clients' faith and spirituality, especially as they pertain to their presenting problems and life aspirations, is an essential aspect of case conceptualization. As we conceptualize our clients, we seek to understand and articulate how their spiritual or religious orientation and issues may be intertwined with their presenting problems. Are their spiritual issues a source of distress, perhaps causing or exacerbating their presenting problems? Is their faith and spirituality potentially a source of strength and a resource that could help them cope with and overcome their problems?

As part of treatment planning, we collaboratively set goals for therapy with our clients that are designed to help them cope with and resolve their presenting concerns and to promote their healing, growth, and long-term well-being. Our treatment plan may include therapeutic goals and interventions in various dimensions of clients' lives, including the biological, psychological, interpersonal, career, and academic. As recommended by Richards and Bergin (2005), we also often include in our treatment plan one or more general spiritual goals, such as helping clients (a) affirm their spiritual identity, (b) live in harmony with their spiritual and religious values, (c) examine their images of God, (d) resolve spiritual and religious issues that may be related to their presenting problems, and (e) explore whether their faith and spirituality may be a resource to assist them in treatment. We also set other specific spiritual goals with clients who wish to do so, tailoring the goals to fit the unique concerns, issues, and preferences of the client.

Case Illustration

As the therapist proceeded with Nick's assessment and case conceptualization, it became clear that he was struggling with a number of interrelated issues. Nick's inability to make decisions for his life was largely influenced by his views about God's role in his life. The perception that he could not gain

God's approval created a state of frenzy for him at times. He also experienced acute feelings of loneliness accompanied by feelings of disconnection from God, which contributed to periods of depression. In these ways, Nick's spiritual struggle was contributing to his emotional dysfunction. In addition, his cyclothymia contributed to his spiritual struggle in that his intense, fast pace made it difficult for him to slow down enough to get in touch with his inner spirituality. Furthermore, his constant state of emotional fluctuation from the cyclothymia made it difficult for him to feel peace and explore a relationship with God. The therapist decided that she would first need to help Nick learn some practices for slowing down and being aware of his inner world. After he learned some basic mood regulation skills (e.g., being aware of his feelings and thoughts), they could begin to work on addressing the areas of his spirituality that were contributing to his cyclothymia. As the cyclothymia regulated, they would be able to explore his spirituality in greater depth.

Early in therapy Nick and the therapist discussed Nick's goals for therapy. His hopes included finding ways to regulate his mood, gain confidence in decision making, develop more lasting relationships, and explore his identity. The therapist asked whether Nick wished to include spirituality in any way in his treatment. He replied, "I think about my life in spiritual ways, so I hope that we can look at my spirituality in therapy. I think it will be a big part of achieving my goals." After listening to Nick's presenting concerns, including his descriptions of the spiritual dimensions of his life, and to his hopes for therapy, the therapist recognized that Nick's spirituality could be an important avenue for gaining insight and creating change. The initial goals for therapy were fairly general and open to adjustment from session to session. The spiritual goals for therapy became more defined as Nick progressed through therapy. Initially, the therapist recognized a potential need to help Nick explore his spiritual identity as they explored his identity overall. She also identified a need for helping Nick create a more positive God image and to address the ways his views of God were affecting his sense of self and others. After addressing some of his initial presenting concerns, Nick's goals for therapy shifted toward a focus on spiritual exploration and change. The goals Nick had for the later half of his therapy included developing a stronger spiritual life, enhancing his relationship with God, and finding greater meaning and purpose for his life.

Authors' Commentary

This case was typical for us in the sense that the client's spiritual and religious issues were an important part of our case conceptualization and treatment planning. Without including the spiritual dimension in our case conceptualizations, we believe that we would often potentially fail to understand our clients' core issues. We find this to be true for most spiritually devout clients. For such clients, we also often find that as therapy progresses the focus on spiritual goals becomes an even more prominent theme in therapy, as was true for Nick. This does not necessarily happen with clients who are less devout or whose spiritual issues are not so closely tied to their presenting concerns, although even with such clients spirituality may still become an important theme. With Nick, we found that understanding his spiritual issues and including some spiritual goals in his treatment plan opened the door to addressing some of his dysfunctional religious beliefs and to accessing the positive resources of his faith during his treatment. Attending to these spiritual issues facilitated his progress in all dimensions of his life, including his relationships, sense of identity, feelings of self-confidence, emotional regulation, and overall sense of meaning and life satisfaction.

TREATMENT IMPLEMENTATION

We combine spiritual perspectives and interventions with mainstream psychological and medical approaches in a multidimensional integrative treatment strategy (Richards & Bergin, 2005). We view addressing issues of faith and spirituality as one important component of a comprehensive treatment plan. It is important to understand those aspects of our clients' spiritual and religious orientation that may be unhealthy or contributing to their presenting problems. We often find that interventions are needed to help clients adopt healthier religious and spiritual beliefs and practices, although when using such interventions we are careful to avoid imposing our own spiritual or religious values on our clients. When our clients regard their faith and spirituality as a potential resource, we design interventions that help them use these resources in their efforts to cope and heal, including recommending client practices such as prayer, meditation and contemplation, reading spiritual writings, repentance and forgiveness, fellowship and altruistic service, worship and ritual, and seeking spiritual direction (Richards & Bergin, 2005). We avoid using spiritual interventions rigidly or uniformly with all clients but seek to implement them in a flexible, treatment-tailoring manner. We pray privately for our clients, encourage them to pray for their own progress in a manner consistent with their beliefs, and seek God's inspiration as we assess and intervene with our clients (O'Grady & Richards, 2004; Richards & Bergin, 2005).

We keep in mind and seek to avoid potential ethical dangers of implementing spiritual interventions in treatment, including dual relationships (religious and professional), displacing or usurping religious authority, imposing religious values on clients, and violating work setting (church-state) boundaries (Richards & Bergin, 2005). Spiritual interventions are not implemented in treatment until we have assessed our clients' psychological functioning, spiritual background and beliefs, and attitude about exploring spiritual issues during treatment. We are careful to work within the value frameworks of our clients and to only recommend interventions that are in harmony with their religious beliefs.

With the majority of our spiritually oriented clients, the incorporation of spiritual perspectives and interventions into the therapeutic process is indicated and enhances both the processes and outcomes of treatment. We have noticed that clients with spiritual beliefs, especially those who live congruently with their spiritual beliefs, seem to make more dramatic gains in the healing process and in maintaining their treatment gains. Many of our clients have shared with us their belief that their own focus on spiritual issues during treatment and their faith in God were some of the most powerful catalysts for positive change. With clients who are not spiritually oriented, we find that it is often still important to address existential and spiritual issues such as life purpose and meaning, values and lifestyle choices, loss and death, and so on.

Case Illustration

Early in therapy, Nick's therapist concluded that before Nick would be able to work on problem solving, mood regulation, or a relationship with God, he may need to slow down his approach to life. In subsequent sessions, the therapist introduced mindfulness exercises in which Nick sat quietly and tried to be aware of his surroundings and how he was experiencing them. He noticed sights, sounds, and sensations. He was able to relax more during sessions after incorporating this level of mindfulness into his life. Next, the therapist focused on helping Nick find a quiet place inside himself and encouraged him to be aware of his inner experience. He reported having difficulty with this stage of mindfulness because he could not picture what an inner self might look like. To help illustrate this idea of an inner, or core self, the therapist showed an illustration of the concept of mortal overlay as described by Richards and Bergin (2005; see Figure 11.1). She explained how the inner self could be conceptualized as the core self or eternal spirit—the part of humans that is constant. Nick and the therapist talked about how this inner self can be obscured by the physical body and accompanying sensations, life experiences, and psychological processes and coping styles. Nick resonated with the idea of an eternal spirit in part because it was consistent with his religious belief that individuals have a soul that extends beyond the life of the body. He also reported that this helped him concentrate on his inner experience and slow down the intensity in which he experienced his life. He said his newfound ability to practice mindfulness was like "stepping through a door into a world that had suddenly slowed down" and that life on that side of the door felt "more real" to him. He said that he liked that world and hoped he could experience it more often.

In addition to practicing awareness, the therapist used moments of silence throughout therapy to help Nick pause and ponder rather than rushing on to the next concern before being aware of what he was experiencing in

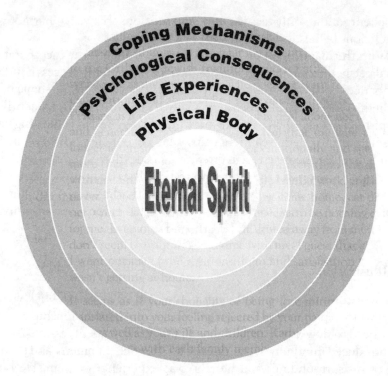

Figure 11.1. Eternal spiritual identity and the mortal overlay.

the present. These times of silence also helped him to feel comfortable with his identity as he faced himself in the silence. Furthermore, silence created space for spiritual insights and experiences to occur, a way to make room for the sacred.

As Nick was better able to "get in touch with himself," he was able to monitor his "down days" and what he was experiencing during those times. He was aware of a deep sense of loneliness and feeling insignificant on those days. He attributed his feelings of insignificance to the belief that he must be flawed in some deep, encompassing way. Nick expressed his belief that if he could feel less lonely in his relationship with God, he would feel less pain and loneliness overall and he might increase in his self-confidence.

Nick's insight into how his spiritual life was affecting his emotional and social well-being seemed worthy of exploration. He also seemed to be expressing part of the solution to his extreme feelings of loneliness. Taking God or a spiritual presence into the loneliness can help clients have courage to face and learn from loneliness. The therapist decided that it could be therapeutic to incorporate Nick's solution into his encounter with his feeling of loneliness. She encouraged Nick to consider what it means to him to feel alone and to record those feelings in his journal. Nick was already in the habit of keeping a journal, so early in therapy, the therapist had encouraged him to record his feelings between sessions. In the following session, Nick shared a journal entry he had written during the week:

> I was in church today and started thinking about life and where I am, what I am doing, and just the way things are going right now. I started thinking about the word *belong* and what it means because sometimes I just do not feel like I belong anywhere. I broke up the word *belong* into *be* and *long*. *Be* means to exist in actuality, have life or reality. *Long* in the verb tense means to have an earnest, heartfelt desire, especially for something beyond reach. Putting those two together, I personally interpret *belong* as meaning having an earnest, heartfelt desire to exist where you are in life or reality.

Nick and the therapist discussed when he feels like he belongs versus when he feels like he does not belong. He expressed that he feels lonely because he does not feel like he belongs anywhere. Then the therapist asked him if he feels like he belongs with God. He replied that he does not feel like he belongs with God but that he deeply wishes that he did. He said that he felt like something was blocking him from feeling that closeness and acceptance with God. Along with feeling sadness about not feeling close to God, he also felt sinful about not feeling close to God. Nick shared some of the mistakes he had made in his life and the regret he felt about the ways that he had handled those experiences in his life. Then he suggested that maybe what was preventing him from feeling a sense of belonging with God was his inability to forgive himself. He said he did not know how to forgive himself. He said he tried to repent and pray for God's forgiveness and to not repeat the same mistakes, but he could not feel forgiven or worthy of God's love.

Nick's perfectionism was making it difficult for him to have a genuine relationship with God and was adding to his feelings of loneliness. It seemed important to help Nick accept his imperfections so he could feel God's love and acceptance and so he could experience greater self-acceptance and increased emotional closeness with others. Encouraging Nick to reconsider the meaning of mistakes and the role of forgiveness helped him feel more willing to emotionally connect with God and others.

Nick and the therapist discussed how inhibiting it can be when we do not forgive ourselves. The therapist also suggested that not forgiving ourselves represented a lack of compassion. She encouraged Nick to picture his 5-year-old niece and to think about how he would feel if she neglected to clean her room before she went out to play. She asked Nick if he would consider severely punishing his niece and berating her for months and years for her failure. Nick replied that he would quickly forgive her and remind her to try to do better next time. The therapist asked if it might be possible that a heavenly father could feel the same about his mistakes. He thought that was possible, given his understanding of God as a perfect father. Next the therapist asked him if he thought it was possible that he could feel that way about his own mistakes. Then Nick and the therapist talked about forgiveness being a process. The therapist shared with him the steps of forgiveness outlined by Richards and Bergin (2005), which include (a) acknowledging shock and denial; (b) developing awareness of the abuse and offense; (c) experiencing the feelings of hurt, grief, and anger; (d) receiving validation that they have been wronged; (e) establishing boundaries to protect from future offense; and (f) beginning the process of forgiving, letting go, and giving up judgment to God. Nick liked considering forgiveness as a process rather than an all-or-nothing pursuit. He expressed that it helped him not feel so overwhelmed by the quest to forgive himself.

Throughout the following week, Nick thought a lot about the idea of forgiving oneself. He returned to the following session and shared a scripture from the Bible, "For if ye forgive men, their trespasses, your heavenly Father will also forgive you: But if ye forgive not men their trespasses, neither will your heavenly Father forgive you" (Mark 6:15). Nick said that for the first time he realized that the commandment to forgive others also applied to his need to forgive himself. He saw himself in the other. The version of the Bible that Nick was reading from included a dictionary that shares orthodox interpretations of various terms. To support his discovery, and to help encourage a compassionate God image, the therapist asked Nick whether he would feel comfortable looking up the word *repent* in his Bible dictionary. He read it out loud in session, "The Greek word of which this is a translation denotes a change of mind, i.e., a fresh view about God, about oneself, and about the world" (Church of Jesus Christ of Latter-day Saints, 1979, p. 760). The therapist and Nick discussed how this view of the repentance process did not include self-berating, or a perfectionistic quest to do everything just right, but rather a seeking after truth and enlightenment about oneself, including oneself in relation to God.

The following session, Nick brought in a journal entry he had written reflecting his journey to understand how self-forgiveness allowed him to feel closer to God and better about himself.

> We are a part of our own forgiveness and repentance process. I have often felt I was not really forgiven for something I have done. Now I realize that when God asks us to forgive others, He is also asking us to forgive ourselves. There have been many times in my life when I have done everything to repent of my failings, but I still don't feel like I am clean and that God has forgiven me. After reading that scripture and the definition of repentance, I realized that my lack of self-forgiveness was the reason I still felt unclean. I was working so hard at correcting things, trying to make them right, forgiving others, and so many other things that I totally forgot that I needed to forgive myself. I would beat myself up over it because I continually wondered why it was that I still felt so blocked from God. Forgiving myself is

not an easy process. As I have begun to work on it though and really start to forgive myself, I have felt more and more clean, and more and more like God has forgiven me and continues to do so.

Over the next few sessions, the therapist and Nick talked about how he was handling the ups and downs of cyclothymia. He reported that he felt more comfortable "riding through" the down days and that he used this time to seek nurturance from himself and from God. He also reported that he was having more success going to bed at regular hours, falling asleep even on his extremely high-energy days, and experiencing fewer depressed days.

During a subsequent session, Nick seemed to feel a great deal of shame as he related for the first time a traumatic childhood event he had experienced. When Nick was in the sixth grade, his family moved to a new community and he became a target for bullies. He described being thrown into bushes, tackled, beaten, and verbally berated repeatedly over a 3-year period of time. Nick reported feeling confused by the constant rejection and abuse. He said he had tried hard to be a good and likable kid, but still others hurt him deeply. Nick was talented at sports and art, and so he had wondered whether the rejection was a result of jealousy. He tried to find some comfort in this attribution, but this was not very consoling. Nick said that from that time in his life until the present, he wondered what big flaws he has that everyone else could see but he could not. He did not share his experiences with anyone as or after they occurred because of the deep shame he experienced. He also stated that he felt that the constant bullying and subsequent shame prevented him from developing open and meaningful relationships in his current life. The therapist shared her feelings of sadness about the abuse that he had experienced, and together they mourned his experience in session. The therapist then encouraged Nick to grieve and mourn for the little boy who was hurt and had felt so alone during the following week.

In the following session, Nick reported that some healing came from mourning the hurt he experienced as a little boy. He said he also recognized more keenly how alone he felt during this period in his life and how alone he continues to feel at times as he keeps others at a distance. He said that he thinks that this period of abuse had affected his ability to feel safe connecting to others in meaningful ways and that he felt abandoned and rejected by God during that time. He spoke again about the hidden flaws that must have brought on the abuse. The therapist asked him if he would describe himself to her at that age in his life. Nick seemed to enjoy describing his 12-year-old self. The therapist asked him how he thought that boy might feel if his 24-year-old brother said, "It's your own fault you are getting hurt so much. You are flawed! No wonder everyone beats you up." The therapist and Nick then discussed the need to give his little boy self another more loving message.

During the following week, Nick decided to communicate new messages to himself about that experience. These messages were messages of understanding, comfort, and encouragement. He also decided to write his 12-year-old self a letter. He brought the letter into session the following week. The first part of the letter recapped the experiences of abuse. He then expressed his compassion and sorrow for his experience, writing,

> Nick, because you have closed yourself off to others, no one has been able to take a look inside and see the real you. They haven't had the chance to accept or reject you because they don't know you. I feel this in even a level deeper than just friends and family. I think it has even gone on to affect your spiritual life. You have talked about feeling abandoned by God, but He does not abandon his children. He loves them and takes care of them. But when you closed your heart to other people, you closed your heart to the Spirit, to Christ, to God. But you have still felt the Spirit in your life. That alone shows you the divine love and incredible power that is there. You have not been open to God's love and guidance, but it has been there. I am sure of it. God would never leave you helpless. Nick, you need to reopen your life. You need to reopen who you are. Open your heart, your mind, your soul, to others. This pain you have felt has lasted a long time, and it is time for it to be taken care of. You want to be healed, trust me; your Father in heaven wants to heal you. You know that if you set your mind to something you can do it. Then set your mind to this. Set your mind to release the pain and allow the light of Christ to fill that space.

Nick expressed feeling pain as he wrote the letter to himself, especially as he revisited the abuse. He said that he also experienced God's love, comfort, and support as he wrote. The following weeks, Nick faced his healing with courage and growth.

It became apparent early in therapy that Nick's psychological and emotional struggles were connected to and influenced by his spiritual struggles and vice versa. Likewise, as Nick worked through his spiritual struggles, his emotional well-being and psychological health improved. For instance, Nick's lack of confidence in decision making was largely influenced by his belief that he was flawed in some fundamental way. This belief had its origins in the bullying and abuse he experienced as a child and in his distorted understandings about how God viewed mistakes. Feeling that he was flawed in some fundamental way made him feel incapable of making choices for his life.

As Nick processed his abuse and assigned more accurate messages to it, his shame decreased and his sense of identity adjusted. Intertwined with this process was an exploration of his God image and his personal understandings about imperfections. As he reconstructed his image of God in a more positive light, his view of self followed. Viewing God as loving, supportive, and forgiving allowed him to consider himself more honestly, accept his failures as a normal part of the human experience, and value his own competencies. Nick's faith in a loving God who could comfort His children, as well as his strengthened sense of identity, reduced the frequency of depressed days and helped him to cope with those days when they did occur with more courage and less distress.

Nick's emotional and psychological struggles minimized his ability to experience a healthy spiritual life. His overly aroused physiological state and his anxious, intense approach to life made it difficult for him to get in touch with the quiet inner place in which spiritual experiences and feelings are most frequently experienced.

As Nick developed a healthier spiritual identity, he came to see himself in a collaborative relationship with God. He described God as being "like a therapist," who listened with compassion and understanding and who did not direct him, but rather gently nudged him to be quiet and to listen to his "heart." This perspective of God's role in his life enhanced Nick's confidence in decision making and his overall sense of himself as a likable and capable human being.

Authors' Commentary

This case illustrates some of the ways that we address spiritual issues in therapy. It shows that spirituality can be both a source of problems and a resource for change and health. The therapist found she needed to address several dysfunctional aspects of Nick's religious beliefs early in therapy (e.g., detached, judgmental God image, diminished spiritual identity). As is often the case in our approach, the therapist referred to the client's sacred scriptures to challenge the dysfunctional aspects of his religious beliefs and to help him clarify his understanding of the doctrines of his church. She followed Nick's lead in the sense that in an earlier session he had brought up scriptures as an important avenue for his religious understandings. As changes in Nick's dysfunctional religious beliefs occurred, his spiritual orientation matured and became more of a healthy resource in his life. The therapist also incorporated and tailored a variety of spiritual interventions into treatment, including the forgiveness process, spiritual identity exploration, spiritual awareness, bibliotherapy, journaling, and prayer.

Because the therapist had educated herself on addressing spiritual issues in psychotherapy, she had an awareness of these interventions. An understanding of how to actually implement these interventions specifically for Nick emerged in an intuitively spiritual way. We believe that some of the therapist's insights about what interventions to use and how to implement them were a result of inspiration (O'Grady & Richards, 2004; Richards & Bergin, 2005). We avoid generic application of "techniques" in therapy, preferring creative approaches that fall within the bounds of ethical and moral practice. At times we do find that our creativity and sensitivity about how and when to use spiritual interventions are enhanced through spiritual means such as inspiration.

As is often the case in our work with clients, the therapist created space for quiet spiritual reflection; we believe that it is in such moments that clients may encounter, wrestle with, and find peace about the most meaningful aspects of their lives (Griffith & Griffith, 2002; Richards & Bergin, 2005; West, 2000).

PREPARING FOR TERMINATION

The duration and nature of therapy influence the way we address the termination stage of therapy. In general, however, we view the termination stage as a time to review our clients' progress, reflect on the role therapy has played in their lives, celebrate their growth, solidify gains made in therapy, and plan for future challenges. When therapy has included a spiritual process, our clients often want to include spirituality in termination to help them feel a sense of closure. Consistent with Aten and coauthors (chap. 10, this volume), when we review our clients' progress, we typically ask them to consider how their spirituality has played a role in the healing process. We may encourage them to share ways in which they think that their spirituality has changed over the course of therapy. This consideration might include reflecting on the following questions:

1. What are some of the ways my spirituality has become more personally meaningful and internalized?
2. How has my God image improved?
3. In what ways am I living more congruently with my values?
4. How has my sense of spiritual identity changed?
5. What role does my spirituality now play in healthy coping?
6. What role did spirituality play in my relationship with my therapist?
7. How does my spiritual growth influence my relationship with others?
8. How is my faith a spiritual resource?
9. What changes do I notice in my religious problem-solving style?
10. How has including spirituality in therapy influenced my healing and growth?
11. How would I describe the change in my relationship with God or a Higher Power?

Often clients rely on their spirituality to make meaning of their therapy and to have confidence to go forward. Their spirituality can provide a sense of peace in the ending of our relationship with them and courage in facing the challenges that lie ahead. Sometimes our clients express gratitude to God for their healing. They may also express hope in their belief that their relationship with God continues and that He will help on the next stage of their journey. As therapists, we too find meaning and strength from being a part of our clients' healing journey. We at times give silent thanks to God for letting us be witnesses to His healing power.

Case Illustration

Nick's therapy lasted 11 months and was a deeply emotional process heavily interlaced with spiritual exploration. Because of the extent of therapy and the depth that was achieved by including the spiritual in his healing, termination had to be handled carefully. The therapist began preparing Nick for termination four sessions before his final session by bringing up the topic and inviting him to begin exploring his feelings about it. The therapist also asked Nick to share in what ways he felt like he had grown during his therapy, including the role he saw spirituality play in his healing. He said that his image of God had altered in dramatic ways. He viewed God as someone who cared, was compassionate and understanding, and was there for him. He described his relationship with God in more collaborative terms and said he felt his spiritual identity had improved. He felt more confident in his abilities and more forgiving of his mistakes. Nick reported that feeling more love and fulfillment in his relationship with God and feeling more loving feelings about himself had helped him be more open to others and their expressions of love. He commented that he was feeling more love toward others and more patience with their mistakes. Nick also stated that he felt that being able to heal the spiritual alongside the emotional had allowed his healing and growth to penetrate more deeply and he hoped in more lasting ways.

In the second-to-last visit, as Nick reflected on his growth, he began to process more fully the therapeutic relationship and said, "You have been such an important part of my spiritual journey that I cannot picture the journey without you." The therapist replied, "Your journey has been important to me too." They experienced the significance of their work together in a few moments of silence. After honoring the relationship in this way, she asked Nick, "Is there anything that we have experienced in our relationship that you can take with you after therapy?" He replied, "I can take the silence with me." Nick stated that during the early stages of therapy, moments of silence felt very uncomfortable for him, but in time he came to appreciate the ways silence helped him feel more spiritually, emotionally, and physically aware and integrated. In response to the therapist's question Nick also stated, "I get to keep all that I have learned. I can take the ways I have grown through our relationship and use it in other relationships. The spiritual strength I have gained in therapy is mine to take with me." In the final session the therapist thanked Nick for allowing her to join him on his healing journey.

In a single follow-up session 6 months after termination, Nick declared that his spirit no longer seemed smaller than his 6 foot 3 inch frame. He also shared a journal entry about his reflections concerning the effect of the therapeutic journey on his life:

> I really know that God is there, that He loves me and wants the best for me. I don't feel alone in my life anymore in that regard. I know that God is there. Now I am not saying that everything has been perfect or anything, because it hasn't. But, I have been so much better at dealing with and handling situations since I have changed the way I look at things in my life. I now better understand how relationships really work. You do what is right, you do what is best, and you let things run their course. Doing so will get you so much further than anything else. I've never felt more alive and ready for life than I do now. It has been the greatest thing for me. And I've started thinking about love and how I do want to share it with others.
>
> It's like right now I could falter, and it wouldn't make a difference. I don't mean that I am going to on purpose or anything, but I am only human and therefore bound to be imperfect. And by not making a difference, I mean that it won't change the way I see myself. Yes, of course there will be guilt and remorse, feeling bad for what was done, but that is part of the repentance process. I will still see myself as a child of God who is trying to improve his life and be the best that he can. I just think that right now I can take on anything and stand strong, and that is a huge step for me in my life.

Authors' Commentary

This case illustrates our approach to termination in the sense that the therapist devoted several sessions to the process of termination, giving the client the opportunity to affirm the progress he had made during treatment, process his feelings about ending the therapeutic relationship, and make plans for how to continue on with his growth process after treatment. As is often the case in our approach, these discussions also included reflections and affirmations about how Nick's faith and spirituality helped him during treatment and how it would continue to be a resource for him after treatment. We often find that terminating the therapy relationship seems to feel less frightening to clients who have felt God's love and support during the treatment process. Their feelings of self-confidence about maintaining their treatment gains and continuing the process of healing and growth are enhanced by their faith that God loves them, will strengthen them, and will continue to walk with them as they face the challenges of their lives. As therapists, in such situations, we recognize that it is time to step out of our role as a source of insight and support for our clients. Having developed a more healthy and collaborative relationship with God, clients feel ready to move on with their lives relying on God's inspiration and support, as well as the loving support of family and friends.

GENERAL COMMENTARY, CONCLUSIONS, AND RECOMMENDATIONS

Although this chapter describes a theistic approach as applied to a theistic client, we find that many aspects of our approach also work well with clients who approach life from Eastern, transpersonal, or humanistic spiritual perspective, as well as with clients who are nonreligious. With such clients, we are careful to work within their beliefs systems, using language and interventions that are compatible with their beliefs. Although discussions about a Supreme Being or God are not helpful with nontheistic clients, it is often helpful to explore with them how their spiritual beliefs may pertain to their presenting problems and concerns, including discussions about their sense of spirituality, meaning and purpose, values, and sources of spiritual support (Richards & Bergin, 2000).

We recognize that in some settings, particularly public settings, therapists may feel constrained from incorporating spirituality into treatment. Although Nick's therapy occurred at a private religious university, the therapist nevertheless still felt some constraints as she sought to include spirituality as part of treatment. This was most obvious during her initial assessment of the client because there was no institutional support available to assist her as a psychologist-in-training in using formalized, written spiritual and religious assessment measures. She also experienced resistance from some members of her supervisory team to the idea of making spirituality such a central focus of treatment. Nevertheless, because her theistic therapeutic orientation affirms the importance of including spirituality in treatment, and because Nick's presenting concerns were so clearly intertwined with his spiritual and religious beliefs, the therapist was able to garner support from her supervisor for her treatment plan.

We hope that therapists in diverse settings and from diverse spiritual traditions and theoretical backgrounds will include spirituality in treatment when it is relevant for their clients. We recognize that doing so can be professionally risky and require much courage, but there is now strong theoretical, empirical, and ethical support for doing so (Richards & Bergin, 2005). We believe that as therapists progress in their ability to incorporate spirituality throughout the therapeutic process, the effectiveness of psychotherapy will be enhanced and public perceptions and support for the profession will grow.

REFERENCES

American Psychiatric Association. (2000). *Diagnostic and statistical manual of mental disorders* (4th ed., text rev.). Washington, DC: Author.

Bergin, A. E. (1980). Psychotherapy and religious values. *Journal of Consulting and Clinical Psychology, 48,* 75–105.

Chirban, J. T. (2001). Assessing religious and spiritual concerns in psychotherapy. In T. G. Plante & A. C. Sherman (Eds.), *Faith and health: Psychological perspectives* (pp. 265–290). New York: Guilford Press.

Church of Jesus Christ of Latter-day Saints. (1979). *The Holy Bible: Authorized King James version.* Salt Lake City, UT: Author.

Crook-Lyon, R. E., O'Grady, K. A., Smith T. B., Jensen, D. R., & Golightly, T. (2005, August). *Should spiritual and religious issues be taught in graduate curricula?* Paper presented at the 113th Annual Convention of the American Psychological Association, Washington, DC.

Fukuyama, M., & Sevig, T. (1999). *Integrating spirituality into multicultural counseling.* Thousand Oaks, CA: Sage.

Griffith, J. L., & Griffith, M. E. (2002). *Encountering the sacred in psychotherapy: How to talk with people about their spiritual lives.* New York: Guilford Press.

Hill, C. H., & Hood, R. W. (1999). *Measures of religiosity.* Birmingham, AL: Religious Education Press.

Lambert, M. J., & Burlingame, G. M. (1996). *The Outcome Questionnaire.* Stevenson, MD: American Professional Credentialing Services.

O'Grady, K. A., & Richards, P. S. (2004, July). *Professional's perceptions of the role of inspiration in science and psychotherapy.* Paper presented at the 112th Annual Convention of the American Psychological Association, Honolulu, HI.

O'Grady, K. A., & Richards, P. S. (2007). God image and theistic psychotherapy. In G. Moriarty & L. Hoffman (Eds.), *God image handbook for spiritual counseling and psychotherapy: Research, theory, and practice.* New York: Haworth Press.

Paloutzian, R. F., & Ellison, C. W. (1991). *Manual for the Spiritual Well-Being Scale.* Nyack, NY: Life Advances.

Pargament, K. I., Murray-Swank, N. A., Magyar, G. M., & Ano, G. G. (2005). Spiritual struggle: A phenomenon of interest to psychology and religion. In W. Miller & H. Delaney (Eds.), *Judeo-Christian perspectives on psychology: Human nature, motivation, and change* (pp. 245–268). Washington, DC: American Psychological Association.

Richards, P. S., & Bergin, A. E. (Eds.). (2000). *Handbook of psychotherapy and religious diversity.* Washington, DC: American Psychological Association.

Richards, P. S., & Bergin, A. E. (2005). *A spiritual strategy for counseling and psychotherapy* (2nd ed.). Washington, DC: American Psychological Association.

Richards, P. S., Hardman, R. K., & Berrett, M. E. (2007). *Spiritual approaches in the treatment of women with eating disorders.* Washington, DC: American Psychological Association

Richards, P. S., & O'Grady K. A. (2005). Working with the religiously committed client. In G. P. Koocher, J. C. Norcross, & S. S. Hill (Eds.), *Psychologist's desk reference* (2nd ed., pp. 338–341). New York: Oxford University Press.

Smith, T. B., & Richards, P. S. (2005). The integration of spiritual and religious issues in racial-cultural psychology and counseling. In R. Carter (Ed.), *Handbook of racial-cultural psychology: Theory and research* (Vol. 1, pp. 132–162). Hoboken, NJ: Wiley.

Stone, C. (2005). Opening psychoanalytic space to the spiritual. *Psychoanalytic Review, 92,* 417–430.

West, W. (2000). *Psychotherapy and spirituality: Crossing the line between therapy and religion.* Thousand Oaks, CA: Sage.

Worthington, E. L., Jr. (1986). Religious counseling: A review of published empirical research. *Journal of Counseling and Development, 64,* 421–431.

Worthington, E. L., Jr., Wade, N. E., Hight, T. L., Ripley, J. S., McCullough, M. E., Berry, J. W., et al. (2003). The Religious Commitment Inventory–10: Development, refinement, and validation of a brief scale for research and counseling. *Journal of Counseling Psychology, 50,* 84–96.

12

TRAINING THERAPISTS TO ADDRESS SPIRITUAL CONCERNS IN CLINICAL PRACTICE AND RESEARCH

EVERETT L. WORTHINGTON JR., STEVEN J. SANDAGE, DON E. DAVIS,
JOSHUA N. HOOK, ANDREA J. MILLER, M. ELIZABETH LEWIS HALL,
AND TODD W. HALL

> The mediocre teacher tells. The good teacher explains. The superior teacher demonstrates. The great teacher inspires.
>
> —William A. Ward

In the previous chapters, strategies for integrating spirituality into each phase of the therapeutic process have been provided. However, little attention has been given to how therapists might develop the proper skills and knowledge to competently address spirituality in therapy. As pointed out in chapter 1, there is also a need for more methodologically sound research to advance the field's understanding of effective treatment approaches for working with the spiritual in counseling and psychotherapy. Therefore, in this chapter, we offer training guidelines for addressing spirituality in clinical practice and research. We suggest that secular programs that train therapists must pay more attention to training in spirituality and religion. On the basis of the existing literature that addresses the integration of faith and practice as well as our collective experience, we offer suggestions for programs that train therapists. We advocate a matching model, in which programs assay their resources and faculty interests against their sense of obligation to develop counselors competent to deal with spirituality and religion issues. Depending on faculty decision, which should be informed by student input, more or less emphasis can be placed on eight sources of learning. We find that direct, authentic faculty who initiate attention to spiritual and religious issues may have the greatest impact on students. Finally, we outline a brief research agenda.

Should spirituality and religion be part of clinical training? Although this might seem a rhetorical question, it is not. In counseling, setting matters. For example, if a therapist is employed by a religious congregation or denomination, and if the clientele see the therapist as a representative of that congregation, then clients might expect topics related to spirituality and religion to be addressed in counseling, and clients might be dissatisfied if that does not occur. However, if a therapist is state licensed and there is no mention of spirituality and religion in the therapist's advertisement or informed consent document, then clients are often uncertain whether they should bring up spiritual- and religious-oriented topics (unless they are absolutely central to the client's concerns). In some cases, a state-licensed therapist explicitly markets the practice as spiritual or religious, and clients may be consented to expect that spirituality and religious issues may be introduced by the therapist. Or clients may withhold their consent for the therapist to deal with such issues unless the clients initiate the discussion. Thus, clients and therapists do not act similarly toward spiritual and religious issues in all settings.

Similarly, the setting in which training occurs affects the way training is conducted. Some doctoral programs are explicitly religiously oriented. Currently, these are mostly explicitly Christian programs (e.g., Biola University), but other spiritual programs (e.g., Institute of Transpersonal Psychology) exist. There are master's-level therapy training programs that explicitly engage spirituality from a variety of traditions. Training in religiously affiliated doctoral programs is expected to be oriented toward integrating the faith that the program promotes into virtually every phase and level of training of the students. Those programs, however, also provide special attention to dealing sensitively with clients who (a) are not of the spiritual or religious faith of most of the therapists, supervisors, and teachers in the program; (b) profess no faith; (c) are antagonistic to any faith tradition; or (d) consider themselves spiritual but not religious. In this chapter, we do not make recommendations about training for such religiously oriented programs. Instead, we focus on secular programs.

Secular programs usually do not have an explicit statement about their stance on spirituality and religion. Some consider spirituality and religion as an area of multicultural diversity; others do not (Hage, 2006; Hage, Hopson, & Siegel, 2006). For instance, Schulte, Skinner, and Claiborn (2002) surveyed directors of counseling training (DCTs) of counseling psychology programs. Only 31% of the program directors said the program discussed spiritual and religious issues as diversity issues. This suggests that spiritual and religious issues are not widely accepted as important to training in counseling psychology, but some programs are more welcoming than are others. Schulte et al. (2002) also found that spiritual and religious knowledge was rarely considered part of the expertise of counseling psychologists. It is important to note that explicit spiritual and religious training occurred infrequently. In addition, 61% of the DCTs thought that approaches to therapy consisting of spiritual and religious elements were legitimate. The 39% of DCTs who did not endorse the potential legitimacy of therapy with spiritual and religious elements represent an interesting group. Perhaps some are trying to be respectful and feel that the sacred is such a sensitive area that therapists should not intrude. However, in therapy, counselors often discuss sensitive areas, and there is empirical evidence that many clients want to discuss spiritual and religious issues (Ganje-Fling, Veach, Kuang, & Houg, 2000; Rose, Westefeld, & Ansley, 2001). Also, some forms of spiritual- and religious-accommodative therapy are evidence based (for a review, see Worthington & Sandage, 2002), and there are effective therapies such as dialectical behavior therapy that build on spiritual traditions (e.g., Zen Buddhism).

We believe that the question posed at the outset of this section—Should spirituality and religious training be undertaken?—does not have a clear answer within the context of the current practices of training programs. However, we proceed by suggesting a model of spiritual and religious training. At the end of the chapter, we invite programs to undertake an analysis of their program and their program's training goals to determine the degree to which all or any of the training model can or should be adopted.

TOWARD A MODEL OF SPIRITUAL AND RELIGIOUS TRAINING

We propose a model of training for therapists. We first present a model describing how highly spiritual and religious clients, therapists, therapists-in-training, supervisors, and university teachers interact in relation to their spiritual and religious values. We then suggest goals for a training program to increase comfort and competence with spiritual and religious issues. To the extent a program finds such goals compatible with its resources, we suggest that mere exposure to spiritual and religious issues in the normal course of training is unlikely to produce comfort and competence with spiritual and religious issues. Thus, we identify eight sources of learning that faculty can focus on to integrate spiritual and religious issues into training.

A Model for Understanding Spiritual and Religious Clients

Worthington (1988) proposed a model for understanding religious clients that has received substantial empirical support (for a review, see Worthington, Kurusu, McCullough, & Sandage, 1996). This model is also generalizable to others who have spiritual or religious commitments, such as therapists, therapists-in-training, supervisors, and university teachers. At the core of Worthington's original model was the idea that highly committed religious people (about one standard deviation higher than the mean of the population) view the world through a religious perspective. He proposed three value dimensions: sacred writings, religious leaders, and religious identity. The values on each dimension, if graphed, could be represented as a point in a value space. We might extend this model to a value on inspirational or sacred writings, spiritual or religious leaders or inspirational figures, and spiritual and religious identity. Because those spiritual and religious values are of central importance to highly religious people, they evaluate a person on whether the other has similar values. On the basis of the degree of similarity, they decide whether to remain in contact with the person. They have a "zone of toleration" (Worthington, 1988, p. 169) of the difference in values they will tolerate. When highly religious people detect someone with values outside of their zone of toleration, social interaction with that person is often curtailed, if possible.

Applied to therapy, clients who are high in spirituality and religion actively discern whether a therapist's spiritual or religious values fit within their zone of toleration. Because spirituality and religious values are important to them, many highly spiritual and religious clients do not passively wait for the therapist to reveal his or her beliefs and values but actively ask or make inferences. If the client detects a therapist whose values are outside of the client's zone of toleration, this inference could result in a weak or ruptured therapeutic bond that might lead to dropping out or seeking referral. Part of what makes up that zone is the value the client places on his or her spiritual and religious identity. Thus, for many religiously fundamentalist clients, for example, only a similar religiously fundamentalist therapist would be acceptable, regardless of how accepting the therapist was of diverse religious clients (Hood, Hill, & Williamson, 2005). This can appear rigid to nonfundamentalists but may also represent a deep loyalty commitment within fundamentalist cultures.

Worthington (1988) suggested that this model could apply to therapists as well as clients. Therapists' spiritual or religious commitments (including commitments to non- or antireligiosity) are reflected by where clients' values fall vis-à-vis the therapist's zone of toleration. Detecting that a client's spiritual or religious values are outside of the therapist's zone of toleration could result in the therapist either referring the client or being ineffective in helping the client. Some trainees can be uncomfortable discussing spiritual and religious issues in therapy; others can be uncomfortable *not* discussing spiritual and religious issues in therapy. Each side of this polarity reflects a potentially limited zone of toleration for client differences that could adversely affect therapy practice.

Besides extending the model of spiritual and religious values to therapists, as we did earlier, we now suggest that a similar model applies to supervisors in dealing with supervisees or their clients who deviate markedly from the supervisors' zones of toleration. Such cases result in supervisors who are uncomfortable dealing with spiritual and religious issues and actively or subtly discourage their discussion. Even if the supervisor is comfortable discussing spiritual and religious issues that are divergent from his or her own position (but within the supervisor's zone of toleration), the supervisor might not be competent to help address spiritual issues.

To a lesser degree, university teachers might respond similarly, feeling antagonistic to students whose spiritual or religious positions are outside of the university teachers' zone of toleration. The teacher may not actively discourage students from dealing with spiritual or religious issues in class assignments but may do so nonverbally. The absence of an enthusiastic encouragement to deal with spiritual and religious issues in classes can be perceived by students, in their low-power position, as discouraging, even if the professor does not intend to discourage. This can be especially true in a training program in which some professors have been harsh, outspoken, or subtly (or not-so-subtly) punitive about spiritual or religious students.

These issues can be especially salient for students who have a strong spiritual commitment, have had a significant spiritual experience (whether positive or negative), or are transitioning from a prior spiritual or religious vocation (e.g., priest, rabbi, chaplain, spiritual director). It is unfortunate when these students are discouraged from exploring spiritual and religious issues, because such students often have valuable experiences and bring unique perspectives on professional roles and issues.

This model of spiritual and religious values in counseling and other relationships, which we described earlier, has implications for training therapists. The following sections outline several key training implications and describe an approach for training therapists.

Goals of Training

One of the goals of training therapists is to broaden the therapist's zone of toleration so that he or she can be comfortable with and effective at forming a working alliance with a wide range of clients. This generally accepted goal should include opportunities for the therapist-in-training to integrate views on spiritual and religious issues into his or her developing professional identity (e.g., to actually discuss spiritual and religious issues in counseling). However, the number and type of opportunities for this are subject to legitimate differences of opinion.

Broadening the therapist's zone of toleration requires two, more specific training goals. The first is to increase the therapist's comfort level by heightening the skills of attunement to spiritual and religious clients (e.g., to discern the spiritual and religious positions of clients and interact sensitively around those areas). Furthermore, for most therapists, who might not have a network of referral sources for all spiritual and religious clients, a second training goal is to build competence with techniques of working with spiritual and religious clients (e.g., spiritual exploration with a client experiencing spiritual struggles) to permit more effective counseling. From our collective experience, we believe that most programs train therapists in such a way that the goals of increasing comfort and competence with diversity issues are endorsed, although the application of these goals to work with spiritual and religious clients may be underdeveloped.

Whereas most secular training programs help students broaden their zone of toleration to accept a more diverse collection of clients, many programs do not provide training that deepens (a) the students' awareness of their spiritual and religious values to achieve comfort with these values and (b) their competence at dealing with spiritual and religious clients. Oftentimes only therapists-in-training who personally identify as spiritual or religious or have communicated their interest in working with spiritual and religious clients are encouraged to build spiritual and religious comfort and competency. However, we believe that all therapists-in-training should be provided with training opportunities aimed at building skills in working with spiritual and religious clients, in line with current ethical guidelines suggesting spirituality and religiosity are important areas of diversity (American Psychological Association [APA], 2002), and to avoid unintentional harm to highly spiritual and religious clients. For example, if a strongly spiritual or religious client were not assessed for spiritual or religious issues, and if his or her beliefs or values were directly implicated in later harm—such as suicide caused by depression over a client's mistaken belief that he or she should be perfect to be acceptable to God—the therapist and supervisor might be culpable and vulnerable to lawsuit.

Competence in spiritual and religious values also becomes an ethical issue when the therapist's values are imposed on the client without consent. It has long been recognized that psychotherapy is not a value-neutral process and that therapist values tend to influence both the goals and the process of therapy (Bergin, 1980). When values are imposed, this shows a lack of respect both for the client's spiritual or religious value system and for the social system represented by the value system (McMinn, 1984). The failure to provide such spiritual and religious training may result in harm to the client or to the therapist-in-training. Just as counseling deals with core beliefs and values of clients, training of therapists does also. Teachers and supervisors have a responsibility to treat students with respect and dignity and not to challenge them beyond their psychological abilities to cope. This requires awareness of trainees' spirituality and religious values.

In addition to training students in spiritual and religious competencies, it is also important to teach students how to (a) deal effectively with resistance to spiritual and religious issues in both clinical and research training settings and (b) articulate support and reasoning for why spiritual and religious issues are necessary to incorporate into their clinical work (e.g., frequency that clients bring up presenting problems related to spiritual and religious issues) and research (e.g., how spiritual and religious issues often influence, mediate, or moderate many variables of interest). This training could be accomplished regardless of whether faculty, supervisors, or counseling staff have personal spiritual or religious commitments.

Having argued for the importance of addressing spiritual and religious issues in training by generalizing Worthington's (1988) model to the training of therapists, we can now address the content required by the two broad goals of training. These two broad goals—achieving comfort with a range of spiritual and religious clients and achieving competence in working therapeutically with them—each involves a number of factors.

Achieving Comfort

Achieving comfort in working with a range of spiritual and religious clients involves, at a minimum, self-awareness of one's own values and their effect on therapy. Shafranske and Malony (1990), in a study of APA members, found that psychologists' spiritual and religious beliefs, rather than clinical training, determined how they approached therapeutic interventions with spiritual and religious clients. Without the benefit of training in these areas, there may be increased risk of intervening in ways that have not been thought through carefully. The therapists' failure to be self-aware of their own spiritual and religious values can lead to therapeutic difficulties, including countertransference issues, acting-out of therapist spiritual and religious value conflicts, and value clashes with clients. Each may lead to failures to establish and maintain a therapeutic relationship and possibly to premature termination.

The possibility of countertransference, positive or negative, deserves special attention. Therapists should be aware of biases and assumptions they may hold regarding those with both similar and different spiritual and religious values. Allport (1954) suggested in his social categorization theory that people make sense of their social world by creating categories of the individuals around them. Therapists' biases often operate unconsciously and automatically as they seek to understand others, including clients, and can lead to erroneous interpretations of behavior or miscommunication. The implication for treatment is that knowing about a client's spiritual and religious values and background is not sufficient unless therapists recognize their own values and the consequent biases. For example, a therapist with strongly held values around gender equality may stereotype a client who self-identifies as a practicing Roman Catholic or Muslim and may misinterpret gender dynamics in the client's relationships. Strategies to reduce stereotypic attitudes and biases include self-reflective exercises to develop awareness of those attitudes and values, effort and practice in changing the automatic perceptions, and increased contact with other spiritual and religious groups (APA, 2002).

Additional skills involving spiritual and religious values are required for supervisors and teachers. Supervisors must be sensitive to parallel processes that can occur in supervision. Teachers must also become self-aware that their self-perceived neutrality, advocacy, or discouragement of dealing with spiritual and religious issues may not be perceived as they intend by students and might in fact harm students.

Students in training programs often face significant challenges, including times of self-doubt, stress, vulnerability, insecurity, and changes in self-definition. It is during times of vulnerability and stress that students can be dislodged from periods of stable spiritual and religious dwelling and tossed into a time of spiritual and religious seeking (Shults & Sandage, 2006; Wuthnow, 1998). Interactions during those times of seeking can strongly influence the life course of students—for psychological and spiritual good or ill. Such transition periods in spiritual development can sometimes include symptoms of depression, anxiety, or frustration, especially if former relational attachments have been challenged (Shults & Sandage, 2006). It is our concern that faculty in many secular training programs give little attention to the effects of such times of vulnerability on students' spiritual and religious lives.

Achieving Competence

In addition to helping therapists feel comfortable with spiritual and religious issues, training programs must also facilitate therapists' competence in working with spiritual and religious clients, which involves the development of a number of skills. Therapists should be familiar with the basic beliefs of the spiritual and religious traditions he or she is most likely to encounter in a given training setting. This knowledge will help the therapist to recognize when the client uses distorted spiritual and religious values or practices. This will also help clarify how spiritual and religious beliefs and values affect the client's perception of the problem and the therapeutic process.

For example, defenses may take the form of psychological mechanisms that are framed in spiritual and religious language, have spiritual and religious content, or are tied in with the client's spiritual and religious experience (Narramore, 1994). Armed with this knowledge, the therapist can enlist the client's spiritual and religious values in the service of the therapeutic progress. Other skills include taking a client's spiritual and religious history and assessing the client's spiritual and religious functioning (see chaps. 3 and 4, this volume), working with the psychological meaning and experience of spiritual and religious issues that arise, and, when congruent with the therapist's and client's values, tailoring psychological interventions and goals to incorporate spiritual and religious values or drawing on explicitly spiritual and religious techniques that are consistent with the client's background and values. Additional skills include recognizing one's own limitations and learning to collaborate with and make effective referrals to spiritual and religious professionals or to clergy. Thus, therapists must be able to develop professional relationships with spiritual and religious people different from themselves. Elaboration on these skill sets may be found in chapters 8 and 9 (this volume).

FACULTY DECISIONS ABOUT SPIRITUAL
AND RELIGIOUS ISSUES

In the following section we present a training model. We suggest that trainees would typically benefit from more attention to spiritual and religious issues. Mere exposure is rarely enough to qualify a trainee to deal with the complexities of cases that he or she will face in practice. However, training is most effective if it is not sequenced willy-nilly in the curriculum but is inserted at times when readiness is high.

A Case for More Rather Than Less Attention to Spiritual and Religious Issues

Therapists-in-training will likely benefit most from systematic training in spiritual and religious issues that does not just expose them to spiritual and religious experience but that intentionally addresses spiritual and religious issues in a variety of contexts, from multiple sources, and throughout training. The premises of our training model are, first, that trainees are exposed to people of diverse beliefs, values, and positions of power and status. Second, trainees are subjected to multiple emotionally charged situations that stretch their own zones of toleration through evaluative classroom situations, client and supervisor interactions around often value-laden issues, and peer interactions. These experiences tug at and push the zones of toleration for therapists-in-training in multiple directions; these tensions demand change in personal values, beliefs, and behaviors. Third, the pushes and pulls from too many people, too strongly, or in too divergent directions can strain personal value systems and result in excessive stress reactions and personal defensiveness of therapists-in-training. Such excesses do not promote optimal learning and change. Fourth, students have a stake in their training, and they should have input into curricular decisions. Taking these four premises into consideration, we suggest that training programs should try to introduce challenging situations in measured doses that therapists-in-training have been prepared to assimilate or that promote manageable accommodations. Programs should consider designing consistent, incremental building of training. Programs must consider the optimal level of challenge to therapists-in-training.

Limitations of Mere Exposure

It might seem that mere exposure to course content, outside speakers who discuss spirituality and religion, or diverse spiritual and religious clients would be helpful. We propose, however, that learning how to integrate one's own spirituality and religion into the practice of counseling, supervision, or research might not be best achieved by mere exposure. Early research on supervision of psychotherapy (Stoltenberg, McNeill, & Crethar, 1994; Wiley & Ray, 1986) showed that therapy skills are not a product of mere therapy experiences. Growth in skill requires supervised therapy experience; this includes experience, guided reflection, and accountability for one's counseling decisions to a more experienced supervisor. Likewise, we hypothesize that mere exposure or experience with spiritual and religious issues—either one's own or with clients, research, or class work—will not effectively train students to deal competently with spiritual and religious issues. The limited effect of exposure will be especially true for students who are particularly defensive about spiritual and religious issues, because mere exposure might reinforce preexisting biases.

Rather, we hypothesize that supervised or mentored experience will be a better way of learning to deal with spiritual and religious issues. This proposition—that providing mere experience is ineffective as a training strategy—has not been empirically tested with spiritual and religious values; however, the principle may be generalized from other research.

Sequencing of Experiences

The timing of points of teaching and training in spiritual and religious sensitivity and competence is important. First, significant impact is often made during teachable moments of stress and vulnerability for trainees when students are seeking knowledge and may be unusually responsive. Yet, if the stress is too high, periods of stress and vulnerability can create defensiveness in which students are threatened in core personal spiritual and religious values and strongly resist new information and new experiential learning.

Second, other teachable moments involve client crises that deal with spiritual and religious issues with which the therapist-in-training is not familiar. Practicum experiences often introduce therapists-in-training to new levels of suffering, vicariously through the lives of clients. This can raise existential questions that register at a spiritual level for some therapists-in-training. The therapist-in-training is often less defensive in such times when he or she needs support and input from a supervisor. The danger is that the therapist-in-training may be especially uncritical and nonanalytic about the suggestions of a supervisor. Although uncritical acceptance may help the therapist-in-training solve the immediate problem, it is not in line with educational goals of having students think critically about their training. Supervisors are wise to attend to the existential effect of clinical practice on therapists-in-training and, without turning supervision into therapy, offer appropriate support and referrals when necessary.

Third, other teachable moments occur in classes. Usually, class interactions, which are focused on content, are times when stress and vulnerability are minimal. Students may ask about the role of religion in psychopathology or may discuss religiously tailored interventions within a course on psychotherapy or empirically supported (or evidence-based) treatments. Students are freed to learn knowledge and skills precisely because they are in a nonthreatening environment in which the emphasis is on information rather than dealing with clients' emotional issues, with their own personal psychological dynamics, or with psychotherapeutic interventions in which the students have invested emotional energy.

SOURCES OF LEARNING

How might therapists-in-training learn how to integrate spiritual and religious skills into their therapeutic practice? We have identified eight sources of learning: (a) coursework, (b) interaction with peers, (c) advising and mentoring, (d) research, (e) personal therapy, (f) practicum experiences (including learning from supervisors, practicum staffing, and clients), (g) predoctoral internship, and (h) postdegree training. We discuss each source subsequently.

Coursework

First, students can learn from coursework. The class material—reading or written assignments (e.g., required assignments, such as a genogram, could include spiritual and religious factors)—expose students to new ideas and ask students to articulate their understanding aloud or in writing. The university teacher also can influence the student through the teacher's actions, responses in class, and responses on written or other evaluative assignments. The classroom contains opportunities to learn, but it also involves evaluative components and power differentials. Typically, students will monitor attitudes of the teacher and will only freely explore controversial topics (which spiritual and religious topics often seem to be) when the student is convinced the teacher's positions mirror the student's (i.e., the student perceives his or her views are within the teacher's zone of toleration). Some assertive spiritual and religious students might challenge teachers to consider spiritual and religious issues, which require teachers to generate a nondefensive response that is both appropriate and educational for the training context.

Sorenson (1997a) reasoned that teachers in programs that explicitly teach how issues of faith are integrated in research and practice during coursework should be expected to be influential in a student's professional life. In Sorenson's (1997a) study, 48 doctoral students sorted 19 doctoral faculty at Rosemead School of Psychology, an institution whose mission is to integrate faith and psychology (as opposed to a secular program), into piles of similarity to each other. Multidimensional scaling was used to uncover underlying dimensions among the faculty. Students implicitly evaluated faculty on four dimensions: (a) how exemplary and helpful the professor was directly to the student to integrate matters of faith and profession or faith and life, (b) evidence of an ongoing process in a relationship with God, (c) emotional transparency, and (d) sense of humor. Staton, Sorenson, and Vande Kemp (1998) replicated the Sorenson (1997a) study at Fuller Theological Seminary with different students and faculty. Staton et al. (1998) concluded the following:

> The most salient dimension to contribute to their own integration was how well they could determine that a given professor had an authentic, lively, and growing relationship with God, coupled with the professor's nondefensive, emotionally unguarded, and even vulnerable relationship with students. (p. 348)

These findings reinforce the idea that professors, and their attitudes toward spiritual and religious issues, are crucial in the acquisition of spiritual and religious comfort and competence.

Interactions With Peers

Peers are hypothesized to provide a substantial (and at this point uninvestigated) source of influence on other students. As personal and professional issues arise, peer interactions occur in one of two settings. First, talk of the spiritual and religious occurs in classes, generally subject to evaluation by faculty who are present. Thus, students in such classes might not be forthright with their comments. Some might harbor competitive motives to put down each other, which could constitute trouble for students on the receiving end of public shaming. Students might therefore be reluctant to share honestly and openly in class.

In the second setting, students spend time together and often share their struggles outside of classes in private dyads or groups. Those presumably more candid and private group or dyadic discussions—without a teacher being present—provide a vehicle for learning. Peers are often an underinvestigated and underrated source of professional socialization.

Advising and Mentoring

Students can learn from their advisors. Students usually are assigned to advisors with the major criterion of similarity of research interests. Thus, often students interested in spiritual and religious research have advisors who share those interests. Still, the relationship with an advisor is often complex. Students share work on publications and are also in personal relationship with research supervisors, and typically this relationship is closer than with most other faculty. Some students might be free to ask about issues concerning the ways that faith intersects practice, personal life, and school dilemmas, whereas for other students, contact with the advisor is more circumscribed and oriented around academic advising and research.

Because the doctoral advisee interacts with the advisor across a broad range of circumstances, the advisee often gets to see the advisor as a person and to know the advisor's strengths and weaknesses, pet peeves, struggles, and triumphs. The student can learn much about faith's position in professional life from an advisor who embraces a personal faith commitment not merely through research and reading but through personal observation. Furthermore, for advisors who do not embrace a faith commitment, students can learn how to deal with spiritual and religious issues, when they arise, as a fair-minded professional.

Research Experiences

How might students learn to integrate spiritual and religious perspectives into their research? Six potential sources are available. First, research mentors might educate students in spiritual and religious research by using an apprentice model. Second, mentors can involve students from the early part of their training in the writing of chapters, and later, as data are collected, in the writing of empirical articles. Third, students can attend spiritual and religious conferences and training workshops. Fourth, students can seek out special interest groups within professional organizations, divisions within organizations (e.g., Division 36 of the APA), and organizations that promote spiritual and religious research (e.g., Society for the Scientific Study of Religion, the Christian Association for Psychological Studies, and others). Fifth, students can be directed in their reading to research articles on spirituality and religion within research teams, relationships with advisors, and interactions with professors who have an interest in spiritual and religious issues. Sixth, places within a program's curriculum might direct reading and research on spiritual and religious issues.

Schulte et al. (2002) found that 83% of DCTs believed that at least one faculty member was willing to supervise student research on spiritual and religious issues, and 90% had some faculty member open to research on spiritual and religious issues in their program. Thus, students interested in conducting spiritual and religious research can usually be supervised in that research.

Personal Therapy

Students can learn from the therapists who counsel them, if they attend therapy. Some programs, especially those deriving from psychoanalytic therapy roots, require students to attend counseling. Most programs do not require training therapy. However, training for most therapists is rigorous and stressful. Because students in the clinically oriented fields value therapy, many attend personal therapy to deal with their stress. As Sorenson (1994, 1997b) observed, personal therapy can promote learning, especially through the unprompted initiation by the therapist of spiritual and religious issues. Therapy can provide a safe environment in which students can learn how to integrate spiritual and religious beliefs into therapy, both through open discussions of their spiritual and religious beliefs and through modeling of the therapist. In addition, much learning in therapy occurs through self-reflection. Some students choose spiritual direction or other forms of spiritual self-care to support their growth during training. Training programs may consider resources and referrals that can be made available to students while also respecting student boundaries.

The potential for personal therapy to substantially influence students regarding spirituality and religion is illustrated by Sorenson, who conducted six programmatic studies on spiritual and religious training within religiously tailored Christian doctoral programs (Sorenson, 1994, 1997a, 1997b; Sorenson, Derflinger, Bufford, & McMinn, 2004; Sorenson & Hales, 2002; Staton et al., 1998). First, students at Rosemead School of Psychology provided written essays on their developmental experiences of God, as well as their experiences with spiritual and religious issues in their own therapy and in their clinical practices (Sorenson, 1994). The most influential person on the students' own clinical handling of spiritual and religious issues was the student's personal therapist.

Second, Sorenson (1997b) compiled a sample of students five times as large as the previous study (Sorenson, 1994). The students' work with others (clients and others) in terms of the integration of issues of personal faith and professional practice was again most related to their own personal therapist's work with them. Third, Sorenson (1997b) identified six therapist behaviors that were critical in the students' development of spiritual and religious issues: (a) treating the student's relationship with God as real; (b) approaching matters of faith and life nondefensively and openly; (c) making connections between the student's life and the student's parents, God, and therapist, and doing so on his or her own initiation rather than being reactive to the student or client; (d) seeing the student's relationship with God as at least partially positive and a resource for healing instead of interpreting it as a projection from family or treating it as pathological or negative; (e) expecting that issues of faith and life would come up and should be part of therapy; and (f) showing a personal openness to the transcendent even if the therapist did not have similar beliefs as the student or client.

Later, Sorenson et al. (2004) replicated the model. They collected data from four APA-accredited doctoral programs at different schools: Rosemead, Fuller Theological Seminary, George Fox University, and Wheaton College. The model identified the same behaviors. Overall, Sorenson's research suggests the importance of a student's personal therapist in shaping how students deal with spiritual and religious issues. This was particularly true when therapists initiated discussions of spiritual and religious issues and were authentic regardless of their own personal spiritual and religious commitments.

Practicum Experiences

Students' practicum experiences include those with supervisors, practicum staff members, and clients. We address each in the subsequent sections.

Experiences With Supervisors

Miller, Korinek, and Ivey (2004) developed the Spiritual Issues in Supervision Scale (SISS) to examine supervisees' perceptions of the degree to which each of several spiritual issues was addressed in supervision of marital and family therapies (MFTs). These issues included gender and identity (e.g., gender, divorce, self-esteem), acceptance (e.g., ethics, power, social support networks), family role (e.g., parenting, sexual intimacy), morality and loss (e.g., abortion, grief, sexual orientation), diversity, value of life (e.g., ethnicity, culture), and supervisory process (e.g., assessment process, treatment planning, supervisory process).

Miller, Korinek, and Ivey (2006) then surveyed 153 master's-level and doctoral-level students from 12 universities, some of whom completed the SISS on more than one supervisor, resulting in 257 cases. A principal-components analysis identified four factors: client system, supervisory system, diversity lens, and lens of meaning and values.

The research studies showed that issues of spirituality arose in supervision of MFTs in talking about client problems, discussing supervisory relationships, and discussing ethnicity and meaning. Spirituality was not encapsulated in silos, that is, spirituality was not addressed merely in explicitly religious conversations with explicitly religious clients on when clients were having an overtly religious or spiritual crisis in faith. Rather, discussions of spirituality and religion arose between supervisors and counselors across a full range of counseling topics, processes, and consideration of life and values. The implication for training in regard to spirituality and religion is this: It is not wise for a training program to think that spiritual issues will be localized. If a training program is serious about responsible mentoring of students in spiritual and religious issues, then these issues will likely be confronted across the spectrum of training.

Typically, practicum experience does not affect students' grades, but evaluation by supervisors clearly affects their future, their ratings in the training program, and their self-concept as a therapist. Clients bring up spiritual issues or present moral dilemmas that have spiritual and religious underpinnings, placing many therapists-in-training in a conflict. Should they bring up the spiritual and religious issues to their supervisors? Not all supervisors are willing to address spiritual and religious issues if they arise. For example,

Schulte et al. (2002) found that although training directors in counseling psychology programs and counseling psychologists are often especially open to multicultural issues, in only 78% of the cases did the directors believe that "practicum supervisors in the program are open to discussing the client's spirituality or religion *if it seems relevant to the case*" (p. 125; [italics added]). It is reasonable to assume that (a) DCTs are more cognizant of the supervisors' positions than are therapists-in-training, and (b) therapists-in-training in practicum are vulnerable. If a maximum of 78% of supervisors are perceived (by DCTs) to be open to discussing spiritual and religious issues when they are relevant to the case, it is reasonable to conclude that many therapists-in-training will simply dodge spiritual and religious issues in supervision. Perhaps trainees will present other aspects of the case but not reveal the spiritual or religious issue. Perhaps they will focus on other cases and describe other issues that are safer than the client's spiritual or religious issues. This does not even consider whether the supervisor is competent to provide wise guidance on spiritual and religious issues or whether the supervisor might differ substantially in spiritual or religious commitment, belief, values, or understanding from counselor and client. Thus, many therapists-in-training must deal with spiritual and religious issues independently because they might not feel safe to do so in supervision.

We might tentatively extend Sorenson's earlier-mentioned programmatic research finding to supervisors, which he did not study. First, spiritual and religious training cannot effectively be dumped at the door of supervisors who are spiritual or religious themselves. Some of the nonspiritual or religious supervisors are likely equally effective trainers. Second, supervisors must tackle spiritual and religious issues with personal authenticity, openness to the students' diversity, and sensitivity to students and clients of the same or different spirituality or religion. Third, and perhaps most important, supervisors must initiate straightforward discussions about spirituality and religion without being hostile or demanding spiritual or religious conformity to their opinions and positions. It is probably not sufficient to assume that most trainees will initiate discussion of spirituality and religion. A few outspoken trainees might indeed initiate discussion, but the chances are most trainees will keep a low profile on this potentially explosive issue. This stems directly from (a) the vulnerable status of the trainee, (b) the lack of spiritual or religious emphasis of most trainers (Bergin & Jensen, 1990), and (c) the finding that programs usually do not encourage discussions of spiritual or religious issues.

Experiences With Practicum Staff Members

Even in practicum staffing, students might be reluctant to present a case that reveals their treatment of a client with a spiritual and religious issue. Even if the supervisor is supportive, some staff members might not be. Thus, students can be intimidated. In Schulte et al. (2002), only two thirds of DCTs said they thought that spiritual and religious issues were discussed in practicum. Given that spiritual or religious issues must be occurring with some clients in virtually any agency, practicum students must not feel completely free to share with staff. Whereas practicum is a source of learning about spiritual and religious issues in therapy, if Schulte et al.'s results are accurate, one wonders how much actual learning is available to students.

Experiences With Clients

Surveys have shown that therapists are not as spiritual or religious as clients (Bergin & Jensen, 1990; Genia, 1994; Kelly, 1994; Shafranske & Malony, 1990). The chances are, then, that some clients will likely present spiritual and religious issues, and therapists-in-training will have to address those issues. The likelihood is that the therapists-in-training (being future therapists) will be mismatched with clients in spirituality and religion and will need assistance in assessing, treating, or referring clients.

In our experience, some client populations have a particular interest in knowing the therapist's spiritual or religious values. For example, conservative Christians, gay and lesbian clients, and adherents of alternative medicine are three populations that frequently have an interest in matching values with a therapist (Worthington, 1991). Beginning therapists sometimes either duck such questions or rush to answer them without adequately understanding the context of the client's concerns. Therapist disclosure about values that fits the client's unique context and concern is more likely to be helpful.

Couple and family systems can raise the degree of complexity in the area of spirituality and religion. For example, couples may be mismatched on spiritual and religious values or beliefs even if they generally subscribe to the same spiritual and religious tradition. In families, it is not uncommon for adolescents to challenge the parents' spiritual and religious values. This immediately puts the therapist in a position of potential triangulation that must be handled with care.

Predoctoral Internship

Little research has been conducted on training of spiritual and religious issues within the predoctoral internship. Stedman (2006) comprehensively surveyed the literature on what is known about the predoctoral internship training; however, spiritual and religious issues were not mentioned in the article. They had not been investigated in prior research and did not appear on Stedman's radar scope as issues that needed to be addressed.

Russell and Yarhouse (2006) surveyed 433 training directors of internship training programs listed on the Association of Psychology Postdoctoral

Internship Centers directory. Of the 32% responding ($N = 139$), only 35.3% ($n = 40$) reported any didactic training in spiritual and religious issues. Of those programs that offered any training, about 50% offered training once a year, about 20% offered it once a semester, and only 6.6% offered spiritual and religious training about monthly. The remaining 25% responded "other" (and follow-up revealed this to mean that some sites had a specifically designated spiritual or religious rotation, or spiritual and religious issues were dealt with as they arose). About 90% of the directors of training said that spiritual and religious issues were dealt with in supervision whenever they arose. Other sources of learning that directors of training listed were consultation, in-services, crisis services, and teaching. Sometimes sites provided workshops, and sometimes sites provided spiritual and religious training as part of multi-cultural training.

Training directors were also asked whether they foresaw training in spiritual and religious issues being conducted at their sites in the future. Of the 139 training directors, 61 left the question blank, 53 reported that they never foresaw it as being offered in their program, and 15 said it might be offered in the next 2 years. Over 90% of the training directors did not see spiritual and religious rotations ever being offered at their sites. Russell and Yarhouse (2006) concluded that spiritual and religious training in internship is almost always dependent on whether the client brings up a relevant issue.

Postdoctoral Training

Postdegree training in spirituality and religion is increasingly available. This can include the postdegree, prelicensure supervision, and training. Some licensed therapists participate in spirituality and religion special-interest groups. All licensed practitioners are required to obtain continuing education. Continuing education oriented toward spiritual and religious issues is available at conventions, through summer institutes (e.g., Cape Cod Institute; http://www.cape.org), online (e.g., http://healthforumonline.com), and through programs offering quizzes on articles within single issues of some journals. Therapists in this category are also encouraged to stay abreast of the current spirituality and religion literature and resources. Similarly, involvement in spiritual and religious professional organizations can provide a wealth of information and opportunities for professional growth as well.

Summary

In surveying the sources of learning, we surmise that, except for doctoral programs that are religiously tailored, a variable amount of spiritual and religious training exists. Most programs seem to be concentrated at the end of the spectrum in which spiritual and religious training happens (a) through faculty or staff who have a personal interest in spiritual and religious issues, (b) when clients bring up an explicit spiritual or religious issue, (c) when trainees have a personal interest in spiritual and religious issues, and (d) haphazardly if specific occasional issues arise in coursework or discussion.

RECOMMENDATIONS FOR SECULAR TRAINING PROGRAMS

Yarhouse and Fisher (2002) identified three training models by which spirituality and religion can be incorporated into training. They described the *integration-incorporation model* as a modest approach that can be tailored to faculty interests and existing courses and training experiences. Yarhouse and Fisher suggested that, at a minimum, this could teach therapists-in-training how to discuss spiritual and religious issues with clients of different spiritual and religious orientations. Specific information about spirituality and religion in ethics, etiology of mental health disorders, diagnosis, and intervention could be worked into a variety of classes without disrupting the ongoing training program. Overall, the integration-incorporation approach, if one can judge by surveys of training programs (Schulte et al., 2002) and internship sites (Russell & Yarhouse, 2006), is most frequently a low-level integration with modest goals, such as increasing counselors' awareness of issues and helping them to develop a more precise vocabulary to discuss the issues.

At a second level, the *certificate-minor model* suggests that students could participate in clearly delineated tracks or minor concentrations in which they craft a subspecialization in spiritual and religious theory and practice. Yarhouse and Fisher (2002) identified two exemplars for such a program: the Illinois School of Professional Psychology and the Minnesota School of Professional Psychology. These programs involve add-ons to the normal curriculum. They permit students interested in spirituality and religion to do additional specialized work in spiritual or religious counseling while earning the same training as other therapists-in-training. The majority of students are exposed unsystematically to spiritual and religious issues in the remainder of the curriculum. Having students with a subspecialization in spiritual and religious counseling does open conversations among peers.

The third level of involvement is the *religious distinctive model*. Such models have been prevalent within the APA's accreditation program for decades. Such programs involve an integrated training program in which students take courses in theology as well as psychology, and they often cannot complete the doctoral degree in the same time frame as do students who are not in a religiously tailored program. Those integrated programs are model programs in that they focus much of the curriculum on integrating psychology and spirituality and require such integration among faculty and students within all courses and practicum experiences.

We observe that there might be at least two additions or changes to Yarhouse and Fisher's (2002) levels of training. First, some programs virtually ignore spiritual and religious issues, relegating their discussion to supervision only if a client brings up the topic or if a crisis arises. We would label such programs as *mimimalist as-needed training models*. Second, we would prefer to subdivide Yarhouse and Fisher's integration-incorporation level of training into *unsystematic* and *systematic* integration-incorporation categories. Many programs seem to use a minimalist level of incorporation of spiritual and religious issues into training that is slightly more intentional than the minimalist as-needed training model. Inclusion of spiritual and religious issues is not an explicit program goal and is thus haphazard. It often depends on the presence of a particular faculty member or members who have spiritual and religious issues as an interest area, and thus the program does not consign spiritual and religious issues to neglect as with the minimalist as-needed training model. We call this the *unsystematic integration-incorporation training model*. There are no program goals or expectations for what students do or do not learn and what competencies they are expected to have by graduation.

Systematic integration-incorporation involves a program that has explicitly decided that spiritual and religious issues are to be integrated in the curriculum. The program is not identified with a religious tradition and does not advocate primarily one approach to religion or spirituality. The two remaining levels in Yarhouse and Fisher's (2002) models—the certificate-minor and religious distinctive models—remain unaltered.

Spiritual and Religious Matching Training Model

In this chapter, we advocate a *spiritual and religious matching training model*. In this model, faculty members assess (a) their own interests and their program's curricular resources, (b) their goals for students, and (c) the sources for input of spiritual and religious information. Curriculum decisions are made by placing all of these considerations together in a matching model.

Many training programs, in theory, view spirituality and religion as an area of diversity, but they have not given special attention to promoting student competencies in dealing with spiritual and religious issues in clients, research, or their own lives. As a general principle of multicultural training, we believe the therapist-trainee is greatly affected by authentic relationships with supervisors and mentors (Sorenson, 1997a, 1997b). Specifically, we hypothesize that clinical supervision will be one of the strongest influences on the therapist's future attitudes, skills, and behaviors toward spiritual and religious issues. If so, Schulte et al. (2002) suggested that too few therapists-in-training are receiving adequate training for competence with spiritual and religious issues. Thus, many therapists-in-training will be unprepared to competently handle this aspect of diversity. We suggest an analysis of the status of training programs in light of Schulte et al.'s article. We fully recognize that such analysis will yield different defensible answers among the programs.

Steps to Increasing Focus on Spiritual and Religious Issues

If a program wishes to change priorities to ensure a higher level of spiritual and religious competencies in students, then we suggest a stepwise approach. The approach begins with consensus building and then progresses to making systematic changes that bring the overall curriculum into line with chosen goals.

First, a program must take a definitive step to decide that it is important to train its students in spiritual and religious issues. An explicit program decision seems to be necessary. If not, faculty members may differ greatly in how they handle spiritual and religious issues as an area of diversity. If the faculty is not clear about their stance, students will, *de facto*, likely be intimidated and discouraged from explicitly dealing with spiritual and religious issues.

Second, we suggest that effective training will not occur by mere counseling experience. It will occur best by intentional inclusion of spiritual and religious issues in practicum, coursework, research, the students' own therapy, interactions with the advisor, and open peer networks that are not mediated by the presence of faculty. If faculty members agree with this premise, then it might be wise to consider their goals for training.

Third, faculty members should work with student representatives to identify competencies that the program considers minimally necessary. These might include competencies in (a) articulation of a student's stance toward addressing spirituality and religion in counseling, (b) assessment of spiritual and religious issues that affect counseling, (c) counseling with emotionally charged spiritual and religious issues without letting the student's beliefs or values negatively affect client outcomes, (d) referrals to a spiritual or religious practitioner, (e) consultation with a spiritual or religious practitioner, (f) recognition of countertransference in spiritual and religious issues, (g) willingness and ability to address spiritual and religious topics forthrightly within practicum and classes, and (h) collaboration with religious leaders.

Fourth, faculty and students should decide on the means for achieving the objectives of the program. Faculty members should strive to be authentic in how they address spiritual and religious issues in their professional lives. Faculty who are authentic—regardless of whether they are personally spiritual or religious—are hypothesized to have the most positive impact on students. Those faculty members who are either critical or non-self-disclosing will inhibit student exploration. Other means, such as invited speakers, commitment to continuing education for faculty members to build their own awareness and skills, and inclusion of spiritual and religious issues in the curriculum when warranted, should be enumerated. Faculty members should make space for students to explore spiritual and religious issues within peer networks. Supervisors should be encouraged to be uniformly open to spiritual and religious issues (without necessarily endorsing a spiritual or religious perspective), or students will likely not share their struggles.

Fifth, faculty and students should establish benchmarks against which student progress and program progress can be measured. What competencies should students develop, and at what level of training? How can the program assess its success in helping students be more aware of and competent in spiritual and religious issues? Then, faculty and students should create an assessment plan that determines whether students are meeting these benchmarks and whether the program is achieving the objectives it has set for itself.

Sixth, faculty and students should strive to create a climate that is not just permissive, addressing issues only as they arise. In this environment, students may not present spiritual or religious issues to supervisors and professors because they are uncomfortable. Thus, reliance on client crises or student initiative to ensure that the program adequately trains in spiritual and religious issues is not the best pathway to excellence in training. Instead, we recommend that programs encourage forthright addressing of spiritual and religious issues, or else students will not take the chances necessary to learn.

PRELIMINARY RESEARCH AGENDA

It is not practical to set forth a detailed and comprehensive research agenda in the current space. However, we aim to suggest briefly some starting points for research in spiritual and religious issues regarding training in secular programs.

First, investigation of our main hypothesis—that mere exposure to experiences with spiritual and religious clients is not effective training—is needed. Second, research regarding how and how often spiritual and religious issues are presented in secular settings needs to be conducted. For example, how often are spiritual and religious issues central to a client's presenting problem (e.g., spiritual or religious crisis) or more subtly relevant (e.g., abortion, divorce, betrayals, loss)? How often are spiritual and religious issues important to the client but not dealt with in therapy? Similarly, how often are clients' personal spiritual and religious beliefs used as effective coping strategies in therapy?

Third, research is needed on how therapists-in-training are currently being trained in spiritual and religious issues from their point of view. For instance, from which sources are students receiving spiritual and religious training (e.g., advisors, readings, supervisors)? How often is spiritual and religious training occurring? Also, how often and how helpful are informal peer discussions of spiritual and religious issues? How many therapists-in-training view spiritual and religious issues as part of being multiculturally competent? How important is spiritual and religious competence to therapists-in-training?

Do therapists feel they have developed competence in minimal skills needed for spiritual and religious issues?

Fourth, would a training program instituting a more intentional effort in training in spiritual and religious issues result in better counselor and client outcomes? Namely, would counselors express more competence and comfort in dealing with spiritual and religious clients? Would posttermination client surveys reveal more satisfied clients?

Fifth, what unwanted effects might occur if a training program made more intentional efforts to highlight spiritual and religious training? Would more students express disgruntlement because they were hostile to spiritual and religious issues or did not believe them to be central in importance to counseling training?

Once this research has been conducted, more complex experiments and studies may be designed. For example, manipulated experiments could be conducted in which some supervisors explicitly initiate discussions of therapist-trainee's spiritual and religious beliefs and client's spiritual and religious beliefs versus other supervisors who do not initiate such discussions.

CONCLUSION: PRIORITY 1 RECOMMENDATION

The fundamental and as yet untested proposition in this chapter is that mere exposure to spiritual and religious experiences—through clients, spontaneous discussions, and almost randomly encountered (and certainly unsystematically organized) reading—will produce little to no improvement in trainees' competencies dealing with spiritual and religious issues in clinical practice (and perhaps in research). This proposition deserves multiple empirical tests, and we believe that its testing deserves the highest priority.

If the proposition is supported, then programs need to determine the degree to which they value explicit training in spiritual and religious issues. If they wish to increase spiritual and religious focus, systematic inclusion of supervised, mentored, and thoughtful experiences must be undertaken. We have provided a training model that can be used to structure programmatic decisions about training regardless of whether a program takes an approach that is primarily as needed, integrative-incorporative, minor emphasis, or religiously tailored in its degree of spiritual and religious training.

REFERENCES

American Psychological Association. (2002). *Guidelines on multicultural education, training, research, practice, and organizational change for psychologists*. Washington, DC: Author.

Allport, G. W. (1954). *The nature of prejudice*. Cambridge, MA: Addison-Wesley.

Bergin, A. E. (1980). Psychotherapy and religious values. *Journal of Consulting and Clinical Psychology, 48*, 95–105.

Bergin, A. E., & Jensen, J. P. (1990). Religiosity of psychotherapists: A national survey. *Psychotherapy, 27*, 3–7.

Ganje-Fling, M., Veach, P. M., Kuang, H., & Houg, B. (2000). Effects of childhood sexual abuse on client spiritual well-being. *Counseling and Values, 44*, 84–91.

Genia, V. (1994). Secular psychotherapists and religious clients: Professional considerations and recommendations. *Journal of Counseling and Development, 72*, 395–398.

Hage, S. M. (2006). A closer look at the role of spirituality in psychology training programs. *Professional Psychology: Research and Practice, 37*, 303–310.

Hage, S. M., Hopson, A., & Siegel, M. (2006). Multicultural spirituality: An interdisciplinary review. *Counseling and Values, 50*, 217–234.

Hood, R. W., Jr., Hill, P. C., & Williamson, W. P. (2005). *The psychology of religious fundamentalism*. New York: Guilford Press.

Kelly, E. W. (1994). The role of religion and spirituality in counselor education: A national survey. *Counselor Education and Supervision, 33*, 227–237.

McMinn, M. R. (1984). Religious values and client–therapist matching in psychotherapy. *Journal of Psychology and Theology, 12*, 24–33.

Miller, M. M., Korinek, A., & Ivey, D. C. (2004). Spirituality in MFT training: Development of the Spiritual Issues in Supervision Scale. *Contemporary Family Therapy, 26*, 71–81.

Miller, M. M., Korinek, A., & Ivey, D. C. (2006). Integrating spirituality into training: The Spiritual Issues in Supervision Scale. *American Journal of Family Therapy, 34*, 355–372.

Narramore, B. (1994). Dealing with religious resistances in psychotherapy. *Journal of Psychology and Theology, 22*, 249–258.

Rose, E. M., Westefeld, J. S., & Ansley, T. N. (2001). Spiritual issues in counseling: Clients' beliefs and preferences. *Journal of Counseling Psychology, 48*, 61–71.

Russell, S. R., & Yarhouse, M. A. (2006). Training in religion/spirituality within APA-accredited psychology predoctoral internships. *Professional Psychology: Research and Practice, 37*, 430–436.

Schulte, D. L., Skinner, T. A., & Claiborn, C. D. (2002). Religious and spiritual issues in counseling psychology training. *The Counseling Psychologist, 30*, 118–134.

Shafranske, E. P., & Malony, H. N. (1990). Clinical psychologists' religious and spiritual orientations and their practice of psychotherapy. *Psychotherapy, 27*, 72–78.

Shults, F. L., & Sandage, S. J. (2006). *Transforming spirituality: Integrating theology and psychology*. Grand Rapids, MI: Baker Academic.

Sorenson, R. L. (1994). Therapists' (and their therapists') God representations in clinical practice. *Journal of Psychology and Theology, 22*, 325–344.

Sorenson, R. L. (1997a). Doctoral students' integration of psychology and Christianity: Perspectives via attachment theory and multidimensional scaling. *Journal for the Scientific Study of Religion, 36*, 530–548.

Sorenson, R. L. (1997b). Transcendence and intersubjectivity: The patient's experience of the analyst's spirituality. In C. Spezzano & G. Gargiula (Eds.), *Soul on the couch* (pp. 166–199). Hillsdale, NJ: Analytic Press.

Sorenson, R. L., Derflinger, K. R., Bufford, R. K., & McMinn, M. R. (2004). National collaborative research on how students learn integration: Final report. *Journal of Psychology and Theology, 23*, 355–365.

Sorenson, R. L., & Hales, S. (2002). Comparing evangelical Protestant psychologists trained at secular versus religiously affiliated programs. *Psychotherapy: Theory, Research, Practice, Training, 39*, 163–170.

Staton, R., Sorenson, R. L., & Vande Kemp, H. (1998). How students learn integration: Replication of Sorenson's (1997) model. *Journal of Psychology and Theology, 26*, 340–350.

Stedman, J. M. (2006). What we know about predoctoral internship training: A review. *Training and Education in Professional Psychology, 8*, 80–95.

Stoltenberg, C. D., McNeill, B. W., & Crethar, H. C. (1994). Changes in supervision as counselors and therapists gain experience: A review. *Professional Psychology: Research and Practice, 25*, 416–449.

Wiley, M. O., & Ray, P. B. (1986). Counseling supervision by developmental level. *Journal of Counseling Psychology, 33*, 439–445.

Worthington, E. L., Jr. (1988). Understanding the values of religious clients: A model and its application to counseling. *Journal of Counseling Psychology, 35*, 166–174.

Worthington, E. L., Jr. (1991). Psychotherapy and religious values: An update. *Journal of Psychology and Christianity, 10*, 211–223.

Worthington, E. L., Jr., Kurusu, T., McCullough, M. E., & Sandage, S. J. (1996). Empirical research on religion and psychotherapeutic processes and outcomes: A ten-year review and research prospectus. *Psychological Bulletin, 119*, 448–487.

Worthington, E. L., Jr., & Sandage, S. J. (2002). Religion and spirituality. In J. C. Norcross (Ed.), *Psychotherapy relationships that work: Therapist contributions and responsiveness to patients* (pp. 383–399). New York: Oxford University Press.

Wuthnow, R. (1998). *After heaven: Spirituality in America since the 1950s*. Berkeley: University of California Press.

Yarhouse, M. A., & Fisher, W. (2002). Levels of training to address religion in clinical practice. *Psychotherapy, 39*, 171–176.

INDEX

Behavioral duties, specification of, 27–28
Behaviorism, 195
Beliefs
    discrepancies between therapist's and client's, 226–227
    global, 123–125
    patients', 30–31
Belief system
    acknowledging client's, 226
    sensitivity to, 17
Benchmarks, 288
Bergin, A. E., 10, 179
Bias
    case study, 34–36
    examining, 168
    therapist's, 44, 273
"Bible counseling," 42–43
Biola University, 268
Boundaries
    of competence, 33
    and countertransference, 57
    interpersonal, 231–233
Brigham Young University, 243
Bruff v. North Mississippi Health Services, Inc., 29, 31–32
Buddha, Gautama, 193
Buddhists, 225

CACREP (Council for Accreditation of Counseling and Related Educational Programs), 18
Callanan, P., 79
Caplan, E., 14
Capps, D. E., 93
Case conceptualizations, 121–140
    case study, 250–252
    client-centered, 139
    developing, 128–131
    functions of, 122
    importance of, 121–122
    meaning-based case studies, 131–139
    meaning-making approach to, 126–139
    and meaning systems, 123–125
    psychoanalytic, 139
    recursive process of developing/using, 122

roles of spirituality/religiosity in, 126–128
Case examples, wisdom of, 28
Case study (of spirituality in therapeutic process), 241–263
    assessment, 246–250
    background information for case, 243
    case conceptualization/treatment planning, 250–252
    commentary/recommendations, 263
    environment of openness/safety, 243–246
    termination preparation, 260–263
    theoretical background, 242
    treatment implementation, 252–260
Casuistry, 28
CBT. See Cognitive behavior therapy
Certificate-minor training model, 285
Child custody, 29, 31
Chirban, J. T., 75
Christian-accommodative cognitive behavior therapy, 201
Christianity, 224
Christian privilege, 196–197
Christians
    evangelical, 188
    fundamentalist, 188–190
    nonjudgmental acceptance of, 184–185
    and protecting against bias, 34–36
Church of Jesus Christ of Latter-Day Saints, 243
Clarification, asking for, 98
"Clearing a space," 68, 69
Clergy. See also Religious leaders
    gathering information from, 111
    help sought from, 17
    intake participation of, 82–83
    and interpersonal boundaries, 231
    referrals from, 82
Client-centered case conceptualization, 139

Sevensky, R. L., 13–14
Sevig, Todd, 9
Shame, 257
Sherman, Allen, 241
Silence, 199, 253, 254, 261
Sin, language about, 184
SISS (Spiritual Issues in Supervision
    Scale), 281
Situational meaning, 124, 125
Skills, spirituality, 198–199
Skinner, B. F., 14
Social categorization theory, 273
Social level, 146
Social support system, 12
Solitude, 199
Special-interest groups, 284
Specification of behavioral duties,
    27–28
Spiritual acceptance, 77–78, 195
Spiritual and religious matching train-
    ing model, 286–287
Spiritual assessment, 93–117, 199
    case study, 44, 115–116
    competent, 44
    creating atmosphere for, 98–99
    extensive, 101–111
    framework of, 93–98
    guidelines for, 46
    implicit, 111–116
    initial, 99–101
    instruments for, 109–111
Spiritual Assessment Inventory, 109
Spiritual assessment model, 83, 84
Spiritual autobiographies, 64–65, 106,
    178–179, 196
Spiritual change experiences, 16
Spiritual changes, 110
Spiritual commitment, 16
Spiritual community
    intervention through, 199
    support from, 12, 229–231
    therapist and client in same,
        231–233
Spiritual coping
    assessment of, 110
    methods of, 94–95
    as protective factor, 83–84

Spiritual distress, 114
Spiritual efficacy, 110
Spiritual emergence, 41
Spiritual emergency, 41
Spiritual flexibility, 110
Spiritual functioning, 145–147
Spiritual genograms, 59–63, 107, 199
Spiritual goals, 77–78, 250
Spiritual history, 199
Spiritual History Scale, 109
Spiritual ideals, 178–180, 189–190
Spiritual intervention guidelines, 46–48
Spiritual interventions, 17
Spiritual Issues in Supervision Scale
    (SISS), 281
Spirituality, 9–19
    APA language on, 16
    awareness of, 3–4, 195–197
    and behaviorism, 195
    best/worst of, 96
    case conceptualization role of, 126–128
    clinical context of, 17–18
    conceptual framework of, 93–98
    cultural context of, 16–17
    definitions of, 9, 11
    extrinsic vs. intrinsic, 11
    global meaning influenced by, 127, 128
    historical context of, 13–16
    importance of, 99
    intake introduction of, 76–77
    and meaning systems, 126–127
    models of, 11–12
    peer-reviewed psychological journals
        on, 15
    positive/negative effects of, 12–13
    presenting problems in relation to, 100
    and religion, 9–11, 196
    research about, 11–13
    as search for the sacred, 94, 95
    solution in relation to, 100
    training context of, 18
    in treatment planning, 145–147
Spiritual life maps, 106
Spiritually accommodative therapy,
    200–201, 269
Spiritually oriented approaches, 200, 201

ABOUT THE EDITORS

Jamie D. Aten, PhD, is an assistant professor of counseling psychology and assistant director of health and mental health research for the Katrina Research Center at the University of Southern Mississippi, Hattiesburg. He has published numerous research articles on religion and spirituality and is a coeditor of a forthcoming book on culture and clinical practice. His current research on the role of the African American church in overcoming rural mental health disparities and mental health disparities among disaster victims is being supported by grants from the U.S. Department of Health and Human Services, Pew Charitable Trusts and Rand Gulf States Policy Institute, and Red Cross/MidSouth Foundation. He also serves as the representative to the Committee on Early Career Psychologists for Division 36 (Psychology of Religion) of the American Psychological Association and as the rural health coordinator for the Mississippi Psychological Association.

Mark M. Leach, PhD, is a professor in the Department of Psychology at the University of Southern Mississippi, Hattiesburg. He has published numerous articles with diversity issues as their foundation, has authored or coedited three books, and has two coedited books forthcoming. He is an associate editor of the journal *Psychology of Religion and Spirituality* of the American Psychological Association Division 36 (Psychology of Religion) and is on the editorial boards of other journals. His primary research interests are in the areas of culture and forgiveness, international counseling issues, spirituality and religion, comparative ethics, and suicide.